ON CALL

PRINCIPLES AND PROTOCOLS

Be on call with confidence!

Successfully managing on-call situations requires a masterful combination of speed, skills, and knowledge. Rise to the occasion with **W.B. SAUNDERS COMPANY's On Call Series!** These pocket-size resources provide you with immediate access to the vital, step-by-step information you need to succeed!

Other titles in the On Call Series

ON CALL
PRINCIPLES AND PROTOCOLS
Third Edition

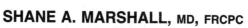

SHANE A. MARSHALL, MD, FRCPC
Director of Cardiac Care
Chief of Medicine
King Edward VIIth Memorial Hospital
Paget, Bermuda

Formerly Chief Resident, Internal Medicine
St. Paul's Hospital
University of British Columbia
Vancouver, British Columbia, Canada

□ □ □

JOHN RUEDY, MD, FRCPC
Dean, Faculty of Medicine
Dalhousie University
Halifax, Nova Scotia, Canada

Formerly Head, Department of Medicine
St. Paul's Hospital
University of British Columbia
Vancouver, British Columbia, Canada

W.B. SAUNDERS COMPANY
A Division of Harcourt Brace & Company
Philadelphia London Toronto Montreal Sydney Tokyo

W.B. SAUNDERS COMPANY
A Division of Harcourt Brace & Company

The Curtis Center
Independence Square West
Philadelphia, Pennsylvania 19106

Library of Congress Cataloging-in-Publication Data

Marshall, Shane A.
On call principles and protocols / Shane A. Marshall, John Ruedy.—3rd ed.

p.   cm.

Includes index.

ISBN 0–7216–5079–1

1. Medical emergencies.   2. Medical consultation.   I. Ruedy,
    John.   II. Title.
    [DNLM: 1. Emergencies handbooks.   2. Emergency Medicine
    handbooks.   WB 39 M369o 2000]

RC86.7.G55 2000   616.02′5—dc21

DNLM/DLC   98-32244

ON CALL PRINCIPLES AND PROTOCOLS   ISBN 0–7216–5079–1

Printed in the United States of America.

Last digit is the print number: 9   8   7   6   5   4   3   2   1

To our families in Bermuda
and Canada

□ □ □

NOTICE

Medicine is an ever-changing field. Standard safety precautions must be followed, but as new research and clinical experience broaden our knowledge, changes in treatment and drug therapy become necessary or appropriate. Readers are advised to check the product information currently provided by the manufacturer of each drug to be administered to verify the recommended dose, the method and duration of administration, and contraindications. It is the responsibility of the treating physician, relying on experience and knowledge of the patient, to determine dosages and the best treatment for the patient. Neither the publisher nor the editor assumes any responsibility for any injury and/or damage to persons or property.

THE PUBLISHER

PREFACE

The responsibility for calls at night is one of the traditional duties of medical students and residents in teaching hospitals. *On Call Principles and Protocols* is designed to facilitate the transition of medical students and residents from the classroom to the hospital setting. We believe that the initiation of the medical student to hospital practice need not be one of trial and error and need not be recalled as a time of stress and uncertainty.

The third edition of *On Call Principles and Protocols* provides referenced updates for the assessment and management of the common problems for which medical students and residents are called at night. The popular On Call Formulary, a quick reference of commonly prescribed medications, has also been expanded and updated. We have been careful to maintain an approach that provides both instruction and reference while emphasizing the rational thought processes required for optimal patient care in specific clinical situations. It is our belief that this structured approach deserves greater emphasis in the undergraduate years, and we are hopeful that it will help in the introduction of students to clinical medicine.

Shane A. Marshall
John Ruedy

ACKNOWLEDGMENTS

We are grateful to the many physicians who provided helpful and detailed comments on individual chapters: Drs. A. Correa, A. Dodek, P. Dodek, L. Halperin, S. Kline, A. Levin, I. Macdonald, J. Martini, A. McLeod, J. Onrot, P. Phillips, J. Russell, S. Stordy, H. Tildesley, A. Uusaro, and S. Whittaker. We would also like to thank Dr. J. Gillies for her major contribution to the first edition of *On Call Principles and Protocols* and to Mr. Ray Kersey for his patience and encouragement during the preparation of the third edition of this book.

STRUCTURE OF THE BOOK

The book is divided into three main sections.

The first section covers introductory material in four separate chapters: Chapter 1, Approach to the Diagnosis and Management of On-Call Problems; Chapter 2, Documentation of On-Call Problems; Chapter 3, Assessment and Management of Volume Status; and Chapter 4, AIDS, HBV, and the House Officer. Volume status is discussed in the introductory section because its assessment is essential in the proper management of many problems in hospitalized patients. A statement on AIDS is included because of the small but finite risk that caring for HIV-infected patients poses to the health care worker.

The second section contains the common calls associated with patient-related problems. Each problem is approached from its inception, beginning with the relevant questions that should be asked over the phone, the temporary orders that should be given, and the major life-threatening problems to be considered as one approaches the bedside:

■ PHONE CALLS

Questions

Pertinent questions asked in order to assess the urgency of the situation.

Orders

Urgent orders to be carried out before the housestaff arrives at the bedside.

Inform RN

RN to be informed of the time the housestaff anticipates arrival at the bedside.

■ ELEVATOR THOUGHTS

The differential diagnosis should be considered by the house-staff while on the way to assess the patient (i.e., while in the elevator).

■ MAJOR THREAT TO LIFE

Identification of the major threat to life is essential in providing focus for the subsequent effective management of the patient.

■ BEDSIDE

Quick Look Test

A rapid visual assessment to place the patient into one of three categories: well, sick, or critical. This helps determine the necessity for immediate intervention.

Airway and Vital Signs

Selective History

Selective Physical Examination

Management

The third section contains the common calls associated with laboratory-related problems.

The Appendices consist of reference items that we have found useful in managing calls.

The On Call Formulary is a compendium of commonly used medications that are likely to be prescribed by the student or resident on call. The alphabetically arranged formulary serves as a quick reference for drug dosages, routes of administration, side effects, contraindications, and modes of action.

COMMONLY USED ABBREVIATIONS

ABD	Abdomen
ABG	Arterial blood gas
AC	*Ante cibum* (before meals)
ACE	Angiotensin-converting enzyme
ACTH	Adrenocorticotropic hormone
ADH	Antidiuretic hormone
AFB	Acid-fast bacillus
AIDS	Acquired immunodeficiency syndrome
AMP	Adenosine monophosphate
ANA	Antinuclear antibody
AP	Anteroposterior
aPTT	Activated partial thromboplastin time
ARDS	Adult respiratory distress syndrome
ASD	Atrial septal defect
AV	Atrioventricular
BID	Twice a day
BP	Blood pressure
BPH	Benign prostatic hypertrophy
Ca	Cancer
CBC	Complete blood (cell) count
CCU	Cardiac care unit
CGL	Chronic granulocytic leukemia
CHF	Congestive heart failure
CLL	Chronic lymphocytic leukemia
CMV	Cytomegalovirus
CNS	Central nervous system
CO	Cardiac output
COPD	Chronic obstructive pulmonary disease

CPK	Creatine phosphokinase
CrCl	Creatinine clearance
C+S	Culture and sensitivity
CSF	Cerebrospinal fluid
CT	Computed tomography
CVA	Costovertebral angle
CVS	Cardiovascular system
CXR	Chest x-ray
D5W	5% dextrose in water
D10W	10% dextrose in water
D20W	20% dextrose in water
D50W	50% dextrose in water
DDAVP	1-desamino-(8-D-arginine)-vasopressin
DIC	Disseminated intravascular coagulation
DKA	Diabetic ketoacidosis
D5NS	5% dextrose in normal saline
DVT	Deep venous (vein) thrombosis
ECF	Extracellular fluid
ECG	Electrocardiogram
EDTA	Disodium edetate
ENDO	Endocrine
ENT	Ears, nose, and throat
ESR	Erythrocyte sedimentation rate
Ext	Extremities
FDP	Fibrin degradation products
FEV$_1$	Forced expiratory volume in 1 second
FFP	Fresh frozen plasma
FIO$_2$	Fraction of inspired oxygen
FTA-ABS	Fluorescent treponemal antibody absorption
FUO	Fever of unknown origin
GERD	Gastroesophageal reflux disease
GI	Gastrointestinal

G-6-PD	Glucose-6-phosphate dehydrogenase
GTT	Glucose tolerance test
GU	Genitourinary
Hb	Hemoglobin
HBV	Hepatitis B virus
HCV	Hepatitis C virus
HEENT	Head, eyes, ears, nose, and throat
HIV	Human immunodeficiency virus
HJR	Hepatojugular reflux
HPI	History of present illness
HR	Heart rate
HS	*Hora somni* (at bedtime)
IBW	Ideal body weight
ICF	Intracellular fluid
ICU	Intensive care unit
ICU/CCU	Intensive care unit/cardiac care unit
IM	Intramuscular
INR	International normalized ratio
ITP	Idiopathic thrombocytopenic purpura
IV	Intravenous
IVC	Intravenous catheter
IVP	Intravenous pyelogram
J	Joule
JVP	Jugular venous pressure
L	Liter
LDH	Lactate dehydrogenase
LLL	Left lower lobe
LLQ	Lower left quadrant
LMWH	Low-molecular-weight heparin
LOC	Level of consciousness
LP	Lumbar puncture
LUQ	Left upper quadrant

LVH	Left ventricular hypertrophy
MAO	Monoamine oxidase
MCV	Mean corpuscular volume
MD	Doctor of Medicine
MHA-TP	Microhemagglutination assay—*Treponema pallidum*
MI	Myocardial infarction
Misc	Miscellaneous
MRI	Magnetic resonance imaging
MSS	Musculoskeletal system
MVP	Mitral valve prolapse
Neuro	Neurologic system
NG	Nasogastric
NMR	Nuclear magnetic resonance (scan)
NPH	Neutral protamine Hagedorn (insulin)
NPO	Nil per os (nothing by mouth)
NS	Normal saline (0.9% saline in water)
NSAID	Nonsteroidal anti-inflammatory drug
NYD	Not yet diagnosed
PA	Posteroanterior
PAC	Premature atrial contraction
PAT	Paroxysmal atrial tachycardia
PC	*Post cibum* (after meals)
Pco_2	Partial pressure of carbon dioxide
PEEP	Positive end-expiratory pressure
PEFR	Peak expiratory flow rate
PMNs	Polymorphonuclear cells
PND	Paroxysmal nocturnal dyspnea
PO	Per os (by mouth)
Po_2	Partial pressure of oxygen
PR	Per rectum
PRN	*Pro re nata* (as needed)

Psych	Psychiatric
PT	Prothrombin time
PTH	Parathyroid hormone
PTT	Partial thromboplastin time
PUD	Peptic ulcer disease
PVC	Premature ventricular contraction
QID	Four times a day
RA	Rheumatoid arthritis
RAD	Right axis deviation
RBBB	Right bundle-branch block
RBC	Red blood cell (count)
Resp	Respiratory system
RLL	Right lower lobe
RLQ	Right lower quadrant
RN	Registered nurse
ROM	Range of motion
RR	Respiratory rate
RTA	Renal tubular acidosis
RUQ	Right upper quadrant
RV	Right ventricle (ventricular)
S_3	Third heart sound
SA	Sternal angle
SAH	Subarachnoid hemorrhage
SBE	Subacute bacterial endocarditis
SC	Subcutaneous
SI	International System of Units
SIADH	Syndrome of inappropriate antidiuretic hormone (secretion)
SL	Sublingual
SLE	Systemic lupus erythematosus
SOB	Shortness of breath
SSRI	Selective serotonin reuptake inhibitor

SSS	Sick sinus syndrome
stat	*Statim* (immediately)
STS	Serologic test for syphilis
SV	Stroke volume
SVT	Supraventricular tachycardia
T$_3$	Triiodothyronine
T$_4$	Thyroxine
TB	Tuberculosis
TBW	Total body water
TIA	Transient ischemic attack
TID	Three times a day
TKVO	To keep the vein open
tPA	Tissue plasminogen activator
TPN	Total parenteral nutrition
TPR	Total peripheral resistance
TSH	Thyroid-stimulating hormone
TTP	Thrombotic thrombocytopenic purpura
URTI	Upper respiratory tract infection
UTI	Urinary tract infection
VIPoma	Vasoactive intestinal polypeptide-secreting tumor
VP	Ventriculoperitoneal
V̇/Q̇	Ventilation-perfusion
VSD	Ventricular septal defect
WBC	White blood cell (count)
WPW	Wolff-Parkinson-White
ZN	Ziehl-Neelsen

CONTENTS

INTRODUCTION

PATIENT-RELATED PROBLEMS: THE COMMON CALLS

LABORATORY-RELATED PROBLEMS: THE COMMON CALLS

APPENDICES

INTRODUCTION

APPROACH TO THE DIAGNOSIS AND MANAGEMENT OF ON-CALL PROBLEMS

Clinical problem solving is an important function required by the physician on call. Traditionally, a physician approaches the diagnosis and management of a patient's problems with an ordered, structured system (e.g., history taking, physical examination, review of available tests, and x-rays) before formulation of the provisional and differential diagnoses and the management plan. The history and physical examination may take 30 to 40 minutes for a patient with a single problem coming to the family physician for the first time, or they may take 60 to 90 minutes for a geriatric patient with multiple complaints. Clearly, if the patient arrives at the emergency department unconscious, having been found on the street, the chief complaint is coma, and the history of present illness (HPI) is limited to the minimal information provided by the ambulance attendants or by the contents of the patient's wallet. In this situation, physicians are trained to proceed concurrently with examination, investigation, and treatment. How this is to be achieved is not always clear, although there is agreement on the steps that should be completed within the initial 5 to 10 minutes.

The physician first confronts on-call problem solving in the final years of medical school. It is at this stage that the structured history taking and physical examination direct the student's approach in evaluating a patient. When on call, the medical student is faced with well-defined problems (e.g., fall-out-of-bed, fever, chest pain) yet feels ill-equipped to begin clinical problem solving unless it involves "the complete history and physical." Anything less than the 60-minute (usually more) "admission history and physical" engenders guilt over a task only partially completed; however, not every on-call problem can involve 60 minutes or more of the physician's time, as unnecessary time spent on patients with relatively minor complaints may deny adequate treatment time to patients who are very ill.

The approach recommended in this book offers a structured system but one that can be logically adapted to most situations. It is intended as a practical guide to assist in efficient clinical problem solving when on call. The clinical chapters are divided into four parts, as follows:

1. Phone call
2. Elevator thoughts

3. Major threat to life
4. Bedside

■ PHONE CALL

Most problems confronting the physician on call are first communicated by telephone. The physician must be able to determine the severity of the problem over the telephone because it is not always possible to immediately assess the patient at the bedside. Patients must be evaluated in order of priority. The phone call section of each chapter is divided into three parts, as follows:

1. Questions
2. Orders
3. Inform RN

The questions are selected to assist in determining the urgency of the problem. Orders that will help expedite the investigation and management of urgent situations are suggested. Finally, the RN is informed of the physician's anticipated time of arrival at the bedside and the responsibilities of the RN in the interim.

■ ELEVATOR THOUGHTS

Because the physician on call is not usually in the immediate vicinity when he or she is informed of a problem that requires assessment, the time spent traveling to the ward (up to 10 minutes in some large hospitals) may be used efficiently to consider the differential diagnosis of the problem at hand. Because time is spent standing still in the elevator, the term "elevator thoughts" has been coined to summarize the directed differential diagnosis. It should be emphasized that the differential diagnosis lists that are offered are not exhaustive but rather focus on the most common or the most serious (life-threatening) causes that should be considered in hospitalized patients.

■ MAJOR THREAT TO LIFE

Identification of the major threat to life that each problem presents provides a focus for the subsequent investigation and management of the patient. The major threat to life posed by each problem follows logically from a consideration of the differential diagnosis. Rather than arriving at the bedside with a memorized list of possible diagnoses, appreciating the one or two most likely threats to life is more useful and relevant in directing one's questions and physical examination. This process serves to ensure that the most serious life-threatening possibility in each clinical scenario is both considered and sought in the initial evaluation of the patient.

■ BEDSIDE

The protocols for what to do on arrival at the bedside are divided into the following parts:

- Quick look test
- Airway and vital signs
- Selective history
- Selective physical examination
- Selective chart review
- Management

The bedside assessment should begin with the quick look test and airway and vital signs. The quick look test is a rapid visual assessment that may enable the physician to categorize the patient's condition into one of three degrees of severity: well (comfortable), sick (uncomfortable or distressed), or critical (about to die). Next is an assessment of the airway and vital signs, which is important in the evaluation of any potentially sick patient. Because of the nature of the various problems that require assessment when on call, the order of the remaining parts is not uniform. For example, Selective Physical Examination may either precede or follow Selective History and Chart Review, and either of these may be superseded by Management if the clinical situation dictates.

Occasionally, the Selective Physical Examination and Management sections are subdivided. This division allows one to focus on the urgent, life-threatening problem, leaving the less urgent problems to be reviewed in the second section.

It is hoped that the principles and protocols offered will provide a logical, efficient system for the assessment and management of common on-call problems.

2

DOCUMENTATION OF ON-CALL
PROBLEMS

Accurate, concise documentation of on-call problems is essential for the continued efficient care of hospitalized patients. In many instances, the patient you are asked to see at night will not be known to you, and you may not be involved in his or her continuing care after your night on call. Some problems can be handled safely over the telephone, but in the majority of situations, a selective history and physical examination will be required to correctly diagnose and treat the problem. Documentation is recommended on every patient you examine. If the problem is straightforward, a brief note is sufficient; however, if the problem is complicated, your note should be concise yet complete.

Begin by recording the date, time, and who you are, e.g., Aug. 10, 2000, 0200H. "Medical student on-call note" or "Resident on-call note."

State who called you and at what time you were called, e.g., "Called to see patient by RN at 0130H because the patient 'fell out of bed.' "

If your assessment is delayed by more urgent problems, say so. A brief one- or two-sentence summary of the patient's admission diagnosis and major medical problems should follow.

This 74-year-old woman with a history of chronic renal failure, type 2 diabetes mellitus, and rheumatoid arthritis was admitted 10 days ago with increasing joint pain.

Next, describe the history of present illness (HPI) of the "fall out of bed" both from the patient's viewpoint and from that of any witnesses. The HPI is no different from the HPI you would document in your admission history. For example,

HPI. The patient was on the way to the bathroom to void, tripped on her bathrobe, and fell to the floor, landing on her left side. She denied palpitations, chest pain, lightheadedness, nausea, and hip pain. There was no difficulty walking unaided and no pain afterward. The fall was not witnessed. The RN found the patient lying on the floor. Vital signs were normal.

If your chart review has relevant findings, include these in your HPI. For example,

Three previous "falls out of bed" on this admission. Patient has no recall of these events.

Documentation of your examination should be *selective*. A call regarding a fall out of bed requires you to examine relevant components of the vital signs, head and neck, and cardiovascular, musculoskeletal, and neurological systems.

It is not necessary to examine the respiratory system or the abdomen unless there is a second separate problem (e.g., you arrive at the bedside and find the patient febrile). On-call problems should not require you to take a complete history and conduct a complete physical examination. These were done when the patient was admitted. Your history, physical examination, and chart documentation should be *directed* (i.e., problem oriented). It may be useful to underline the positive physical findings both for yourself (it aids your summary) and for the housestaff who will be reviewing the patient in the morning.

Physical Examination

Vitals	BP 140/85
	HR: 104/min
	RR: 36/min
	Temp: 38.9 PO
HEENT	No tongue or cheek lacerations
	No hemotympanum
CVS	Pulse rhythm normal; JVP 2 cm > SA
MSS	No skull or face lacerations or hematomas
	Spine and ribs normal
	Full, painless ROM of all 4 limbs
	7- × 9-cm hematoma left thigh
	Reflexes ⎫
	Motor ⎬ Normal
	Sensory ⎭
Neuro	Alert. Oriented to time, place, and person

Relevant laboratory, electrocardiographic (ECG), or x-ray findings should be documented. Again, it is useful to underline abnormal findings. For example,

- Glucose   7.2 mmol/L
- Sodium   141 mmol/L
- Potassium   3.9 mmol/L
- Calcium   Not available
- Urea   12 mmol/L
- Creatinine   180 mmol/L

Your diagnostic conclusion regarding the problem for which you were called must be clearly stated. It is not enough to write "patient fell out of bed." The RN could have written that without even consulting you. The information gathered must be synthesized to achieve the highest level of diagnostic integration possible. This provisional diagnosis should be followed by a differential diagnosis in order of the most likely alternative explanations. For the patient who fell out of bed, your diagnostic conclusion might be as follows.

1. "Fall out of bed" due to difficulty reaching the bathroom to void (?diuretic-induced nocturia, ?contribution of sedation)

2. Large hematoma (7 × 9 cm) left thigh

Your plan must be clearly stated—both the measures taken during the night and the investigations or treatment you have organized for the morning. Avoid writing "Plan–see orders." It is not always obvious to the staff taking over the next day why certain measures were taken. If you informed the intern, resident, or attending physician of the problem, document with whom you spoke and the recommendations given. Record whether any of the patient's family members were informed of the problem and what they were told. Finally, sign or print your name clearly so the staff know who to contact should they have any questions about the management of this patient the following day.

3

ASSESSMENT AND MANAGEMENT
OF VOLUME STATUS

The assessment of volume status is an integral part of the physical examination. You will find in your years as a medical student and intern and later as a practicing physician that this skill plays a key role in helping to choose the appropriate investigation and management in many clinical situations.

Ideally, this skill is best learned at the bedside. However, some background knowledge will help you in the accurate assessment and interpretation of a patient's volume status.

First, terminology must be clarified. The human body is composed mostly of water (Fig. 3–1). In fact, *total body water* (TBW) makes up 60% of the weight of the adult male. Of this, two thirds is *intracellular fluid* (ICF) and one third is *extracellular fluid* (ECF) (i.e., water that is outside of cells). Of the ECF, two thirds is *interstitial fluid*, such as fluid bathing the cells, cerebrospinal fluid, and intraocular fluid. Only 7% of total body weight is *intravascular fluid* (plasma). Clinically, it is the extracellular fluid, consisting of intravascular and interstitial fluids, that one is trying to assess when determining the volume status of a patient.

■ ASSESSMENT OF VOLUME STATUS

There are only three basic states of volume status that a patient can have: volume depleted, normovolemic (euvolemic), and volume overloaded. On approaching the bedside, ask yourself whether the patient is volume depleted, normovolemic, or volume overloaded.

Quick Look Test

Does the patient look well (comfortable), sick (uncomfortable or distressed), or critical (about to die)?

In most instances as you enter the patient's room and first see the patient, it will be apparent whether there is a serious fluid balance abnormality. Patients who are seriously volume depleted look wan, drawn, and tired, whereas patients who are volume overloaded look uncomfortable, anxious, and restless. Of course, these are general guidelines only, and a more detailed physical examination is required.

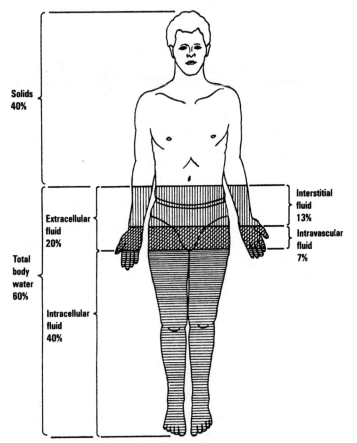

Figure 3–1 □ Body fluid compartments.

Vital Signs

In most cases, simply taking the patient's vital signs will help you determine whether there is significant volume depletion.

Measure the heart rate (HR) and blood pressure (BP) first with the patient supine and then after the patient stands for 1 minute. If the patient is unable to stand alone, ask for assistance or have the patient sit up and dangle his or her legs over the side of the bed. If the patient is hypotensive in the supine position, this maneuver is not necessary.

An increase in HR of > 15 beats/min, a fall in systolic BP of > 15 mm Hg, or any fall in diastolic BP signifies the presence of postural hypotension, which may indicate *intravascular volume depletion.*

A patient with autonomic dysfunction (e.g., beta blockers, diabetic neuropathy, Shy-Drager syndrome) may also have a pronounced postural fall in BP but without the expected degree of compensatory tachycardia. Also, unlike in the volume-depleted patient, there should be no other features of ECF deficit in the patient with uncomplicated autonomic dysfunction.

A *resting tachycardia* may be seen with either volume depletion or volume overload. *Volume depletion* results in a low stroke volume. As can be seen from the following formula, the patient must therefore generate a tachycardia to maintain cardiac output.

$$\text{Cardiac output} = \text{Heart rate} \times \text{Stroke volume}$$
$$\text{CO} = \text{HR} \times \text{SV}$$

The volume-overloaded patient also generates a tachycardia in an effort to increase forward flow and thereby relieve the lungs of venous congestion. A normovolemic patient without other complicating features will have a normal HR.

Measure the respiratory rate. The most important feature to look for when measuring the respiratory rate is tachypnea, which may be seen in the volume-overloaded patient in whom pulmonary edema has developed.

Selective Physical Examination

HEENT   *Look at the oral mucous membranes.* The adequately hydrated patient has moist mucous membranes. It is normal for a small pool of saliva to collect at the undersurface of the tongue in the area of the frenulum, and this should be looked for.

Resp   *Listen for crackles.* Pulmonary edema with bilateral basilar crackles and, occasionally, wheezes or pleural effusions may be a manifestation of the volume-overloaded patient.

CVS   *Look at the neck veins.* Examination of the internal jugular veins is one of the most helpful components of the volume status examination. The JVP may be assessed with the patient at any inclination from 0 to 90 degrees, but it is easiest to begin looking for the JVP pulsation with the patient at a 45-degree inclination. If, at 45 degrees, you are unable to visualize the neck veins, this usually signifies that the JVP is either very low (in which case you will need to lower the head of the bed) or very high (in which case you may need to sit the patient upright to see the top of the column of blood in the internal jugular vein). Once the

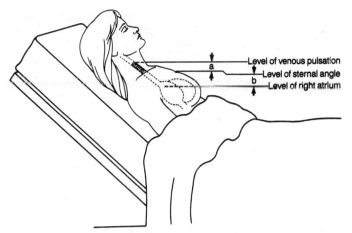

Level of venous pulsation
Level of sternal angle
Level of right atrium

Figure 3–2 □ Measurement of jugular venous pressure. a, The perpendicular distance from the sternal angle to the top of the column of blood. b, The distance from the center of the right atrium to the sternal angle, commonly accepted as measuring 5 cm, regardless of inclination.

internal jugular vein pulsation is identified, measure the perpendicular distance from the sternal angle to the top of the column of blood (Fig. 3–2). This distance represents the patient's JVP in cm of H_2O above the sternal angle. Its value represents a composite of the volume of venous return to the heart, the central venous pressure, and the efficiency of right atrial and right ventricular emptying. A JVP of 2 to 3 cm above the sternal angle is normal in the adult patient. A significantly volume-depleted patient will have flat neck veins, which may fill only when the patient is placed in the Trendelenberg position. A volume-overloaded patient will usually have an elevated JVP of > 3 cm above the sternal angle.

Listen for an S_3. An S_3 is most often associated with the volume-overloaded state and sometimes may be heard only in the left lateral position.

ABD   *Examine the liver.* An enlarged, tender liver and a positive hepatojugular reflux may be manifestations of the volume-overloaded state.

Skin   *Check the skin turgor.* Evaluation of the skin turgor in an adult is best performed by raising a fold of skin from the anterior chest area over the sternal angle. In a normovolemic patient, the skin should return promptly to its usual position. A sluggish return suggests an interstitial fluid deficit. Taut, nonpliable skin that cannot be raised in a fold suggests interstitial fluid excess. Look at the skin creases and check for edema. Accentuated skin creases from bedsheets pressing against the posterior thorax and sacral or pedal edema indicate interstitial fluid excess.

Selective Chart Review

Sometimes, it is difficult to decide at the bedside whether a patient's volume status is normal. There are a few items in the chart that may guide you in a difficult case.

1. Look at the creatinine-to-urea ratio. A ratio of < 12 (calculated in SI units) is suggestive of volume depletion.
2. Examine the fluid balance records. Unfortunately, fluid balance records often are notoriously inaccurate. However, if well-kept records are present, a number of clues may be found. A patient who is taking in very little fluid (whether orally or intravenously) may well be volume depleted. A patient whose urine output is > 20 ml/hr probably is not volume depleted. A net positive intake of several liters over a few days may be indicative of fluid retention with concomitant volume overload.
3. Look for a change in weight. A gain or loss of several pounds since admission may indicate a significant fluid gain or loss, respectively.
4. In the volume-depleted patient, look at the chart for contributing causes.

Gastrointestinal (GI) losses	Vomiting
	Nasogastric suction
	Diarrhea
Urinary losses	Diuretics
	Osmotic diuresis (hyperglycemia, mannitol administration, hypertonic intravenous [IV] contrast material)
	Postobstructive diuresis
	Diabetes insipidus
	Recovery phase of acute tubular necrosis
	Adrenal insufficiency
Surface losses	Skin (increased sweating due to fever, evaporation in burn patients)
	Respiratory tract (hyperventilation, nonhumidified inhalation therapy)
Fluid sequestration	Pancreatitis
	Ileus

	Burns
Blood losses	GI tract
	Surgical
	Trauma
	Iatrogenic (laboratory sampling)
Other	Inadequate oral or parenteral intake

■ CLASSIC STATES OF VOLUME STATUS

It is a rare occasion when a patient has every feature of volume depletion or volume overload. Still, it is useful when examining a patient to carry a mental picture of the three "classic" states of volume status.

The Classic Volume-Depleted Patient

Quick Look Test

The patient looks wan, tired, and drawn.

Vital Signs

HR	Resting tachycardia
	Postural rise in HR of > 15 beats/min
BP	Normal or low resting BP
	A postural drop in systolic BP of > 15 mm Hg or
	any drop in diastolic BP
RR	Normal
HEENT	Dry oral mucous membranes
Resp	Clear
CVS	JVP flat
	No S_3
ABD	Normal
Skin	Poor turgor
	No edema

The Classic Volume-Overloaded Patient

Quick Look Test

The patient looks sick and short of breath. Often, he or she will be sitting upright and appear uncomfortable, anxious, and restless.

Vital Signs

HR	Resting tachycardia
	Postural rise in HR of < 15 beats/min
BP	May be low, normal, or high

	No postural fall in systolic or diastolic BP
RR	Tachypnea
Resp	Crackles bilaterally at bases
	± Wheezing
	± Pleural effusions
CVS	JVP > 3 cm above the sternal angle
	S_3 present
ABD	Positive hepatojugular reflux
	± Enlarged tender liver
Ext	Accentuated skin creases on posterior thorax
	Sacral or pedal edema

The Classic Patient with Normal Volume Status

Quick Look Test

The patient looks well.

Vital Signs

HR	Normal
	Postural rise in HR of < 15 beats/min
BP	Normal
	Postural fall in systolic BP of < 15 mm Hg and no fall in diastolic BP
RR	Normal
HEENT	Moist oral mucous membranes
Resp	Clear
CVS	JVP 2 to 3 cm above the sternal angle
	No S_3
ABD	Normal
Ext	No edema

■ CHOOSING THE CORRECT INTRAVENOUS FLUID

Selection of an appropriate IV fluid for a particular clinical situation need not be a guessing game. A basic understanding of physiology will help to make your fluid management decisions rational and effective.

Water is important in the body because it serves as a *solvent* for a variety of solutes. *Solutes* can be either electrolytes or non-electrolytes.

Electrolytes are substances that dissociate into charged components (ions) when placed in water, and they include the following commonly measured substances:

$$\left.\begin{array}{l}\text{Sodium}\\\text{Potassium}\\\text{Calcium}\\\text{Magnesium}\end{array}\right\}\quad\text{Cations}$$

$$\left.\begin{array}{l}\text{Chloride}\\\text{Bicarbonate}\end{array}\right\}\quad\text{Anions}$$

In physiologic solutions, the total number of cations always equals the total number of anions.

Nonelectrolytes are solutes that have no electrical charges, and they include such substances as glucose and urea.

As mentioned previously, intravascular volume is mostly made up of *water*, which acts as a solvent to dissolve and transport electrolytes and nonelectrolytes. Water is able to move from one body compartment to the next by the process of *osmosis*. When two solutes are separated by a semipermeable membrane, such as a cell membrane, water will tend to flow across the membrane from the solution of lower concentration to that of higher concentration, with the net effect being to equalize the solute concentration on each side of the membrane (Fig. 3–3).

Suppose you were seeing a patient in whom you had decided to infuse a liter of pure water without any solutes. What would happen to the patient's red blood cells (RBCs)? Understanding the process of osmosis allows you to reason that because the solute concentration inside the RBCs is vastly higher than that in the water infused, water would move across the cell membrane into the RBCs (Fig. 3–4). There is a limit to how much the RBC membrane can stretch, and eventually the RBCs would burst. Similarly, you can see that if a hypertonic solution was infused

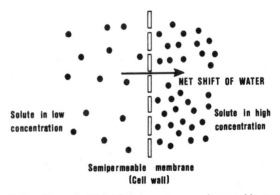

Figure 3–3 □ Osmosis. Water flows across a semipermeable membrane to equalize solute concentrations on each side of the membrane.

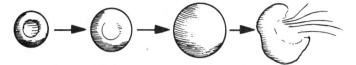

Figure 3–4 □ Osmosis. Effect of infusion of pure water on RBC volume.

directly into the patient's vein, the RBCs would shrink (crenate) as water moved out of the RBCs and into the surrounding solution.

For these reasons, most IV solutions that are prepared for hospital use are usually close to isotonic—that is, they have the same solute concentration as blood—to minimize such fluid shifts. Although cell membranes allow water to pass freely by the process of osmosis, such membranes limit the passage of solutes to varying degrees. Some solute molecules cross membranes more readily than others, depending on their size and physical properties.

In hospitalized patients, there are only three solutes that you need to know about to effectively diagnose and treat disorders of fluid balance. *Glucose* distributes widely throughout both intracellular and extracellular spaces, whereas *sodium* is limited primarily to the extracellular space. *Albumin* remains largely within the intravascular space. The distribution of these three solutes is a fundamental principle you will find useful in guiding your decisions about choice of fluid therapy.

D5W consists of 50 g of dextrose dissolved in 1 L of water. It has an osmolality of 252 mOsm/L, which will prevent the patient's RBCs from shrinking or swelling. Dextrose can be expected to equilibrate rapidly among the intravascular, interstitial, and intracellular spaces, and water will follow along quickly by osmosis.

Normal saline (NS) is another commonly used IV solution. It has an osmolality of 308 mOsm/L, and although slightly hypertonic, it is not sufficiently different from blood tonicity to cause cell shrinkage. NS will stay predominantly in the extracellular space longer than a glucose infusion because sodium does not readily move intracellularly.

Albumin and *plasma* will stay in the intravascular space for many hours because albumin is a large molecule that does not easily traverse the endothelial pores of the blood vessels. The half-life of albumin within the intravascular space is 17 to 20 hours.

With this knowledge of solutes and their membrane permeability, it will be easy to make logical choices regarding fluid management.

In patients with *intravascular volume depletion*, the goal of treatment is to correct and maintain adequate intravascular volume and tissue perfusion. Hence, the volume-depleted patient could be treated with IV NS, albumin, or plasma. Because NS is more readily available and much less expensive, it is the treatment of choice for the initial resuscitation of the volume-depleted patient. Infusion of D5W would be of little benefit because the glucose and water would rapidly distribute throughout the intravascular, interstitial, and extravascular spaces.

In patients with *intravascular volume excess*, the goal of treatment is to improve and maintain adequate cardiac function and tissue perfusion. This usually requires the use of preload reducing measures, as outlined in Chapter 24, pages 273 to 274. However, because these patients often are critically ill, they require IV access for medication administration. The best choice of fluid to give, usually at a TKVO (to keep the vein open) rate, is D5W, which will very quickly leave the intravascular space. Infusion of NS or albumin could worsen the patient's condition by further increasing intravascular volume. This is why cardiac patients, who are at risk for volume overload, usually are given an IV infusion of D5W when IV access is required for administration of medication. An alternative is to use a Heplock at the IV site.

Another IV solution, "2/3 1/3," contains 33 g/L glucose and 512 mmol/L sodium and chloride and is approximately isotonic at 269 mOsm/L. Although there is no particular physiologic basis for its use, it has been popularized as a maintenance IV solution for patients in whom oral intake cannot be met.

■ REMEMBER

1. Volume status abnormalities should be corrected at a rate similar to the rate at which they developed. Biological systems are more responsive to rates of change than to absolute amounts of change. It is safest to correct half the deficit and then reevaluate. There is no substitute for frequent repeated examination of the patient when trying to effect changes in volume status.

2. Occasionally, you will be faced with a patient in whom there is a discrepancy between the two compartments of the extracellular fluid, such as the patient with a decreased intravascular volume but an excess of interstitial fluid (i.e., edema). This discrepancy is most commonly seen in states of marked hypoalbuminemia.

   Fluid transfer from the intravascular space to the interstitial space depends on the permeability of the capillary bed, how much hydrostatic pressure is being exerted to force fluid out of the intravascular space, and the difference in *oncotic pressure* between the intravascular and interstitial spaces (Fig. 3–5).

   Oncotic pressure is exerted by *plasma protein* (i.e., albu-

Hydrostatic pressure

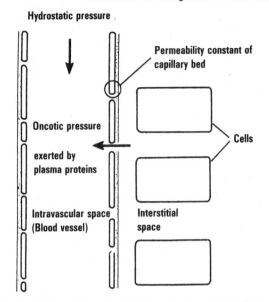

Figure 3–5 □ Factors influencing fluid transfer between the intravascular and extravascular spaces.

min). There is little, if any, protein in the interstitium, and hence the intravascular oncotic pressure exerted by albumin tends to draw water out of the interstitium and into the intravascular space. This knowledge becomes important in the occasional patient who has intravascular volume depletion as assessed by your clinical examination, together with interstitial fluid excess (i.e., edema). To help shift fluid from the interstitium to the intravascular space in such a patient, a logical choice is to administer IV albumin. Artificial plasma expanders (e.g., *gelofusine, polygeline,* dextran, hetastarch) also may be used. They are high-molecular-weight glucose polymers that remain in the intravascular space because of their large size.

Remember that oncotic pull comes from albumin. It does not come from sodium, so NS is not an appropriate fluid to give in this situation. It does not come from RBCs, so a blood transfusion is an equally inappropriate choice. Note that albumin is available in two concentrations—5% and 25%. The 25% albumin is the preferred concentration when trying to effect a shift in fluid from the interstitial space to the intravascular space.

Unfortunately, albumin, plasma, and artificial plasma ex-

Table 3-1 □ COMMONLY USED INTRAVENOUS FLUIDS

	Glucose (g/L)	Na (mmol/L)	Cl (mmol/L)	K (mmol/L)	Ca (mmol/L)	Lactate (mmol/L)	Approximate Osmolality (mOsm/L)
D5W	50	—	—	—	—	—	252
D10W	100	—	—	—	—	—	505
D20W	200	—	—	—	—	—	1010
D50W	500	—	—	—	—	—	2525
"2/3 1/3"	33	51	51	—	—	—	269
0.45% NaCl (1/2NS)	—	77	77	—	—	—	154
0.9% NaCl (NS)	—	154	154	—	—	—	308
D5NS	50	154	154	—	—	—	560
D5/0.2% NS	50	34	34	—	—	—	321
Ringer's lactate	—	130	109	4	3	28	272
Albumin	—	145	145	Available in 5% concentrations (50, 250, or 500 ml) or 25% concentrations (20, 50, or 100 ml)			
Fresh frozen plasma (FFP)	200–250 ml of plasma that has been separated from whole blood and frozen within 8 hours of collection. FFP contains all coagulation factors.						
Stored plasma	200–250 ml of plasma that has been separated from whole blood and frozen 8–72 hours after collection. Contains all coagulation factors but with reduced levels of factors V and VIII.						

panders are expensive, and their effect in removing edema fluid is transient. Hence, their continued use for this indication is controversial. Certainly, the best way to correct edema in a patient with a decreased intravascular volume but an excess of interstitial fluid is to correct the underlying cause of interstitial volume excess. In most cases, the cause is hypoproteinemia (e.g., malabsorption, liver disease, nephrotic syndrome, protein losing enteropathy).

In summary, most disorders of fluid balance can be treated logically and successfully with the simple principles of water and solute transfer across cell membranes. Table 3–1 provides a listing of the commonly used IV fluids.

4

AIDS, HBV, AND THE HOUSE OFFICER

The risk of transmission of human immunodeficiency virus (HIV) from patient to health care worker is extremely low. The rate of transmission is < 0.5% after direct inoculation of infected blood through a needlestick puncture and even lower after other types of exposure.[1] Circumstances that may increase the risk of seroconversion include procedures involving a needle placed directly in a vein or artery, a deep injury, the presence of visible blood on the device, or a high viral load in the source patient (i.e., at the time of seroconversion and in the terminal stages of acquired immunodeficiency syndrome [AIDS]).[2]

Hepatitis B virus (HBV) represents a risk of transmission that is many times that of HIV. In the United States, thousands of health care workers become infected with HBV each year.[3] Hepatitis B vaccination is strongly recommended for all staff.

Strict adherence to universal precautions, also referred to as blood and body fluid precautions, will minimize these risks (Table 4–1).

Despite attention to safe practices, you may, in the course of your training, have accidental exposure to potentially infectious blood or body fluids. Your hospital should have an established policy for helping you, and you should contact the appropriate individual if you have been accidentally exposed.

The following general guidelines are recommended if you have been exposed to blood or body fluids.

■ FIRST AID

1. Seek assistance from a more senior member of staff.
2. Immediately cleanse the contaminated site.
   a. Needlestick
      - Allow the puncture site to bleed.
      - Thoroughly scrub the site for 2 to 4 minutes with a povidone-iodine–based detergent or solution (e.g., Betadine).
   b. Skin contamination
      - Open wound: flush the area with water or saline; cleanse with Betadine.
   c. Mucous membrane or eye contact

Table 4–1 □ UNIVERSAL PRECAUTIONS TO PREVENT TRANSMISSION OF HIV

Universal Precautions

Because a medical history and physical examination cannot reliably identify all patients infected with HIV or other blood-borne pathogens, blood and body fluid precautions should be consistently used for all patients, especially those in emergency care settings in which the risk of blood exposure is increased and the infection status of the patient is usually not known.

1. Use appropriate barrier precautions to prevent skin and mucous membrane exposure when exposure to blood, body fluids containing blood, or other body fluids to which universal precautions apply (see below) is anticipated. Wear gloves when touching blood or body fluids, mucous membranes, or nonintact skin of all patients; when handling items or surfaces soiled with blood or body fluids; and when performing venipuncture and other vascular access procedures. Change gloves after contact with each patient; do not wash or disinfect gloves for reuse. Wear masks and protective eyewear or face shields during procedures that are likely to generate droplets of blood or other body fluids to prevent exposure of mucous membranes of the mouth, nose, and eyes. Wear gowns or aprons during procedures that are likely to generate splashes of blood or other body fluids.

2. Wash hands and other skin surfaces immediately and thoroughly following contaminations with blood, body fluids containing blood, or other body fluids to which universal precautions apply. Wash hands immediately after gloves are removed.

3. Take care to prevent injuries when using needles, scalpels, and other sharp instruments or devices, when handling sharp instruments after procedures, when cleaning used instruments, and when disposing of used needles. Do not recap used needles by hand; do not remove used needles from disposable syringes by hand; and do not bend, break, or otherwise manipulate used needles by hand. Place used disposable syringes and needles, scalpel blades, and other sharp items in puncture-resistant disposal containers, which should be located as close to the use area as is practical.

4. Although saliva has not been implicated in HIV transmission, the need for emergency mouth-to-mouth resuscitation should be minimized by making mouthpieces, resuscitation bags, or other ventilation devices available for use in areas in which the need for resuscitation is predictable.

5. Health care workers with exudative lesions or weeping dermatitis should refrain from all direct patient care and from handling patient care equipment until the condition resolves.

Universal precautions are intended to supplement rather than replace recommendations for routine infection control, such as hand washing and use of gloves to prevent gross microbial contamination of hands. In addition, implementation of universal precautions does not eliminate the need for other category- or disease-specific isolation precautions, such as enteric

Table continued on following page

precautions for infectious diarrhea or isolation for pulmonary tuberculosis. Universal precautions are not intended to change waste management programs undertaken in accordance with state and local regulations.

Body Fluids to Which Universal Precautions Apply

Universal precautions apply to blood and other body fluids containing visible blood. Blood is the single most important source of HIV, hepatitis B virus, and other blood-borne pathogens in the occupational setting. Universal precautions also apply to tissues, semen, vaginal secretions, and the following fluids: cerebrospinal, synovial, pleural, peritoneal, pericardial, and amniotic.

Universal precautions do not apply to feces, nasal secretions, sputum, sweat, tears, urine, and vomitus unless they contain visible blood. Universal precautions also do not apply to human breast milk, although gloves may be worn by health care workers in situations in which exposure to breast milk might be frequent. In addition, universal precautions do not apply to saliva. Gloves need not be worn when feeding patients or wiping saliva from skin, although special precautions are recommended for dentistry, in which contamination of saliva with blood is predictable. The risk of transmission of HIV, as well as hepatitis B virus, from these fluids and materials is extremely low or nonexistent.

Use of Gloves for Phlebotomy

Gloves should be effective in reducing the incidence of blood contamination of hands during phlebotomy (drawing of blood samples), but they cannot prevent penetrating injuries caused by needles or other sharp instruments. In universal precautions, all blood is assumed to be potentially infectious for blood-borne pathogens. Some institutions have relaxed recommendations for the use of gloves for phlebotomy by skilled health care workers in settings in which the prevalence of blood-borne pathogens is known to be very low (e.g., volunteer blood donation centers). Institutions that judge that routine use of gloves for all phlebotomies is not necessary should periodically reevaluate their policy. Gloves should always be available for those who wish to use them for phlebotomy. In addition, the following general guidelines apply:

1. Use gloves for performing phlebotomy if cuts, scratches, or other breaks in the skin are present.
2. Use gloves in situations in which contamination with blood may occur—for example, when performing phlebotomy on an uncooperative patient.
3. Use gloves for performing finger or heel sticks on infants and children.
4. Use gloves when training persons to do phlebotomies.

From Rubin RH: Acquired immunodeficiency syndrome. Scientific American Medicine, Vol 2. Rubenstein E, Federman DD, Eds. Scientific American, Inc., New York, 1990, Section 7, Subsection XI, p. 1. All rights reserved.

Table 4-2 □ PROPHYLAXIS AFTER PARENTERAL EXPOSURE TO HBV

Exposed Person	Treatment*	Comment
Unvaccinated	1 dose of HBV hyperimmune globulin; vaccine (primary series)	A substantial proportion of health care workers at high risk for exposure to blood (10–40% in some studies) may be immune or may be chronic carriers of natural infection. Screening for antibody to hepatitis B core antigen will identify these persons; if the test result is available within 24–72 hours after exposure, unnecessary treatment can be avoided.
Known response to previous vaccination		
Serum anti-HBsAg titer ≥ 10 mIU/ml	No treatment	
Serum anti-HBsAg titer < 10 mIU/ml	1 booster dose of vaccine	
Serum anti-HBsAg titer unknown	1 booster dose of vaccine	
No response to previous vaccination	2 doses of HBV hyperimmune globulin 1 month apart	If reimmunization with an additional 1 or more doses of vaccine has not been attempted, HBV vaccine (up to 3 doses) should be provided.
Previously vaccinated but response unknown		
Serum anti-HBsAg titer ≥ 10 mIU/ml	No treatment	
Serum anti-HBsAg titer < 10 mIU/ml	1 dose of HBV hyperimmune globulin; 1 booster dose of vaccine	Consider giving a second dose of HBV hyperimmune globulin in 1 month if risk factors† for a lack of response are present.
Serum anti-HBsAg titer unknown	1 booster dose of vaccine	Consider giving HBV hyperimmune globulin if risk factors† for a lack of response are present.

*The following doses are recommended: 0.06 ml of HBV hyperimmune globulin per kilogram of body weight IM, 1 ml of vaccine IM as a booster, and 1 ml of vaccine IM at 0, 1, and 6 months for the primary series.
†Obesity, immunosuppression, age > 50 years, smokers.

Reproduced in modified form by permission from Gerberding JL: Management of occupational exposures to blood-borne viruses. N Engl J Med 1995;332:445. Copyright 1995 Massachusetts Medical Society. All rights reserved.

Table 4–3 □ HIV PROPHYLAXIS AFTER EXPOSURE

Source	Exposed Person
HIV antibody positive	1. Do baseline HIV antibody. 2. Counsel regarding risks, sex, and health care. 3. Advise to report mono/flu-like illness over next 6 months. 4. Repeat HIV antibody at 6 and 12 weeks and 6 and 12 months. If symptomatic, consider HIV antibody stat and then monthly for 6 months. 5. Antiretroviral therapy* should be recommended.
High risk	Obtain informed consent to do HIV antibody.† If positive, treat as above for HIV antibody positive. If negative, treat as simple puncture wound (e.g., needlestick).
Low risk	Do baseline HIV antibody. Repeat at 6 and 12 months on request of exposed employee.
Unknown source	Do baseline HIV antibody. Repeat at 6 and 12 months on request of exposed employee.

*The reporting of needlesticks or other exposure to HIV-contaminated fluids should not be delayed. Therapy should be initiated as soon as possible, preferably within 1 to 2 hours after exposure. One recommended dosing regimen is *zidovudine* (AZT) 200 mg PO every 4 hours (6 times a day) for 3 days and then 100 to 200 mg every 4 hours (5 times a day) for the next 25 days.[4] Potential side effects include headache, nausea, myalgia, insomnia, anemia, neutropenia, and nail pigmentation. Alternatively, combination therapy (*zidovudine* 200 mg PO three times a day and *lamivudine* 150 mg PO twice daily)[5, 6] has been proposed to increase antiretroviral activity, and to provide activity against AZT-resistant HIV strains. A protease inhibitor (e.g., *indinavir* 800 mg PO three times a day) may be added for exposures with the highest risk of transmission, or if the source patient is already receiving AZT or lamivudine.

†Local laws regarding informed consent for testing source blood should be followed.

- Mouth: Rinse with an oxygenating agent such as 3% hydrogen peroxide for 30 seconds. Repeat several times.
- Eyes: Rinse well with water for 3 to 5 minutes.
3. Save the instrument, without washing, in a sharps container.
4. Report immediately to the designated officer responsible for helping you.

■ IMMEDIATE MANAGEMENT

Treatment of parenteral exposure (i.e., nonintact skin, mucous membrane, or skin puncture) may include

1. Tetanus prophylaxis—*tetanus toxoid* 0.5 ml, if indicated.
2. HBV prophylaxis after exposure (Table 4–2).
3. HIV prophylaxis after exposure (Table 4–3). Procedures regarding assessment of the source person vary among institutions. Zidovudine (AZT) prophylaxis has been subjected to a case-control study that suggests that the risk of HIV conversion after percutaneous exposure can be reduced with AZT prophylaxis.[2] Because combination therapy has been shown to reduce viral load more effectively than AZT alone, it is possible that combination therapy may provide more effective prophylaxis.[7] Therapy should be initiated as soon as possible, preferably within 1 to 2 hours after exposure.

References

1. Gerberding JL: Management of occupational exposures to blood-borne viruses. N Engl J Med 1995;332:444–451.
2. Centers for Disease Control and Prevention: Case control study of HIV seroconversion in health-care workers after percutaneous exposure to HIV-infected blood—France, United Kingdom, and United States, January 1988–August 1994. MMWR 1995;44:929–933.
3. Alter MJ, Hadler SC, Margolis HS, et al: The changing epidemiology of hepatitis B in the United States. JAMA 1990;263:1218–1222.
4. New drugs for HIV infection. Med Lett Drugs Ther 1996;38:35–37.
5. McLeod A, Beardsell A: Management of accidental exposure to HIV in blood and body fluids: An update of the previous guideline. BC Med J 1997;39:324–327.
6. Update: Provisional Public Health Service recommendations for chemoprophylaxis after occupational exposure to HIV. MMWR 1996;45:468–473.
7. Gerberding JL, Henderson DK: Management of occupational exposures to bloodborne pathogens: Hepatitis B virus, hepatitis C virus, and human immunodeficiency virus. Clin Infect Dis 1992;14:1179–1185.

PATIENT-RELATED PROBLEMS: THE COMMON CALLS

5

ABDOMINAL PAIN

Many patients complain of abdominal pain during their hospital stays. It is essential to distinguish the acute abdominal emergency from the recurrent nonemergency. The former requires urgent medical or surgical intervention, whereas the latter requires thorough, but less urgent, investigation. Avoid ordering analgesic agents until a preliminary diagnosis is made. Narcotic analgesic agents may mask the physical findings of an acute abdomen, thereby delaying recognition and treatment of a serious intra-abdominal disorder.

■ PHONE CALL

Questions

1. **How severe is the pain?**
2. **Is the pain localized or generalized?**
3. **What are the vital signs?**
   Fever and abdominal pain are suggestive of intra-abdominal infection or inflammation.
4. **Is this a new problem?**
5. **What was the reason for admission?**
6. **Is the patient on steroids?**
   Steroids may mask the pain and fever attendant with inflammatory processes, tricking you into underestimating the nature or severity of a patient's abdominal pain. If the patient is on steroids, even mild abdominal pain should be assessed soon.

Orders

If the abdominal pain is mild and the vital signs are normal, ask the RN to call immediately if the pain becomes worse before you are able to assess the patient.

Inform RN

"Will arrive at bedside in . . . minutes."
Abdominal pain of acute onset, severe abdominal pain, or pain associated with fever or hypotension requires you to see the patient immediately. Mild recurrent abdominal pain is a less urgent problem and may be attended to in an hour or two if other patient problems of higher priority exist.

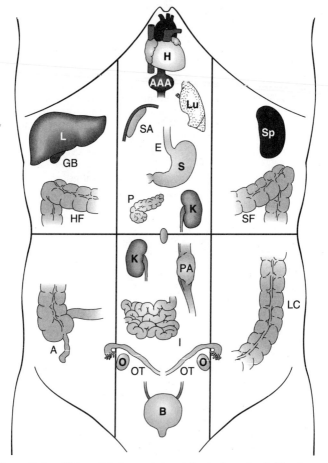

Figure 5–1 □ Differential diagnosis by abdominal quadrant. (See key on opposite page.)

■ ELEVATOR THOUGHTS
(What causes abdominal pain?)

The causes of *localized abdominal pain* are numerous. A useful system for approaching the problem is "diagnosis by location." Figure 5–1 illustrates a differential diagnosis by location.

The causes of *generalized abdominal pain* are fewer. Disorders producing either localized or generalized pain are indicated by an asterisk, and additional causes of generalized abdominal pain alone are listed in the legend to Figure 5–1.

Key to Figure 5–1

Right upper quadrant
  L, Liver (hepatitis, abscess, perihepatitis)
  GB, Gallbladder (cholecystitis, cholangitis, choledocholithiasis)
  HF, Hepatic flexure (obstruction)
Right lower quadrant
  A, Appendix (appendicitis,* abscess)
  O, Ovary (torsion, ruptured cyst, carcinoma)
Left upper quadrant
  Sp, Spleen (rupture, infarct, abscess)
  SF, Splenic flexure (obstruction)
Left lower quadrant
  LC, Left colon (diverticulitis, ischemic colitis)
  O, Ovary (torsion, ruptured cyst, carcinoma)
Epigastrium
  H, Heart (myocardial infarction, pericarditis, aortic dissection)
  AAA, Abdominal aortic aneurysm
  Lu, Lung (pneumonia, pleurisy)
  SA, Subphrenic abscess
  E, Esophagus (gastroesophageal reflux disease)
  S, Stomach and duodenum (peptic ulcer)
  P, Pancreas (pancreatitis)
  K, Kidney (pyelonephritis, renal colic)
Hypogastrium
  K, Kidney (renal colic)
  PA, Psoas abscess
  I, Intestine (infection,* obstruction,* inflammatory bowel disease*)
  O, Ovary (torsion, ruptured cyst, carcinoma)
  OT, Ovarian tube (ectopic pregnancy, salpingitis, endometriosis)
  B, Bladder (cystitis, distended bladder)
Generalized abdominal pain
  1. See conditions marked with an asterisk.
  2. Peritonitis (any cause)
  3. Diabetic ketoacidosis
  4. Sickle cell crisis
  5. Acute intermittent porphyria
  6. Acute adrenocortical insufficiency due to steroid withdrawal

■ MAJOR THREAT TO LIFE

- Perforated or ruptured viscus
- Ascending cholangitis
- Necrosis of viscus
- Exsanguinating hemorrhage

A *perforated* or *ruptured viscus* may result in hypovolemic shock (from third space losses), septic shock (from bacterial peritonitis), or both. Progression of infection from an initial localized site (e.g., *ascending cholangitis*) to septic shock may occur rapidly (i.e., within hours of the patient's first presenting symptom). *Necrosis of a viscus,* as in severe pancreatitis, intussusception, volvulus, strangulated hernia, or ischemic colitis, may cause hypovolemic or septic shock and electrolyte and acid-base disturbances. *Exsanguinating hemorrhage* with hypovolemic shock may result from a leaking abdominal aortic aneurysm, a ruptured ectopic pregnancy, or a splenic rupture; occasionally it may have an iatrogenic cause, such as a liver or renal biopsy or a misdirected thoracentesis.

Patients with myocardial infarction and aortic dissection occasionally present with abdominal pain. These diagnoses should be considered, especially if no local abdominal signs can be identified.

■ BEDSIDE

Quick Look Test

Does the patient look well (comfortable), sick (uncomfortable or distressed), or critical (about to die)?

Appearances are often deceptive in acute abdominal disease. If the patient has recently received narcotic analgesics or high-dose steroids, he or she may appear well despite a serious underlying problem.

Patients with severe colic are often restless, in contrast to those with peritonitis, who lie immobile, avoiding movement that exacerbates the pain. With peritonitis, patients may have their knees drawn up to reduce abdominal tension.

Airway and Vital Signs

What is the blood pressure (BP)?

Hypotension associated with abdominal pain is an ominous sign suggestive of impending hypovolemic, hemorrhagic, or septic shock.

Are there postural changes (lying and standing) in the BP and heart rate (HR)?

If the supine BP is normal, recheck the BP and HR with the patient standing. A drop in BP that is associated with an increased heart rate (> 15 beats/min) suggests volume depletion.

What is the temperature?

Fever associated with abdominal pain is suggestive of intra-abdominal infection or inflammation. However, the lack of fever in the elderly patient or in the patient receiving an antipyretic or immunosuppressive drug does not rule out infection.

Selective History and Chart Review

Diagnosis is often dependent on a careful history addressing (1) the pain at onset and its subsequent progression, (2) any associated symptoms, and (3) the past history.

Pain

Is the pain localized?

The location of maximum intensity of the pain can provide a clue to the site of origin (see Fig. 5–1). Remember that a patient may complain of diffuse abdominal pain, but on careful examination, the pain will be found to be localized.

How is the pain characterized (e.g., severe or mild, burning or knifelike, constant or waxing-and-waning, as in colic)?

There are characteristic descriptions of pain associated with certain diseases as follows: the pain of peptic ulcer tends to be burning; that of a perforated ulcer is sudden, constant, and severe; that of biliary colic is sharp, constricting ("taking one's breath away"); that of acute pancreatitis is deep and agonizing; and that of obstructed bowel is gripping, with intermittent worsening.

Did the pain develop gradually or suddenly?

The severe pain of colic (renal, biliary, or intestinal) develops within hours. An acute onset with fainting suggests perforation of a viscus, ruptured ectopic pregnancy, torsion of an ovarian cyst, or a leaking abdominal aortic aneurysm.

Has the pain changed since its onset?

A ruptured viscus initially may be associated with localized pain, which subsequently shifts or becomes generalized, with the development of chemical or bacterial peritonitis.

Does the pain radiate?

Pain radiates to the dermatome or cutaneous areas supplied by the same sensory cortical cells as the deep-seated structure (Fig. 5–2). For example, the diaphragm is supplied by the cervical roots C3, C4, and C5. Many upper abdominal or lower thoracic conditions that cause irritation of the diaphragm refer pain to the cutaneous supply of C3, C4, and C5 (i.e., the shoulder and the neck). The liver and gallbladder are derived from the right 7th and 8th thoracic segments. Thus, biliary colic frequently refers pain to the inferior angle of the right scapula. The pain of pancreatitis may radiate to the midback or scapula.

Are there any aggravating or alleviating factors?

Pain that increases with meals, decreases with passage of bowel movements, or both suggests a hollow gut origin. An exception is pain from duodenal ulcer, which is often relieved by the ingestion of food. The pain of pancreatitis is often worsened after eating and may be relieved by sitting up or leaning forward. Pain that increases with inspiration suggests pleuritis or peritonitis, and pain that is aggravated by micturition suggests a urogenital cause.

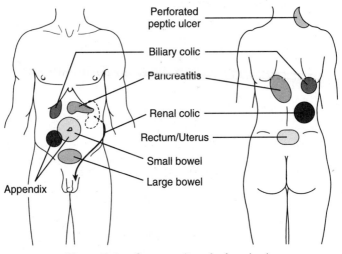

Figure 5–2 □ Common sites of referred pain.

Associated Symptoms

Is there nausea or vomiting?

Vomiting occurring with the onset of pain frequently accompanies acute peritoneal irritation or perforation of a viscus. It is also commonly associated with acute pancreatitis or obstruction of any muscular hollow viscus. Pain relieved by vomiting suggests hollow gut origin (e.g., bowel obstruction). Vomiting many hours after the onset of abdominal pain may be a clue to intestinal obstruction or ileus.

What is the nature of emesis?

Brown, feculent emesis is pathognomonic of bowel obstruction, either paralytic or mechanical. Frank blood is suggestive of an upper gastrointestinal (GI) bleed. Vomiting food after fasting is consistent with gastric stasis or gastric outlet obstruction.

Is there diarrhea?

Diarrhea and abdominal pain are seen in infectious gastroenteritis, ischemic colitis, appendicitis, and partial small bowel obstruction. Diarrhea alternating with constipation is a common symptom of diverticular disease.

Is there fever or chills?

Check the temperature record since admission. Check the medication sheet for antipyretic, steroid, or antibiotic drugs because fever may be masked by the administration of these medications.

Past History and Chart Review

Is there a history of peptic ulcer disease or antacid ingestion?
Peptic ulcer disease is a chronic, recurring disease. History repeats itself!

Is there a history of blunt or penetrating trauma to the abdomen? Has there been a liver or kidney biopsy or a thoracentesis since admission?
A subcapsular hemorrhage of the spleen, liver, or kidney may result in hemorrhagic shock 1 to 3 days later.

Is there a history of alcohol abuse and ascites?
Spontaneous bacterial peritonitis must always be considered in the alcoholic patient with ascites and fever.

Is there a history of coronary or peripheral vascular disease?
Atherosclerosis is a diffuse process and may affect the vascular supply to several body systems. In addition to the possibility of a myocardial infarction presenting with abdominal pain, a leaking abdominal aortic aneurysm, an aortic dissection, and ischemic colitis due to atherosclerosis of the mesenteric arteries should be considered.

If the patient is a premenopausal woman, ask the date of the last normal menstrual period.
Abdominal pain associated with a missed period raises the possibility of an ectopic pregnancy. Hypotension in this situation suggests a ruptured ectopic pregnancy, a life-threatening situation.

Is there a history of previous abdominal surgery?
Adhesions are responsible for 70% of bowel obstructions.

Is the patient anticoagulated?
Intra-abdominal hemorrhage may occur in the anticoagulated patient, especially if there is a history of peptic ulcer disease.

Is there a history of use of aspirin or nonsteroidal anti-inflammatory drug (NSAID), alcohol, or other ulcerogenic drug?

Selective Physical Examination

Vitals	Repeat now
HEENT	Icterus (cholangitis, choledocholithiasis)
	Spider nevi (risk of spontaneous bacterial peritonitis if ascites is present)
Resp	Generalized or localized restriction of abdominal wall movement in respiration (localized or generalized peritoneal inflammation)
	Stony dullness to percussion, decreased breath

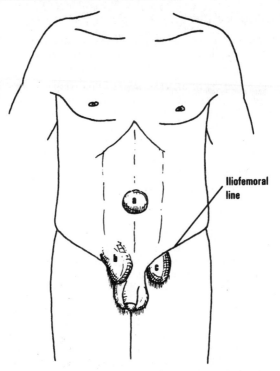

Figure 5–3 □ Hernial orifices. a, Umbilical hernia; b, inguinal hernia; c, femoral hernia. Note that the "bulge" of the inguinal hernia begins superiorly to the inguinal ligament, whereas the "bulge" of the femoral hernia originates inferiorly to the inguinal ligament.

	sounds, decreased tactile fremitus (pleural effusion)
	Dullness to percussion, diminished or bronchial breath sounds, crackles (consolidation and pneumonia)
CVS	Decreased JVP (volume depletion)
	New onset of dysrhythmia or mitral insufficiency murmur (myocardial infarction)
ABD	Before examining the abdomen, make sure your hands are warm and make sure the head of the bed is flat. It may be helpful to flex the patient's hips to relax the abdominal wall. When examining for tenderness, begin in a nonpainful region. Watch the patient's face as you examine.

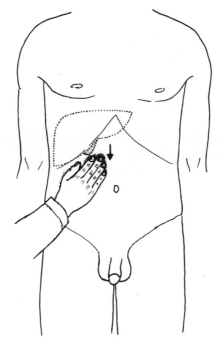

Figure 5–4 □ Murphy's sign. A positive Murphy's sign is manifested by pain and inspiratory arrest when the patient takes a deep breath while the examiner applies pressure against the abdominal wall in the region of the gallbladder. A positive Murphy's sign is often seen in the presence of cholecystitis.

	Visible peristalsis (bowel obstruction)
	Bulging flanks (ascites)
	Loss of liver dullness (perforated viscus)
	Localized tenderness, masses (see Fig. 5–1)
	Rigid abdomen, guarding, rebound tenderness (peritonitis)
	Shifting dullness, fluid wave (ascites)
	Absent bowel sounds (paralytic ileus or late bowel obstruction)
	Check all hernia orifices (strangulated hernia) (Fig. 5–3)
	Murphy's sign (cholecystitis) (Fig. 5–4)
	Psoas sign (appendicitis) (Fig. 5–5)
	Obturator sign (appendicitis) (Fig. 5–6)
Rectal	Tenderness (retrocecal appendicitis, prostatitis)
	Mass (rectal carcinoma)

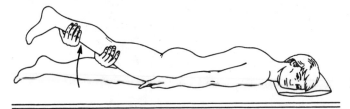

Figure 5–5 □ Psoas sign. A positive psoas sign is manifested by abdominal pain in response to passive hip extension. (This test also may be performed with the patient lying on his or her side.) This sign is often present in patients with appendicitis or a psoas abscess.

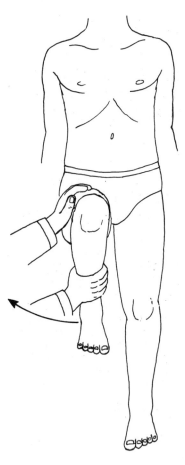

Figure 5–6 □ A positive obturator sign is manifested by abdominal pain in response to passive internal rotation of the right hip from the 90-degree hip/knee flexion position, when the patient is supine. This sign is often present in patients with appendicitis.

Rectal fissure (Crohn's disease)
Stool positive for occult blood (ischemic colitis, peptic ulcer)

Pelvic   Tenderness (ectopic pregnancy, ovarian cyst, or pelvic inflammatory disease)
Mass (ovarian cyst or tumor)

Management

Your assessment and investigation thus far may not have led you to a specific diagnosis of the etiology of the patient's abdominal pain. You will, however, have determined from your physical examination whether the patient has developed shock, the most serious complication from disorders that cause abdominal pain.

Shock. The initial treatment of either *hypovolemic* or *septic shock* is the same and is aimed at immediate expansion of the intravascular volume.

1. Rapid volume repletion can be achieved using normal saline (NS) or Ringer's lactate (500 to 1000 ml IV as rapidly as possible, followed by an intravenous rate titrated to the JVP and vital signs). In this situation, IV fluids should be given through a large-bore peripheral IV or central line.
2. Blood should be drawn for a stat crossmatch for 4 to 6 units of packed red blood cells (RBCs), hemoglobin (Hb), prothrombin time (PT), activated partial thromboplastin time (aPTT), and platelet count. Baseline values of electrolytes, urea, creatinine, blood glucose, amylase, and white blood cell (WBC) and manual differential also are useful. Two sets of blood cultures should be drawn if septic shock is suspected.
3. If hemorrhagic shock is suspected, packed red blood cells (RBCs) should be given in place of, or in addition to, the crystalloid, NS, or Ringer's lactate as soon as the crossmatch has been completed. In extreme circumstances O-negative blood may be used while waiting for the crossmatched supply.
4. When shock occurs in the setting of a disorder causing abdominal pain, urgent surgical consultation is almost always required. Ensure that the patient is NPO (nothing by mouth). Consider inserting a nasogastric (NG) tube if the patient is vomiting.
5. As resuscitation measures are being initiated, additional investigations can be arranged, as follows:
   a. Order three radiographic views of the abdomen (anteroposterior [AP] abdomen supine and erect or lateral decubitus and posteroanterior [PA] chest erect). If the patient

looks unwell or critical, these x-rays will need to be done on a stat portable basis.

(1) *Toxic megacolon* is manifested by an increase in diameter of the midtransverse colon (> 7 cm) and a mucosal pattern of thumbprinting or thickening. This condition is a medical or surgical emergency.

(2) Look for air under the diaphragm in the chest film or between the viscera and subcutaneous tissue in the lateral decubitus film. This sign is indicative of a perforated viscus.

(3) Look for air/fluid levels that suggest bowel obstruction or ileus.

(4) Look for calcified gallstones, which could be a cause of cholecystitis or pancreatitis.

(5) Pancreatic calcifications, if present, may be a clue that the patient is having a recurrent attack of chronic pancreatitis.

b. If septic shock is suspected, specimens for Gram's stain, culture, and sensitivity testing should be obtained immediately from sputum, if available; urine, which may require catheterization; and wounds. If there is ascites, an immediate diagnostic paracentesis should be performed.

6. Once culture specimens have been obtained in a case of suspected septic shock, empiric, broad-spectrum antibiotics (e.g., a third-generation cephalosporin, plus metronidazole) should be started immediately to treat infection due to coliforms and gut anaerobes.

Acute "Surgical" Abdomen. If the patient is not in shock or has been successfully resuscitated from shock, you must consider the possible underlying conditions responsible for the complaint of abdominal pain. Of utmost importance at this point is to determine whether the patient has an acute "surgical" (i.e., requiring surgery) abdomen.

PERFORATED OR RUPTURED VISCUS. Finding air under the diaphragm on the upright chest x-ray (CXR) or between the viscera and subcutaneous tissue on the lateral decubitus film indicates a perforated or ruptured viscus. Immediate surgical consultation is required. Ensure that the patient is NPO.

INTRA-ABDOMINAL HEMORRHAGE. Abdominal pain due to an intra-abdominal hemorrhage almost always requires immediate surgical consultation. Ensure that the patient is kept NPO and that blood has been sent for a stat crossmatch for 4 to 6 units of packed RBCs.

RUPTURED INTRA-ABDOMINAL ABSCESS. An intra-abdominal abscess that has ruptured often results in acute peritonitis and, if left untreated, may progress to septic shock. Urgent surgical consultation for proper drainage is required. Ensure that the patient is kept NPO.

NECROSIS OF A VISCUS. Necrosis of an intra-abdominal viscus due to intussusception, volvulus, strangulated hernia, or ischemic colitis requires urgent surgical consultation. Ensure that the patient is kept NPO.

Other Conditions. Other specific conditions that may not cause an acute surgical abdomen are common and should be considered if none of the above-mentioned conditions are present. Each has features requiring specific attention for the physician on call.

PANCREATITIS. Pancreatitis should be suspected in any patient with abdominal pain but with no evidence of an upper GI bleed or ascites. The abdominal x-ray films may reveal a sentinel loop, colonic distention, a left pleural effusion, or calcification within the pancreas (Fig. 5–7). An elevated serum amylase or lipase level supports the diagnosis, but normal levels do not exclude the possibility of pancreatitis. The patient should be NPO. IV fluids with NS should be ordered to replace any losses. Narcotic analgesic agents usually are required. *Meperidine* (Demerol) 50 to 150 mg IM or SC every 3 to 4 hours PRN is the drug of choice because morphine can cause spasm of the sphincter of Oddi. If the patient develops a fever, an abdominal ultrasound or a computed tomography (CT) scan should be ordered to search for a possible pancreatic abscess. In cases of severe pancreatitis with sepsis, abscess formation, or generalized peritonitis, broad-spectrum antibiotics directed against bowel flora (see page 42, point 6) are appropriate.

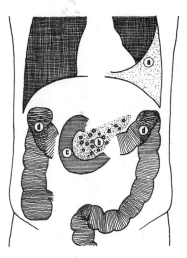

Figure 5–7 □ Radiographic features of pancreatitis. a, Left pleural effusion; b, calcification within the pancreas; c, sentinel loop; d, colonic distention.

INTRA-ABDOMINAL ABSCESS. A contained intra-abdominal abscess will require delineation by either ultrasound or CT scan. This can be arranged in the morning provided the patient is otherwise stable. Abscesses may be treated with ultrasound-guided percutaneous drainage, surgical drainage, or antibiotics alone, depending on the circumstance.

PEPTIC ULCER DISEASE OR GASTROESOPHAGEAL REFLUX DISEASE (GERD). Cases of suspected peptic ulcer disease or gastroesophageal reflux disease (GERD) should be considered for endoscopy. H_2 blockers are common initial therapy for both conditions, and once-daily dosing may be as effective as more frequent dosing. Commonly used agents include *cimetidine* (Tagamet) 800 mg PO at bedtime, *ranitidine* (Zantac) 300 mg PO at bedtime, *famotidine* (Pepcid) 40 mg PO at bedtime, and *nizatidine* (Axid) 300 mg PO at bedtime. Proton pump inhibitors such as *omeprazole* 20 mg PO daily and *lansoprazole* 15 mg PO daily are very effective antisecretory agents but more expensive than the H_2 antagonists. Antacids may be given (e.g., *Gelusil* 30–60 ml PO four times a day) during the acute phase but are contraindicated if endoscopy is to be performed because they coat the lining of the stomach and may obscure the endoscopist's view of mucosal lesions.

Helicobacter pylori infection is the cause of peptic ulcer disease in many patients. Eradication of this organism increases the rate of healing and decreases the likelihood of recurrence. Many effective regimens exist for the treatment of *H. pylori* and are commonly referred to as "triple therapy." Such regimens usually include an antisecretory agent (an H_2 antagonist or proton pump inhibitor) and two antimicrobial drugs (e.g., *metronidazole* 500 mg PO twice a day and *amoxicillin* 1 g PO twice a day). Unfortunately, it is not possible to distinguish which patients with peptic ulcer disease are infected on the basis of symptoms alone. When presented at night with a patient in whom peptic ulcer disease is suspected, empiric triple therapy for *H. pylori* is not recommended and should be reserved for patients with peptic ulcer disease confirmed by endoscopy.

PYELONEPHRITIS. Pyelonephritis requires empiric IV antibiotics (ampicillin and an aminoglycoside) until the specific organism has been identified.

RENAL STONES. Patients with renal stones may be managed medically with narcotic analgesic agents and/or with *diclofenac* 75 mg IM or IV or 100 mg PR. Surgical removal, basket extraction, or lithotripsy may be required if the stone has not passed within a few days or if an associated persistent infection is present.

INFECTIOUS GASTROENTERITIS. Infectious gastroenteritis may require specific antibiotics if the stool culture results reveal a bacterial cause. Viral gastroenteritis is treated supportively with IV fluids and antiemetics. *Clostridium difficile* infection should be suspected in any patient developing diarrhea during or after a course of antibiotics. Sigmoidoscopy may reveal a characteristic pseudomembrane, in which case *metronidazole* 500 mg PO every 6 hours or *vancomycin* 125 to 500 mg every 6 hours may be instituted before confirmation by *C. difficile* culture or toxin assay.

OVARIAN CYST, TUMOR, OR SALPINGITIS. These are best managed by referral to a gynecologist.

■ ABDOMINAL PAIN IN THE AIDS OR IMMUNOSUPPRESSED PATIENT

Symptoms such as chronic abdominal pain, nausea, and vomiting are common in the critically ill acquired immunodeficiency syndrome (AIDS) or immunosuppressed patient. Many AIDS patients already appear chronically ill, and this must be factored into one's assessment of the cause of abdominal pain. Many also will already have abnormalities in baseline laboratory values, making *changes* in laboratory parameters more important than absolute values.

The following features are pertinent in the evaluation of abdominal pain in the AIDS or immunosuppressed patient:

1. Fever is a sensitive sign of infection in the AIDS patient with abdominal pain. Unfortunately, it is a nonspecific finding in the AIDS patient and may be due to nonabdominal occult infections or due to human immunodeficiency virus (HIV) itself. AIDS patients with temperatures ≥ 38.5°C should have blood cultures drawn twice, although frequently no etiologic agent is isolated.

2. AIDS and immunocompromised patients commonly have leukopenia due to the effect of HIV suppression of the bone marrow and to drugs. Thus, even a normal WBC level, especially if accompanied by a left shift, should be interpreted as a sign of possible infection in the AIDS patient with fever and abdominal pain.

3. Bowel wall ulceration or perforation due to *cytomegalovirus (CMV)* infection is a common cause of an acute surgical abdomen in the AIDS patient. Hepatitis, pancreatitis, and gastritis may also be seen in this patient population.

4. Causes of small bowel obstruction that should be considered include bulky lymphadenopathy due to tuberculosis or to *Mycobacterium avium-intracellulare* and tumors such as bowel lymphoma.

5. Pancreatitis is an unusual cause of abdominal pain in AIDS patients and, when seen, may be a side effect of *pentamidine*

or *trimethoprim-sulfamethoxazole,* two drugs used to treat *Pneumocystis carinii* pneumonia.

■ ABDOMINAL PAIN IN THE ELDERLY

The investigation and management of abdominal pain in the elderly patient should proceed along the same lines as for other patient groups. Of note in the elderly is that abdominal pain may be very mild despite the presence of an acute abdomen. One should not underestimate the seriousness of mild abdominal pain in the elderly, especially if associated with acute confusion, fever, an elevated WBC level, or a metabolic acidosis.

Two conditions causing abdominal pain that are usually unique to the elderly are *colonic perforation* due to diverticular disease and *mesenteric ischemia* due to atherosclerosis.

6

CHEST PAIN

In developed countries, in which coronary artery disease is the leading cause of death, it is not surprising that when a patient complains of "chest pain," you will wonder whether the patient is having angina or, worse yet, a heart attack. There are, however, several other equally serious causes of chest pain that may go undiagnosed if not specifically looked for. In the assessment of chest pain, history taking is your most powerful tool.

■ PHONE CALL

Questions

1. How severe is the pain?
2. What are the vital signs?
3. What was the reason for admission?
4. Does the patient have a past history of angina or myocardial infarction (MI)? If yes, is the pain similar to their usual angina or previous MI?

Orders

If MI is suspected:
1. Electrocardiogram (ECG) stat
2. Oxygen by face mask or nasal prongs at 4 L/min. If the patient is a CO_2 retainer, you will have to be cautious when giving oxygen (maximum FIO_2 0.28 by mask or 2 L/min by nasal prongs).
3. Nitroglycerin 0.3 to 0.6 mg sublingually (SL) every 5 minutes, provided the systolic blood pressure (BP) is > 90 mm Hg
4. Ask the RN to take the patient's chart to the bedside.

Inform RN

"Will arrive at bedside in . . . minutes."

Most causes of chest pain are diagnosed by history. It is impossible to obtain an accurate and relevant history by speaking to the RN over the telephone; the history must be taken first-hand from the patient. Because some causes of chest pain represent medical emergencies, the patient should be assessed immediately.

■ ELEVATOR THOUGHTS
(What causes chest pain?)

Cardiac	Angina
	Myocardial infarction
	Aortic dissection
	Pericarditis
Resp	Pulmonary embolism or infarction
	Pneumothorax
	Pleuritis (± pneumonia)
GI	Esophageal spasm, reflux, dysmotility; esophagitis
	Peptic ulcer disease
MSS	Costochondritis
	Tietze's syndrome
	Arthropathies
	Xiphodynia
	Rib fracture
Skin	Herpes zoster
Psych	Panic disorder
	Anxiety disorder

■ MAJOR THREAT TO LIFE

- Myocardial ischemia or MI
- Aortic dissection
- Pneumothorax
- Pulmonary embolus

Cardiogenic shock or fatal dysrhythmias may occur as a result of *myocardial ischemia or infarction. Aortic dissection* may result in death from cardiac tamponade, aortic rupture, acute aortic insufficiency, or MI and may damage other organ systems by compromising vascular supply. A *pneumothorax* may cause hypoxia by compressing the ipsilateral lung. A tension pneumothorax may also result in hypotension as a result of positive intrathoracic pressure decreasing venous return to the heart. *Pulmonary embolism* may cause hypoxia and, in more severe cases, may result in acute right ventricular failure.

■ BEDSIDE

Quick Look Test

Does the patient look well (comfortable), sick (uncomfortable or distressed), or critical (about to die)?

Most patients with chest pain from MI or myocardial ischemia look pale and anxious. Patients with pericarditis, a pneumothorax, or pulmonary embolism involving the pleural surface look apprehensive and breathe with shallow, painful respirations. If the patient looks well, suspect esophagitis or a musculoskeletal problem, such as costochondritis.

Airway and Vital Signs

What is the BP?

Most patients with chest pain will have a normal BP. Hypotension may be seen with MI, massive pulmonary embolism, an aortic dissection resulting in cardiac tamponade, or tension pneumothorax. Hypertension, occurring in association with myocardial ischemia or aortic dissection, should be treated urgently (see Chapter 16, pages 162 to 163).

A wide pulse pressure should raise the suspicion of aortic insufficiency, which may be seen as a complication of a proximal aortic dissection.

A pulsus paradoxus (see page 269) may be a clue to the presence of a pericardial effusion, which may be seen with an aortic dissection or with pericarditis.

What is the HR?

Does the patient have tachycardia? Severe chest pain of any cause may result in sinus tachycardia. Heart rates of > 100 beats/min should also alert you to the possibility of a tachydysrhythmia such as atrial fibrillation, other supraventricular tachycardias, or ventricular tachycardia, which may require immediate cardioversion.

Does the patient have bradycardia? Bradycardia in a patient with chest pain may represent sinus or atrioventricular (AV) nodal ischemia (as may be seen with MI) or beta blockade or calcium channel blockade due to drugs. Immediate treatment of bradycardia is not required unless the rate is extremely slow (< 40 beats/min) or the patient is hypotensive (see Chapter 18, pages 177 to 178).

What is the breathing pattern?

Tachypnea may accompany any type of chest pain. Shallow, painful breathing suggests a pleural (pleuritis, pneumothorax, pericarditis, pulmonary embolism) or musculoskeletal cause.

What does the ECG show?

The ECG should be reviewed immediately after taking the vital signs to avoid delays in administering thrombolytic therapy if the patient is having an acute MI. Because thrombolysis is most effective when given within the first 4 hours of chest pain, if an MI is suspected based on the ECG, call your resident *immediately* to assess the patient for possible thrombolytic therapy. Remember, a normal ECG does not rule out the possibility of angina or MI.

The ECG in a case of aortic dissection may look perfectly normal. The presence of left ventricular hypertrophy (LVH) may provide a clue to long-standing hypertension, which is a risk factor for a dissection.

The most common ECG finding in a patient with pulmonary embolism is sinus tachycardia, but a rightward axis should also be looked for.

The ECG in a patient with pericarditis may show diffuse, usually mild, ST elevations and sometimes PR depression.

Management I

Is the patient receiving oxygen?

Ensure that the patient is receiving oxygen at an appropriate concentration. If you have access to a pulse oximeter, attach the patient, and keep the oxygen saturation level ≥ 93%.

Does the patient have chest pain now? If myocardial ischemia is suspected, proceed as follows.

Chest Pain and Systolic BP of > 90 mm Hg

- If the last dose of SL nitroglycerin was given > 5 minutes ago, give another dose immediately. If, after an additional 5 minutes, the pain is still present, give a third nitroglycerin dose.
- If the pain continues despite three doses of nitroglycerin, ask the RN to draw 10 mg (1 ml) of morphine into a syringe diluted with 9 ml of normal saline (NS). Give the *morphine* in 2- to 4-mg aliquots IV until the pain is relieved, provided the systolic BP is > 90 mm Hg.

  Morphine sulfate may cause hypotension or respiratory depression. Take the patient's BP and respiratory rate (RR) before each dose is given. If necessary, *naloxone hydrochloride* (Narcan) 0.2 to 2 mg IV or SC may be given every 5 minutes to a total of 10 mg to reverse these side effects. Nausea or vomiting may also occur and can usually be controlled with *dimenhydrinate* 25 mg IV or 50 mg PO every 4 hours as needed.
- If the chest pain requires the administration of morphine, arrange for assessment by the intensive care unit/cardiac care unit (ICU/CCU) team as soon as possible.

Chest Pain and Systolic BP of < 90 mm Hg

- What is the patient's normal BP? If the systolic BP is normally 90 mm Hg, you may proceed cautiously with nitroglycerin 0.3 mg SL, as described, provided there is no further drop in the BP.

- If the hypotension is an acute change, establish IV access immediately with a large-bore IV catheter (size 16 if possible). (Refer to Chapter 18, page 180, for management of hypotension.)

If the Patient Looks Sick or Critical

Establish IV access using D5W if not already done.
Draw arterial blood gases (ABG) sample.
Attach to pulse oximeter.

Selective History and Chart Review

How does the patient describe the pain?
Crushing, squeezing, vise-like pain or pressure is characteristic of MI. Severe tearing or ripping pain is characteristic of an aortic dissection.

Is the pain the same as the patient's usual angina?
If the patient recognizes the current discomfort as his or her usual angina, he or she is probably right.

Is the chest pain worse with deep breathing or coughing?
Pleuritic chest pain suggests pleuritis, pneumothorax, rib fracture, pericarditis, pulmonary embolism, pneumonia, or costochondritis.

Does the pain radiate?
Radiation of the pain to the jaw, shoulders, or arms is suggestive of myocardial ischemia or infarction. Radiation of pain to the back suggests myocardial ischemia, MI, or aortic dissection distal to the left subclavian artery. Dissection proximal to the left subclavian artery characteristically causes nonradiating anterior chest pain. A burning sensation that radiates to the neck and is accompanied by an acid taste in the mouth is suggestive of esophageal reflux.

Is there any associated nausea, vomiting, diaphoresis, or lightheadedness?
Cardiogenic nausea and vomiting are associated with larger MIs but do not suggest a particular location, as was previously thought.

Is the chest pain worse with swallowing?
Chest pain that is made worse by swallowing suggests an esophageal disorder or pericarditis.

Selective Physical Examination

Vitals	Repeat now
Body habitus	Does the patient look marfanoid? (A tall, thin patient with long limbs and arachnodac-

tly may have a connective tissue disorder predisposing him or her to an aortic dissection.)

HEENT	White exudate in oral cavity or pharynx (thrush with possible concomitant esophageal candidiasis)
Resp	Asymmetric expansion of the chest (pneumothorax)
	Deviation of the trachea to one side (large pneumothorax on the side opposite the deviation)
	Hyperresonance to percussion (on the side of a pneumothorax)
	Diminished breath sounds (on the side of a pneumothorax)
	Crackles (CHF secondary to acute MI, pneumonia)
	Consolidation (pulmonary infarction or pneumonia)
	Pleural rub (pulmonary embolism, pneumonia)
	Pleural effusion (pulmonary embolism, pneumonia, ruptured aortic dissection)
Chest wall	Tender costal cartilages (costochondritis)
	Erythema, swelling of costal cartilages (Tietze's syndrome, arthritis)
	Tender xiphoid process (xiphodynia)
	Localized rib pain (rib fracture)
CVS	Unequal carotid pulses (aortic dissection)
	Unequal upper limb BP or diminished femoral pulses (aortic dissection)
	Elevated JVP (right ventricular failure secondary to MI or pulmonary embolism; tension pneumothorax)
	Right ventricular heave (acute RV failure secondary to pulmonary embolism)
	Left ventricular heave (CHF)
	Displaced apical impulse (away from the side of a pneumothorax)
	Loud P_2 (acute cor pulmonale), S_3 (CHF)
	Mitral insufficiency murmur (papillary muscle dysfunction due to ischemia or infarction)
	Aortic stenosis murmur (angina)
	Aortic insufficiency murmur (proximal aortic dissection)
	Pericardial rub (pericarditis)
	Pericardial rubs are biphasic or triphasic

scratching sounds that vary with position

ABD   Guarding, rebound tenderness (perforated ulcer)

Epigastric tenderness (peptic ulcer disease)

Generalized abdominal pain (mesenteric infarction from aortic dissection)

CNS   Hemiplegia (aortic dissection involving a carotid artery)

Skin   Unilateral maculopapular rash or vesicles in a dermatomal pattern (herpes zoster)

Look at the Chest X-ray

Review the CXR as soon as possible.

If a pneumothorax is suspected, upright inspiratory and expiratory films should be ordered. A pneumothorax is identified by a peripheral hyperlucent area indicating free air in the pleural space and partial or complete collapse of the affected lung (Fig. 6–1). A tension pneumothorax is a medical emergency and should be treated urgently as outlined in Chapter 20, page 207.

The CXR may be normal in a patient with angina or an MI. Sometimes pulmonary venous congestion will be seen if there is significant associated left ventricular dysfunction.

If an aortic dissection is suspected, look specifically for a widened mediastinum or prominent aortic knuckle (Fig. 6–2). Suspected aortic dissection requires you to proceed urgently with the appropriate investigation and management (see page 55).

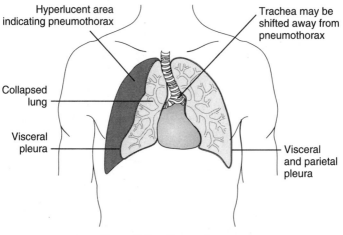

Figure 6–1 □ Pneumothorax.

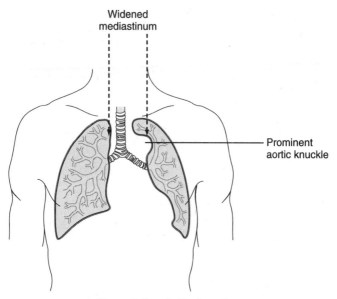

Figure 6–2 □ Aortic dissection.

The CXR may be normal in a patient with pericarditis, unless significant pericardial fluid has accumulated, in which case the cardiac silhouette may be enlarged.

The CXR of a patient with suspected pulmonary embolism may be entirely normal or may show any of the features illustrated in Figure 24–3.

Management II

Angina. If *angina* has been relieved with 1 to 3 nitroglycerin tablets, review the precipitating cause. An adjustment in the anti-anginal medication may be required and should be made in consultation with your resident and attending physician. However, if the angina occurred at rest or this is the first episode of angina, the patient should be assessed by the ICU/CCU staff regardless of whether the pain was relieved with ≤ 3 nitroglycerin tablets.

If the angina required more than three doses of nitroglycerin or IV morphine, serial cardiac enzymes and ECGs should be ordered. If the clinical impression is of possible MI, the patient should be transferred to the ICU/CCU for continuous ECG monitoring.

Myocardial Infarction. If an MI is suspected based on history or ECG changes (see Appendix D, page 409), the patient should be transferred to the ICU/CCU as soon as possible. The patient also should be evaluated immediately for possible thrombolytic therapy. Ongoing myocardial ischemia may also require treatment with aspirin, IV nitroglycerin, heparin, or beta blockers.

Aortic Dissection. Suspicion of aortic dissection requires urgent investigation and management as follows.

1. Arrange for an urgent CT scan of the thorax or a transesophageal echocardiogram.

   If neither of these can be performed within the next hour, a transthoracic echocardiogram may detect a dilated aortic root, aortic valvular insufficiency, or a pericardial effusion, any of which may be a clue to the presence of a dissection. Occasionally, an aortic dissection flap also is directly visualized with this test.

2. Draw blood for a stat crossmatch for 6 to 8 units of packed red blood cells (RBCs), electrolytes, urea, creatinine, glucose, complete blood cell count (CBC) and differential, prothrombin time (PT), and activated partial thromboplastin time (aPTT).

3. Review the ECG for evidence of an acute MI. This finding suggests aortic dissection involving the coronary ostia.

4. The patient should be transferred to the ICU/CCU as soon as possible for careful control of BP (see Chapter 16, page 162).

5. Surgical consultation should be obtained early if the diagnosis of dissection is apparent. The diagnosis can be confirmed by nuclear MRI or aortography.

Pericarditis. Patients with suspected pericarditis should have nonurgent echocardiograms performed to look for pericardial effusions or signs of hemodynamic compromise. *Indomethacin* (Indocin) 50 mg PO three times a day or *aspirin* 650 mg PO four times a day is helpful.

Nonsteroidal anti-inflammatory drugs (NSAIDs) are contraindicated in the patient who has the syndrome of aspirin sensitivity, nasal polyps, and bronchospasm; in the patient who is anticoagulated; and in the patient who has active peptic ulcer disease. Because of their sodium-retaining properties, caution should be used in giving NSAIDs to patients in CHF. NSAIDs should also be used with caution in patients with renal insufficiency because these drugs may inhibit renal prostaglandins, which are responsible for maintaining renal perfusion in those with prerenal conditions; sulindac (Clinoril) may not have this effect.

Pulmonary Embolus. The management of pulmonary embolus is discussed in Chapter 24, page 277.

Pneumothorax. A pneumothorax may require chest tube drainage depending on its size. If the patient develops a tension pneumothorax, immediate treatment is necessary to relieve the pressure using a 16-gauge IV catheter as described on page 207.

Pneumonia. Suggested antibiotics for pneumonia are discussed in Chapter 24, pages 280 to 282, and should be chosen according to the Gram's stain results and patient's characteristics.

Esophagitis. The pain of esophagitis may be temporarily treated with antacids. Choose carefully. Magnesium-containing antacids (Gelusil, Maalox) may cause diarrhea, whereas antacids containing solely aluminum (Amphogel, Basalgel) may cause constipation. Do not substitute one GI complaint for another! *Gelusil* 30 to 60 ml at 1 and 3 hours after meals and at bedtime is a standard antacid order. More frequent doses may be required if the pain is severe. An alginate such as Gaviscon 10 to 20 ml PO or 2 to 4 tablets (chewed) after meals and at bedtime followed by a glass of water may also be used. Elevation of the head of the bed and avoidance of nighttime snacks may also be helpful.

An H_2 blocker such as *cimetidine* (Tagamet) 400 mg PO twice a day, *ranitidine* (Zantac) 150 mg PO twice a day, *famotidine* (Pepcid) 20 mg PO twice a day, or *nizatidine* (Axid) 150 mg PO twice a day should also be started to aid in the long-term treatment of this disease.[1] *Omeprazole* (Losec) 20 mg PO daily is more expensive than H_2 blockers but is usually effective in erosive esophagitis resistant to the usual agents. *Cisapride* (Prepulsid) 20 mg PO twice a day is a useful prokinetic agent that may help minimize reflux.

Esophageal candidiasis will not respond to antacids. Immunocompromised patients may experience severe chest pain from this condition. Diagnosis should be confirmed by endoscopy. Although useful in thrush, Mycostatin is not effective in esophageal candidiasis. In the AIDS or immunocompromised patient, *fluconazole* (Diflucan) has been shown to be more effective than *ketoconazole* (Nizoral) in eradicating *Candida* from the esophagus but to provide no better symptomatic relief.[2] Doses are *fluconazole* 100 to 200 mg or *ketoconazole* 200 to 400 mg PO once daily. An alternative is *itraconazole* (Sporanex) 100 to 200 mg PO daily. Ketoconazole is the least expensive.

Peptic Ulcer. The pain of peptic ulcer disease may be temporarily treated with antacids. *Gelusil* 30 to 60 ml at 1 and 3 hours after meals and at bedtime is a standard antacid order. More frequent doses may be required if the pain is severe. An H_2 blocker such as *cimetidine* (Tagamet) 300 mg PO every 6 hours, *ranitidine* (Zantac) 150 mg PO twice a day, *famotidine* (Pepcid) 20 mg PO twice a day, or *nizatidine* (Axid) 150 mg PO twice a day may help in the long-term treatment of this disease. *Omeprazole* (Losec) 20 to 40 mg PO daily is more expensive but may be useful in ulcers resistant to H_2 blockade. A patient with suspected peptic ulcer disease should be referred for a possible endoscopic evaluation in the morning.

Costochondritis. Costochondritis may be treated with an NSAID, such as *naproxen* (Naprosyn) 250 mg PO twice a day (see precautions, page 55).

Herpes Zoster. Unilateral chest pain in a dermatomal distribution may precede the typical skin lesions of herpes zoster ("shingles") by 2 or 3 days. The rash begins as a reddened, maculopapular area, which rapidly evolves into vesicular lesions. Treatment of acute herpes zoster neuritis may be difficult and often requires narcotic *analgesics, amitriptyline hydrochloride,* and in some cases, *steroids.* Topical preparations of *capsaicin* (Zostrix) may also provide temporary relief of neuralgic pain but should not be applied directly to open skin lesions. Antiviral agents such as *acyclovir* 800 mg PO every 6 hours may reduce the severity and duration of localized herpes zoster. Immunocompromised patients may require larger doses such as 800 mg PO five times a day or 10 mg/kg IV every 8 hours.

Panic and Anxiety Disorders. *Panic attacks* are defined as "discrete periods of discomfort or fear" and are often associated with chest pain, dyspnea, diaphoresis, and dizziness. These symptoms may also be accompanied by feelings of depersonalization and a fear of dying, of "going crazy," or of "losing control." Chest pain may also be a feature of an *anxiety disorder.* Because of the possibility of a life-threatening cause of chest pain, panic and anxiety disorders should be diagnoses of exclusion. Short-acting benzodiazepines such as *alprazolam* 0.5 mg PO daily or *lorazepam* 1 to 2 mg PO three times a day as needed may be helpful in the short-term treatment of these disorders.

References

1. Pope CE: Acid-reflux disorders. N Engl J Med 1994;331:656–660.
2. Laine L, Dretler RH, Conteas CN, et al: Fluconazole compared with ketoconazole for the treatment of *Candida esophagitis*: A randomized trial. Ann Intern Med 1992:117:655–660.

7

COMBATIVENESS—THE OUT-OF-CONTROL PATIENT

Every once in a while, you will be paged by an exasperated nurse who has been trying to reason with an out-of-control patient. We are not referring here to the moody or uncooperative patient—we are referring to the hostile individuals whose temporary behavior poses a real physical threat to themselves, other patients, or hospital staff. Your job is not to act as the strong-arm of the hospital law. Your role is to deem which medical reasons, if any, are responsible for the patient's behavior and to administer appropriate treatment.

■ PHONE CALL

Questions

1. What was the reason for admission?
2. What medications is the patient taking now?
3. Is there an obvious reason for the patient's combative behavior?
4. What measures have been used thus far to calm or reason with the patient?
5. What additional hospital personnel are there to help you now?
6. What is the patient's estimated height and weight?

Orders

1. Ask the RN to call the hospital's security personnel now, if not already done. Your job is not to hurry to the ward to help hold down the patient. Your role is to determine the cause of the patient's behavior and to institute appropriate treatment.

2. *Haloperidol* (Haldol) 1 to 10 mg IM stat. By the time the RN has called you, he or she has usually wrestled with the patient for 10 to 20 minutes, enlisted the aid of orderlies, and tried everything at his or her immediate disposal. The RN by this time is desperate for a medication order, and providing the patient is not allergic, haloperidol is a good choice.

   The initial dose depends on the patient's height and body weight: 1 mg IM may suffice for the elderly patient of slight build, whereas 10 mg IM may be necessary for the young, large football player.

Inform RN

"Will arrive at the bedside in . . . minutes."
The out-of-control patient requires your immediate attention.

■ ELEVATOR THOUGHTS
(What causes dangerously combative
behavior?)

Any confusional state due to an acute or a chronic medical or psychiatric condition can result in temporary hostile or combative behavior. How an individual reacts in a given situation is often a reflection of his or her premorbid personality. The most common out-of-control patient is a young individual who feels frustrated, confined, and overwhelmed by the illness and the hospital environment. A second common out-of-control patient is the elderly person who becomes disoriented and combative, particularly at night (the sundown phenomenon).

Numerous other medical conditions may set off this behavior in any hospitalized patient and should be carefully looked for, including intracranial disease, systemic disorders (drugs, organ failure, metabolic and endocrine disorders, infections and inflammation), and psychiatric disorders. Once the patient is safely approachable, these conditions should be carefully sought (see Chapter 8, pages 63 to 64).

■ MAJOR THREAT TO LIFE

- Physical injury

  Patients who are acutely agitated and hostile are not reasoning properly and appear to be "looking for a fight." The typical out-of-control patient will have pulled out the intravenous (IV) lines, nasogastric (NG) tubes, or Foley catheter and will be cursing, threatening, and pummeling any hospital personnel within striking distance. The patient loses regard for his or her own safety and risks both new injury and worsening of the underlying medical condition that necessitated the hospitalization.

■ BEDSIDE

Quick Look Test

Does the patient look well (comfortable), sick (uncomfortable or distressed), or critical (about to die)?

The combative patient looks very much alive, agitated, and (often) ready for a fight!

Stand back from the situation for a moment and observe the patient. You must judge from a distance how dangerous the patient is and what immediate measures will be required to calm the patient and regain control. Look for any obvious signs or conditions that may require specific treatment.

- Is the patient cyanotic or having difficulty breathing (hypoxia)?
- Does the patient appear to be hallucinating (drug intoxication or withdrawal)?
- Is the patient in pain?

Management

The first priority is to calm the patient and regain control of the situation. In performing this task, the first rule is to remain calm yourself. It is not necessary to jump into the brawl, and you will be far more effective by using your head in this situation.

1. Some patients will become calm simply because "the doctor" has arrived, and they will feel less helpless and more in control of themselves with a physician there to address their immediate concerns. You will be able to judge within the first 30 seconds whether you are lucky enough for this to be the situation.
2. Some patients are so completely out of control that calm reasoning is futile. These patients may require temporary physical restraints while medication is being given. You may try to explain to the patient that you are going to give him or her "a shot" to calm the patient down and make the patient feel better. If he or she does not allow you to approach because of aggressive behavior, the patient will need to be held down while medication is administered. Continued restraint may be required until the medication takes effect. Should you need to physically restrain a violent individual, the general rule is to have at least one person per limb plus one.
   - If the patient has already been given the haloperidol that you ordered over the telephone and is still out of control, physical restraints may be necessary. Allow adequate time for the medication administered to take effect. If the patient remains agitated, you may give additional doses of *haloperidol* 1 to 3 mg PO or IM until adequate sedation is achieved. Always use the lowest effective dosage.
   - The two main acute side effects of haloperidol are hypotension and the occasional acute dystonic reaction (spasm of the face, tongue, back, or neck). The hypotension is usually postural, and once the patient is cooperative, he or she should be assisted when initially going from the

supine to the upright position. Acute dystonic reactions usually respond to *diphenhydramine* 25 to 50 mg PO, IM, or IV or *benztropine mesylate* 1 to 2 mg PO, IM, or IV.

- If haloperidol is not available, a good alternative choice is *chlorpromazine* (Thorazine) 25 to 50 mg PO or IM every 3 to 4 hours.
- Hypotension may be particularly pronounced with IM chlorpromazine and may respond to fluid administration with normal saline (NS). The treatment for acute dystonic reactions is the same as for haloperidol.

3. Benzodiazepines or barbiturates should be avoided because although they have valuable sedative properties, they tend to cloud consciousness and may actually compound the behavioral problem.

4. Call the patient's family, explain what has happened, and see if the family can shed any light on the patient's behavior. If physical restraints (wrist and ankle restraints or a posey) have been required, inform the family immediately and reassure them that you anticipate that the restraints will be required only temporarily. Emphasize that these measures are being used only temporarily to protect the patient from injuring himself or herself. There is no better way to upset an uninformed and unsuspecting family than to have them walk into their loved one's room the next day and find the patient "tied down" to the bed.

5. Once the acute crisis is over, a thorough evaluation for underlying causes of confusion (any of which may lead to combative behavior) should be undertaken (see Chapter 8). Once the patient is safely approachable, a directed physical examination looking for life-threatening (see page 65) or correctable causes (see page 67) of confusion should be performed. You will have to use your judgment because sometimes these patients are best left alone to sleep for a while. Just as often, however, the recently out-of-control patient will be grateful for the additional attention received from a concerned medical student or physician.

8

CONFUSION/DECREASED LEVEL OF CONSCIOUSNESS

Confusion is a common problem in hospitalized patients, especially among the elderly. Unfortunately, the terms *delirium, toxic psychosis, acute brain syndrome,* and *acute confusional state* often are used interchangeably to refer to any cause of confusion. When the term *metabolic encephalopathy* is used, it implies that the confusion is not due to psychiatric disorders or structural intracranial lesions.

The two recommended terms are delirium and dementia. *Delirium* is characterized by restlessness, agitation, clouding of consciousness, and, in some patients, bizarre behavior, hallucinations, delusions, and illusions. *Dementia* refers to a state of irreversible loss of memory and a global cognitive deficit. The level of consciousness is an important distinguishing feature between delirium and dementia. Delirium is characterized by a clouding of consciousness (a decreased clarity of awareness of the environment), whereas dementia is associated with a normal level of consciousness. Also, the signs of delirium fluctuate, whereas the confusion seen with dementia is more constant.

Drowsiness, stupor, and *coma* refer to various degrees of unresponsiveness or diminished levels of consciousness.

■ PHONE CALL

Questions

1. **Clarify the situation. In what way is the patient confused?**
2. **What are the vital signs?**
3. **Has there been a change in the level of consciousness?**
4. **Have there been previous episodes of confusion?**
5. **What was the reason for admission?**
6. **Is the patient diabetic?**
   Confusion can be caused by either too much or too little sugar in the blood. Hypoglycemia (due to excess insulin or oral hypoglycemic agents) and marked hyperglycemia (due to inadequate insulin or oral hypoglycemic dosage) are prime considerations when confusion occurs in the diabetic patient.
7. **How old is the patient?**
   A 30-year-old patient is much more likely to have a serious yet reversible cause of confusion than an 80-year-old patient receiving multiple medications.

Orders

1. Blood glucose, Chemstrip, or glucose meter reading—hypoglycemia is a rapidly reversible cause of confusion.
2. O_2 saturation, if pneumonia or a respiratory disorder was the reason for admission—this can be measured by attaching a pulse oximeter to the patient.

Inform RN

"Will arrive at the bedside in . . . minutes."

Confusion in association with fever, decrease in the level of consciousness, or acute agitation (see Chapter 7) requires you to see the patient immediately.

■ ELEVATOR THOUGHTS (What causes confusion or a decreased level of consciousness?)

Many disorders that begin with confusion may lead to a diminished level of consciousness and, ultimately, coma (note items marked with an asterisk in the following lists). To cause a diminished level of consciousness, both cerebral hemispheres must be affected (e.g., drugs or toxins) or there must be suppression of the brainstem reticular activating system.

Central Nervous System (Intracranial)

1. Dementia
    a. Alzheimer's disease
    b. Multi-infarct dementia
    c. Parkinson's disease
    d. Normal pressure hydrocephalus*
2. Malignancy (primary central nervous system [CNS] tumor, CNS metastasis, paraneoplastic syndrome)
3. Head trauma (subdural and epidural hematoma, concussion, cerebral contusion)*
4. Postictal state*
5. Transient ischemic attack (TIA)/stroke*
6. Hypertensive encephalopathy*
7. Wernicke's encephalopathy (thiamine deficiency)
8. Vitamin B_{12} deficiency

---

*Indicates disorders that may begin with confusion but may lead to a diminished level of consciousness or coma.

Systemic

Drugs

1. Alcohol withdrawal—confusion in the alcoholic patient may occur when the patient is intoxicated, during early withdrawal, or later as part of delirium tremens
2. Narcotic and sedative drug excess* or withdrawal—even "normal" doses of these drugs frequently cause confusion in the elderly
3. Nonsteroidal anti-inflammatory drugs (NSAIDs), including aspirin
4. Antihypertensives (methyldopa, beta blockers)
5. Psychotropic medications (tricyclic antidepressants, lithium, phenothiazines, monoamine oxidase [MAO] inhibitors, benzodiazepines, selective serotonin reuptake inhibitors [SSRIs])*
6. Miscellaneous (steroids, cimetidine, antihistamines, anticholinergics)

Organ Failure*

1. Respiratory failure (hypoxia, hypercapnia)
2. Renal failure (uremic encephalopathy)
3. Liver failure (hepatic encephalopathy)
4. Congestive heart failure (CHF) (hypoxia), hypertensive encephalopathy

Metabolic*

1. Hyperglycemia, hypoglycemia
2. Hypernatremia, hyponatremia
3. Hypercalcemia

Endocrine

1. Hyperthyroidism or hypothyroidism*
2. Hyperadrenocorticism or hypoadrenocorticism

Infection or Inflammation

1. Meningitis,* encephalitis,* brain abscess*
2. Lyme disease
3. Cerebral vasculitis (systemic lupus erythematosus [SLE], polyarteritis nodosa)*

Psychiatric Disorders

1. Mania, depression
2. Schizophrenia

---

*Indicates disorders that may begin with confusion but may lead to a diminished level of consciousness or coma.

■ MAJOR THREAT TO LIFE

- Intracranial mass
- Delirium tremens
- Meningitis

Patients with an *intracranial mass* (e.g., subdural or epidural hematoma, brain abscess, tumor) may initially present with confusion. Patients with untreated *delirium tremens* can have a mortality rate of up to 15%. *Meningitis* must be recognized early if antibiotic medication is to be effective.

■ BEDSIDE

Quick Look Test

Does the patient look well (comfortable), sick (uncomfortable or distressed), or critical (about to die)?
Most patients with delirium look sick, whereas most patients with dementia look well.

Airway, Vital Signs, and Chemstrip Results

Is the patient receiving oxygen?
An F_{IO_2} of > 0.28 given to a patient with chronic obstructive pulmonary disease (COPD) may depress the respiratory center, resulting in confusion from hypercapnia.

What is the BP?
Hypertensive encephalopathy is rare; diastolic blood pressure (BP) is usually > 120 mm Hg. Confusion in association with a systolic BP of < 90 mm Hg may be due to impaired cerebral perfusion secondary to shock. Drug overdose, adrenal insufficiency, and hyponatremia are metabolic causes that should be considered in the hypotensive, confused patient.

What is the HR?
A tachycardia suggests sepsis, delirium tremens, hyperthyroidism, or hypoglycemia, but it may also occur in any agitated, anxious patient.

What is the temperature?
Fever suggests infection, delirium tremens, or cerebral vasculitis.

What is the respiratory rate?
Confusion in association with tachypnea should alert you to the possibility of hypoxia. Tachypnea with confusion and petechiae in a young patient with a femoral fracture is a classic presentation of fat embolism syndrome.

What is the blood glucose result?

Hypoglycemia is most commonly seen in the patient with diabetes mellitus who has received the usual insulin dose but has not eaten. Rarely, an incorrect dose of insulin, surreptitious insulin use, or an insulinoma is the cause (see Chapter 32, page 352, for the management of hypoglycemia and pages 347 to 350 for the management of hyperglycemia).

Selective Physical Examination I

Is there evidence on physical examination of one of the major threats to life?

HEENT	Nuchal rigidity (meningitis)
	Papilledema (hypertensive encephalopathy, intracranial mass)
	Pupil size and symmetry

HEENT   Nuchal rigidity (meningitis)

Papilledema (hypertensive encephalopathy, intracranial mass)

Pupil size and symmetry

Dilated pupils suggest increased sympathetic outflow, such as may be seen in delirium tremens or cocaine ingestion, whereas pinpoint pupils suggest narcotic excess or recent application of constricting eyedrops.

Palpate the skull for fractures, hematomas, and lacerations (subdural or epidural hematoma, concussion)

Hemotympanum or blood in the ear canal (basal skull fracture)

Neuro   General appearance—behavior and attitude

Level of consciousness—alert, drowsy

Mood, affect—depressed, agitated, restless

Form of thought—flight of ideas, circumstantiality, loosening of associations, perseveration

Thought content—delusions, concrete thinking

Perceptions—illusions, hallucinations (auditory, visual)

Mental status: A detailed mental status examination is required in the assessment of the confused patient. However, if the patient has a decreased level of consciousness or is agitated or uncooperative, not all the categories discussed subsequently will be appropriate.

Orientation—time, place, and person

Registration—name 3 objects (e.g., apple, pencil, car) and have the patient repeat them

Attention and calculation—serial 7s

Recall—ask for the 3 aforementioned objects (apple, pencil, car)

Language—point to and identify objects; follow a 3-stage command; write a sentence

Long-term memory—birthdate, name of home town

Judgment—test hypothetical situations

A full neurologic examination is required (within the limits posed by the mental status examination).

Is there any tremor (delirium tremens, Parkinson's disease, hyperthyroidism)?

Is there any asymmetry of pupils, visual fields, eye movement, limbs, tone, reflexes, or plantars? Asymmetry suggests structural brain disease.

Management I

Bacterial Meningitis. If there is a suspicion of bacterial meningitis, refer immediately to Chapter 12, pages 98 to 99, for further investigation and management.

Intracranial Lesion. A structural intracranial lesion (e.g., stroke, tumor, subdural hematoma, or epidural hematoma) should be suspected in the patient with new findings of asymmetry on neurologic examination. An urgent computed tomography (CT) head scan will help define the intracranial lesion. Prompt referral to a neurosurgeon will be required for a subdural or an epidural hematoma and for a cerebellar hemorrhage.

Delirium Tremens. Delirium tremens (confusion, fever, tachycardia, dilated pupils, diaphoresis) and alcohol withdrawal must be treated urgently with sedation. Benzodiazepines are of proven benefit. The loading dose of *diazepam* (Valium) is 5 to 10 mg IV at a rate of 2 to 5 mg/min every 30 to 60 minutes until the patient is sedated (i.e., drowsy but rouses when stimulated). The maintenance dose is 10 to 20 mg PO four times a day, with subsequent tapering. Alternatively, *chlordiazepoxide* 100 mg PO four times a day for several days, with subsequent gradual tapering of the dose, may be used. *Thiamine* 100 mg PO, IM, or IV daily for up to 3 days, if not already administered during this hospitalization, should be given to prevent the development of Wernicke's encephalopathy in the alcoholic or malnourished patient. If necessary, IV D5NS then may be given to correct volume depletion after the initial dose of thiamine.

Selective Physical Examination II

Are there other correctable causes of confusion?

Vitals   Hypertension and bradycardia may signify rising intracranial pressure

	Hypothermia suggests myxedema or alcohol, barbiturate, or phenothiazine intoxication
HEENT	Subhyaloid hemorrhage (subarachnoid hemorrhage)
	Conjunctival and fundal petechiae (fat embolism syndrome) (Fig. 8–1)
	Lacerated tongue or cheek (postictal)
	Goiter (hyperthyroidism or hypothyroidism)
Resp	Cyanosis (hypoxia)
	Barrel chest (COPD with hypoxia or hypercapnia)
	Bibasilar crackles (CHF with hypoxia)
CVS	Elevated JVP ⎫ S_3 ⎬ CHF Pitting edema ⎭
ABD	Costovertebral angle tenderness (pyelonephritis)
	Liver, spleen, or kidney tenderness (infection)
	Guarding, rebound tenderness (intra-abdominal infection)
	Shifting dullness, dilated superficial veins, caput medusa (liver failure)
Neuro	Argyll Robertson pupils, i.e., accommodate but do not react to light (syphilis) (Fig. 8–2)
	Cranial nerve palsies (Lyme disease)
	Asterixis, constructional apraxia (liver failure) (Fig. 8–3)
Skin	Axillary fold, neck, upper chest petechiae (fat embolism syndrome)

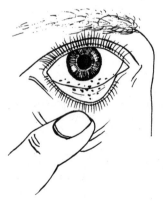 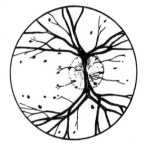

Figure 8–1 □ Conjunctival and fundal petechiae seen in fat embolism syndrome.

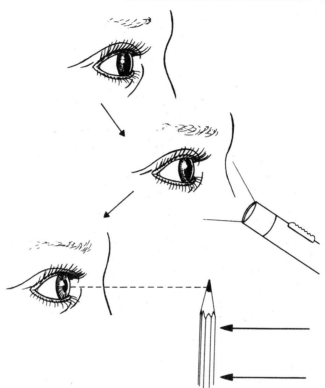

Figure 8–2 □ Argyll Robertson pupils. Pupils do not react to light, but they accommodate.

Selective History and Chart Review

What drugs is the patient receiving?

Remember, even the "usual" doses of some drugs can cause confusion in the elderly because of alterations in intestinal, renal, or hepatic blood flow; drug protein binding; or changes in body fluid compartments.

Is there a history of alcohol abuse?

It is important to establish when alcohol was last ingested because withdrawal symptoms are unlikely after 1 week of abstinence.

Is the patient postoperative?

Postoperative patients are predisposed to confusion because of central nervous system (CNS) effects of anesthetic and

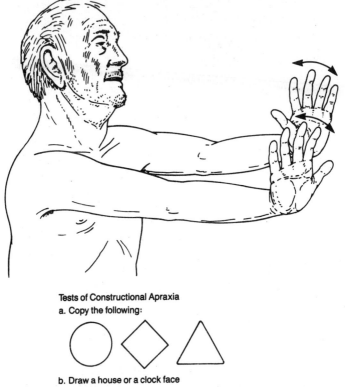

Tests of Constructional Apraxia
a. Copy the following:

b. Draw a house or a clock face
c. Write signature

Figure 8–3 □ *Top*, Asterixis. Wrist flapping seen when the arms are outstretched. *Bottom*, Tests of constructional apraxia.

analgesic medications, nutritional deficiencies (e.g., thiamine), and fluid and electrolyte disturbances. These physiologic abnormalities may be exacerbated in the elderly patient because of sensory impairment (reduced visual or auditory acuity), psychological factors, and cultural expectations.

If there is a decreased level of consciousness, has the change been gradual or sudden?

A sudden decrease in the level of consciousness is usually due to drug ingestion or an acute intracranial catastrophe (hemorrhage, trauma). Gradually developing unresponsiveness (over days or weeks) is usually due to a preceding systemic medical disorder (e.g., metabolic or endocrine disorders, hepatic or renal failure).

Does the patient have acquired immunodeficiency syndrome (AIDS)?

Human immunodeficiency virus (HIV) infection may result in cognitive impairment in the otherwise asymptomatic patient with AIDS. Patients in the more advanced stages of AIDS may suffer a wide variety of neurologic problems associated with confusion, including HIV-1–associated cognitive-motor complex (impaired concentration, slowness of hand movements, and difficulty walking), CNS opportunistic infections (e.g., toxoplasmosis, cryptococcal meningitis), and neoplasms (e.g., primary lymphoma of the brain).

Examine the most recent laboratory test results for those that may indicate the reason for confusion in the patient. Not all of the tests listed will be available or pertinent.

- Blood glucose (hypoglycemia, hyperglycemia)
- Urea, creatinine (renal failure)
- Liver function (liver failure)
- Sodium (hyponatremia, hypernatremia)
- Calcium (hypercalcemia)
- Hemoglobin (Hb), mean corpuscular volume (MCV), red blood cell (RBC) morphology (anemia with oval macrocytes suggests vitamin B_{12} or folate deficiency)
- White blood cell count (WBC) and differential (infection)
- Arterial blood gasses (ABG) (hypoxia or CO_2 retention)
- T_4, T_3, TSH (hyperthyroidism, hypothyroidism)
- Antinuclear antibody (ANA), rheumatoid factor, erythrocyte sedimentation rate (ESR), C3, C4 (vasculitis)
- Drug levels (digoxin, lithium, aspirin, antiepileptic drugs)

Management II

Drugs. If the confusion is secondary to drugs, stop the medication.

If reversal of postoperative narcotic depression is indicated, give *naloxone* (Narcan) 0.2 to 2.0 mg IV, IM, or SC every 5 minutes (maximum total dose, 10 mg) until the desired improved level of consciousness is achieved. Maintenance doses every 1 to 2 hours may be required to maintain reversal of the CNS depression. Naloxone should be used with caution in patients known to be physically dependent on opiates.

Reversal of the benzodiazepine effect can be achieved by administering *flumazenil* 0.2 mg IV over 30 seconds, followed by 0.3 mg IV at 1 minute, 0.5 mg IV at 2 minutes, and continued doses of 0.5 mg IV q1minute until the desired effect is achieved or a total of 3 mg IV is given.

Dementia. Dementia is a diagnosis of exclusion. The following investigations are required to rule out a treatable cause of dementia.

- Complete blood cell count (CBC), electrolytes, urea, creatinine
- Calcium, phosphorus
- Liver function tests
- Serum vitamin B_{12}, folate
- T_4, T_3, TSH
- Serologic test for syphilis (STS)
- CT or magnetic resonance imaging (MRI) head scan

Renal and Hepatic Failure. In *end-stage* renal and liver failure, ensure that the problem has not been compounded by hepatotoxic or nephrotoxic medications. Aggressive treatment of the renal failure (dialysis if necessary) or the liver failure (lactulose, neomycin) should be undertaken when indicated.

Hyponatremia or Hypernatremia. For the management of hyponatremia or hypernatremia, refer to Chapter 34.

Hypercalcemia. For the management of hypercalcemia, see Chapter 30.

Vitamin B_{12} Deficiency. Suspected vitamin B_{12} deficiency needs to be confirmed with a serum vitamin B_{12} level.

Mania, Depression, or Schizophrenia. Suspected mania, depression, or schizophrenia requires psychiatric consultation for confirmation of diagnosis. Agitation in a confused patient may require *haloperidol* 1 to 5 mg PO or IM every 4 to 6 hours.

Cerebral Vasculitis. Cerebral vasculitis is rare. High-dose steroid therapy is the accepted initial treatment.

Fat Embolism. Fat embolism syndrome can have a mortality rate of up to 8%. The mainstay of treatment is oxygen therapy. If the patient requires an FIO_2 of > 0.5, transfer to the ICU/CCU for probable intubation and mechanical ventilation with postive end-expiratory pressure (PEEP) is recommended.

9

DECREASED URINE OUTPUT

Decreased urine output is a problem frequently seen on both medical and surgical services. Proper management of these patients calls on your skills in assessing volume status.

■ PHONE CALL

Questions

1. **How much urine has been passed in the last 24 hours?**
   Urine output of < 400 ml/day (< 20 ml/hr) is *oliguria*. *Anuria* suggests a mechanical obstruction of the bladder outlet or a blocked Foley catheter.
2. **What are the vital signs?**
3. **What was the reason for admission?**
4. **Is the patient complaining of abdominal pain?**
   Abdominal pain is a clue to the possible presence of a distended bladder, as may be seen with bladder outlet obstruction.
5. **Does the patient have a Foley catheter?**
   If the patient has a Foley catheter in place, the urine output assessment usually can be assumed to be accurate. If not, you will have to ensure that the total volume of voided urine has been collected and measured.
6. **What is the most recent serum potassium level?**

Orders

1. If a Foley catheter is in place and the patient is anuric, ask the nurse to flush the catheter with 20 to 30 ml normal saline (NS) to ensure patency. A Foley catheter clogged with sediment is a common problem and a satisfying one to treat before beginning a more detailed investigation for decreased urine output.
2. Serum electrolytes, urea, creatinine. A serum potassium level of > 5.5 mmol/L indicates that hyperkalemia is present. This is the most serious complication of renal insufficiency. A serum HCO_3 measurement of < 20 mmol/L suggests metabolic acidosis due to renal insufficiency. A serum HCO_3 of < 15 mmol/L should prompt you to determine the arterial pH. Elevations in serum urea and creatinine levels can

be used as guidelines to assess the degree of renal insufficiency present.

Inform RN

"Will arrive at bedside in . . . minutes."

Provided that the patient is not in pain and a recent serum potassium level is not elevated, an assessment of decreased urine output can wait 1 or 2 hours if other problems of higher priority exist.

■ ELEVATOR THOUGHTS (What causes decreased urine output?)

Prerenal causes (underperfusion of kidney)	Volume depletion
	Reduced cardiac output (congestive heart failure [CHF], constrictive pericarditis, cardiac tamponade)
	Drugs that reduce effective glomerular perfusion (diuretics, angiotensin-converting enzyme inhibitors, nonsteroidal anti-inflammatory drugs [NSAIDs], cyclosporine)
	Hepatorenal syndrome
Renal causes	Glomerulonephritic syndromes (acute glomerulonephritis, subacute bacterial endocarditis [SBE], systemic lupus erythematosus [SLE], other vasculitides)
	Tubulointerstitial problems
	Acute tubular necrosis due to
	Hypotension
	Nephrotoxins
	Exogenous (aminoglycosides, amphotericin B, IV contrast materials, chemotherapy)
	Endogenous (myoglobin, uric acid, oxalate, amyloid, Bence Jones protein)
	Acute interstitial nephritis due to drugs (penicillin, other beta-lactam antibiotics, NSAIDs, diuretics), autoimmune disease (e.g., SLE), infiltrative diseases, infection
	Vascular problems
	Emboli (from aortic atheromas, SBE, or left heart thrombi)
	Renal artery thrombosis

Postrenal causes	Bilateral ureteric obstruction (obstruction) (e.g., stones, clots, sloughed papillae, retroperitoneal fibrosis, retroperitoneal tumors)
	Bladder outlet obstruction (e.g., prostatic hypertrophy, carcinoma of the cervix, stones, clots, urethral strictures)
	Blocked Foley catheter

■ MAJOR THREAT TO LIFE

- Renal failure
- Hyperkalemia

Decreased urine output from any cause may result in or may be a manifestation of progressive renal insufficiency, leading to renal failure. Of the complications of renal failure, hyperkalemia is the most immediately life threatening because it may lead to potentially fatal cardiac dysrhythmias.

■ BEDSIDE

Quick Look Test

Does the patient look well (comfortable), sick (uncomfortable or distressed), or critical (about to die)?
A sick- or critical-looking patient suggests advanced renal insufficiency. A restless patient suggests pain from a distended bladder. However, both of these conditions can be present in a patient who appears to be deceptively well.

Airway and Vital Signs

Check for postural changes. A postural rise in HR of > 15 beats/min, a fall in systolic BP of > 15 mm Hg, or any fall in diastolic BP suggests significant hypovolemia. *Caution:* A resting tachycardia alone may indicate decreased intravascular volume. Fever suggests concomitant urinary tract infection.

Selective Physical Examination I

Examine for *prerenal* (volume status), *renal*, or *postrenal* (obstructive) causes of decreased urine output. *Caution:* More than one cause may be present at any time.

HEENT	Jaundice (hepatorenal syndrome)
	Facial purpura ⎫ Amyloidosis
	Enlarged tongue ⎭

Resp	Crackles, pleural effusions (CHF)
CVS	Pulse volume, JVP
	Skin temperature, color
ABD	Enlarged kidneys (hydronephrosis secondary to obstruction, polycystic kidney disease)
	Enlarged bladder (bladder outlet obstruction, neurogenic bladder, blocked Foley catheter)
Rectal	Enlarged prostate gland (bladder outlet obstruction)
Pelvic	Cervical or adnexal masses (ureteric obstruction secondary to cervical or ovarian cancer)
Skin	Morbilliform rash (acute interstitial nephritis)
	Livedo reticularis on lower extremities (atheromatous embolic renal failure)

Selective Chart Review

Review the patient's history and hospital course, looking specifically for factors that may predispose to prerenal, renal, or postrenal causes of decreased urine output (see Elevator Thoughts).

Look for recent blood urea and creatinine values. A creatinine-to-urea ratio of < 12 suggests a prerenal cause. A urine specific gravity of > 1.020 or urine sodium concentration of < 20 mmol/L also suggests a prerenal cause.

Look for specific combinations of factors that may predispose to renal failure, such as a patient receiving both angiotensin-converting enzyme inhibitors and diuretics, aminoglycosides in a septic patient, IV contrast material in a patient receiving an angiotensin-converting enzyme inhibitor, or a patient with CHF who was given an NSAID.[1]

Management I

Your job becomes simpler when you can find a *prerenal* or *postrenal* cause for decreased urine output.

Prerenal. First ensure that the intravascular volume is normal. If the patient is in CHF, initiate diuresis as discussed in Chapter 24, pages 273 to 274. If the patient is volume depleted, replenish the intravascular volume with NS. Add *no* potassium supplement to the IV solution until the patient passes urine. Do not give Ringer's lactate because it contains potassium.

Postrenal. Lower urinary tract obstruction can be adequately excluded by passage of a Foley catheter into the bladder.
1. If there has been bladder outlet obstruction, the initial urine volume on catheterization usually will be > 400 ml, and the patient will experience immediate relief. Remember to listen

carefully for heart murmurs before catheterizing the patient. If there is documented evidence of a cardiac valvular abnormality requiring bacterial endocarditis prophylaxis, refer to Chapter 21, pages 246 to 247. After catheterization, watch for the development of postobstructive diuresis by monitoring urine volume status carefully for the next few days.

2. If a Foley catheter is already in place, ensure that flushing the catheter with 20 to 30 ml of NS allows free flow of fluid from the bladder. This maneuver will exclude an intraluminal blockage of the Foley catheter as a cause of postrenal obstruction.

3. The presence of a Foley catheter in the bladder rules out only lower urinary tract obstruction. If the preceding two steps fail to restore urine output, a *renal ultrasound* examination should be ordered first thing in the morning to exclude upper urinary tract obstruction. Although bilateral ureteric obstruction is rare, additional useful information, such as documentation of the presence of both kidneys and an estimate of renal size, also may be obtained.

Renal. If prerenal and postrenal factors are not operative in causing the patient's decreased urine output, you are left in the murky waters of renal causes of decreased urine output. A search for the renal causes of decreased urine output can wait until some more important questions are answered (see Management II).

Management II

Regardless of the causes of decreased urine output (prerenal, renal, or postrenal), you must now answer the following four questions.

1. Are any of the following five life-threatening complications of decreased urine output present?
   - Hyperkalemia (the most immediately serious problem)
     - Order a stat serum potassium level, if not already done.
     - Review the chart for a recent serum potassium level.
     - Order a stat electrocardiogram (ECG) if suspicion of hyperkalemia exists. Peaked T waves are early signs of hyperkalemia (Fig. 9–1). More advanced ECG manifestations include depressed ST segments, prolonged PR intervals, loss of P waves, and wide QRS complexes.
     - Discontinue any potassium supplements.
     - Treat as outlined in Chapter 33, pages 354 to 356.
   - CHF
     CHF is suggested by tachypnea, elevated JVP, crackles on pulmonary auscultation, an S_3, and sacral or pedal edema. Refer to Chapter 24, pages 273 to 274, for management of CHF.

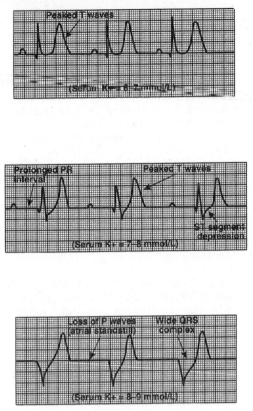

Figure 9–1 □ Progressive electrocardiographic features of hyperkalemia.

□ Severe metabolic acidemia (pH < 7.2)
   Metabolic acidemia is suggested by the presence of (compensatory) hyperventilation and confirmed by arterial blood gas (ABG) measurement. Investigation should take place as outlined in Chapter 28, page 317.
□ Uremic encephalopathy
   Uremic encephalopathy manifests itself as confusion, stupor, or seizures and is managed by dialysis. If seizures occur, they should be managed as outlined in Chapter 23 until dialysis can be initiated.
□ Uremic pericarditis
   Uremic pericarditis is suggested by the presence of pleuritic chest pain, pericardial friction rub, or diffuse ST segment elevation on the ECG. It is managed best with dialysis.

2. Is the patient receiving any drugs that may worsen the situation?
   - Potassium supplements
   - Potassium-sparing diuretics (spironolactone, triamterene, amiloride)
   - Nephrotoxic drugs (NSAIDs, aminoglycosides)

   Review the need for these agents and discontinue immediately if possible. If aminoglycosides are required, doses will need to be adjusted based on serum levels.

3. Is the patient in oliguric renal failure?

   If the patient has produced < 400 ml/day urine (< 20 ml/hr), the patient has oliguric renal failure. Although this has a higher mortality rate than nonoliguric renal failure, there is little evidence to support efforts to convert oliguric to nonoliguric renal failure through the aggressive use of diuretics. In fact, diuretics may worsen the situation if the renal failure has been caused by IV contrast agents.[2] In general, loop diuretics should be used in this situation only if there is coexisting CHF.

4. Does the patient need dialysis?

   If the patient does not pass urine despite high doses of diuretics, the indications for urgent dialysis are as follows:
   - Hyperkalemia
   - CHF
   - Metabolic acidemia (pH < 7.2)
   - Severe uremia (urea level of > 35 mmol/L; creatinine level of > 800 mmol/L) ± uremic seizures
   - Uremic pericarditis

   If the patient is in renal failure and if one or more of these conditions are present, request an urgent nephrology consultation to dialyze the patient. While awaiting the nephrologist's arrival, all of the following problems can be temporarily treated with nondialysis measures:
   - *Hyperkalemia.* Glucose with insulin infusion, $NaHCO_3$, calcium, sodium polystyrene sulfonate. (Refer to Chapter 33 for treatment of hyperkalemia.)
   - *CHF.* Preload measures (sit the patient up, morphine, nitroglycerin ointment). Give O_2 (refer to Chapter 24, pages 273 to 274).
   - *Metabolic acidemia* $NaHCO_3$ (refer to Chapter 28, page 317, for assessment of metabolic acidosis).
   - Patients with *uremic encephalopathy* should be kept calm and at bedrest until dialysis can be initiated.
   - Patients with *uremic pericarditis* may be treated symptomatically for pain with an NSAID until dialysis can be initiated.

Once these questions have been addressed, you can sit down

and think about possible *renal causes* of decreased urine output. The majority of renal causes are diagnosed by history, physical examination, and laboratory findings. Occasionally, a renal biopsy is required. A simple urinalysis can often provide valuable clues to the diagnosis.

- *Urine dipstick.* Hematuria and proteinuria together suggest *glomerulonephritis.* A positive orthotoluidine test result for blood may represent red blood cells (RBCs), free hemoglobin, or myoglobin. Suspect *rhabdomyolysis* if there is a positive orthotoluidine test result on dipstick but few or no RBCs on urine microscopy. (In this case, order tests of serum for creatine phosphokinase [CPK], Ca, and PO_4 and of urine for myoglobin.)

A positive test result for urinary protein alone should prompt you to do a serum albumin and 24-hour urine collection for protein and creatinine clearance to identify the *nephrotic syndrome*, if present.

- *Urine microscopy.* RBC casts are diagnostic of *glomerulonephritis.* WBC casts, particularly eosinophil casts, may be seen in cases of *acute interstitial nephritis.* Pigmented granular casts may be seen with *acute tubular necrosis.* Oval fat bodies are suggestive of *nephrotic syndrome.*
- *Urine for eosinophils.* Ask for this test if there is a suspicion of *acute interstitial nephritis.*

In most cases, beyond these simple tests, no further investigation is required at night. Ensure, however, that for any suspected *renal* cause of decreased urine output, prerenal and postrenal factors are not additional contributors to the poor urine output.

■ REMEMBER

All medications that the oliguric or anuric patient is receiving should be reviewed, and any potential nephrotoxins should be discontinued if possible. Drugs that depend on renal excretion (e.g., digoxin, aminoglycosides) also may require dosage adjustment.

References

1. Thadhani R, Pascual M, Bonventre JV: Acute renal failure. N Engl J Med 1996;334:1448–1460.
2. Solomon R, Werner C, Mann D, et al: Effects of saline, mannitol, and furosemide on acute decreases in renal function induced by radiocontrast agents. N Engl J Med 1994;331:1416–1420.

10

DIARRHEA

Avoid treating diarrhea as a diagnosis. Diarrhea is always a symptom of another underlying disorder and seldom warrants nonspecific "antimotility therapy." Your job at night is to determine what the likely cause of diarrhea is, whether additional investigations should be performed, and whether complications have arisen that require treatment.

■ PHONE CALL

Questions

1. **What are the vital signs?**
2. **What was the reason for admission?**
3. **Is this a new problem? If not, has a diagnosis of the reason for diarrhea been made?**
4. **Has the patient had recent surgery?**
5. **Is the patient HIV positive?**
6. **Is there blood, pus, or mucus in the stool?**
   Bloody stools with pus or mucus suggest inflammation, as may be seen with infection, inflammatory bowel disease, or ischemic colitis.
7. **Does the patient have abdominal pain?**
   Moderate or severe abdominal pain suggests ischemic colitis, diverticulitis, or inflammatory bowel disease.

Orders

None

Inform RN

"Will arrive at the bedside in . . . minutes."

A single episode of diarrhea in an otherwise well patient does not usually require bedside assessment. If the diarrhea is frequent, severe, or associated with passage of blood, the patient should be evaluated at the bedside as soon as possible. If the patient is hypotensive, tachycardic, or febrile, he or she should be assessed immediately.

■ ELEVATOR THOUGHTS
(What causes diarrhea?)

Acute Diarrhea
(Diarrhea of < 2 Weeks' Duration)

"The Four I's"

Infection	Inflammation and toxins (Table 10–1)
Iatrogenic	Drugs (laxatives, stool softeners, magnesium-containing antacids, sorbitol-containing liquid dosage forms, digoxin, quinidine, colchicine, and xanthines) and surgery (gastrectomy, vagotomy, cholecystectomy, intestinal resection)
Ischemia	Mesenteric thrombosis, vascular embolus to the mesenteric artery, volvulus
Impactions	Fecal impaction

Chronic Diarrhea
(Diarrhea of > 2 Weeks' Duration)

"The Five I's and Two M's"

Infection	Amebiasis, giardiasis, *Clostridium difficile*
Inflammatory bowel disease	Ulcerative colitis, Crohn's disease, collagenous colitis, lymphocytic colitis, radiation enteritis or colitis
Infiltrative disorders	Amyloid, lymphoma
Irritable bowel syndrome	
Intake	Laxative abuse, caffeine, sweeteners (sorbitol, fructose, xylitol)
Malabsorption	Celiac disease, short bowel syndrome, bacterial overgrowth
Metabolic/hormonal	Enzyme deficiencies (lactase deficiency, pancreatic insufficiency)
	Hormone production (gastrinoma, carcinoid, VIPoma, villous adenoma, medullary carcinoma of the thyroid)
	Endocrinopathies (diabetic diarrhea, hyperthyroidism, Addison's disease)

Any of the causes of acute diarrhea, if left untreated, may also cause chronic diarrhea.

Table 10–1 □ **ETIOLOGIC AGENTS IN INFECTIOUS DIARRHEA**

Inflammatory

Bacterial

Salmonella sp.
Shigella sp.
Campylobacter sp.
Yersinia enterocolitica
Vibrio parahemolyticus (uncooked shellfish)
Plesiomonas shigelloides (uncooked shellfish)
Aeromonas hydrophilia (untreated wellwater, brackish water)
Mycobacterium avium-intracellulare*
Mycobacterium tuberculosis*
Chlamydia*
Escherichia coli†

Protozoal

Entamoeba histolytica*
Giardia lamblia*
Cryptosporidium sp.*
Isospora belli*
Enterocytozoon bieneusi (Microsporidia)*
Cyclospora sp.*

Viral

Norwalk virus
Rotavirus
Cytomegalovirus*
Herpes simplex*
Epstein-Barr virus*
HIV enteropathy*

Nematodes

Strongyloides stercoralis*

Toxins

Toxins produced in vivo

Clostridium difficile (after antibiotic administration)
Clostridium perfringens (beef, poultry)
Vibrio cholerae
Bacillus cereus (fried rice)
Enterotoxigenic E. coli (hamburger)†

Preformed toxins

Staphylococcus aureus (potato salads, mayonnaise, puddings)
Bacillus cereus (fried rice)

---

*Prevalence in HIV-positive patients.
†Enteroinvasive (EIEC), enterohemorrhagic (EHEC), and enteroaggregative (EAggEC) E. coli strains produce an inflammatory diarrheal illness. Enteropathogenic E. coli (EPEC) produces a noninflammatory diarrheal illness by attachment to intestinal brush border, resulting in a disaccharidase deficiency and loss of absorptive surface. Enterotoxigenic E. coli (ETEC) attaches to the small intestinal mucosa and produces toxins that result in a secretory diarrhea.[2]

■ MAJOR THREAT TO LIFE

- Intravascular volume depletion; electrolyte imbalance
- Systemic infection

Volume depletion and *electrolyte disturbances* are the reasons that many children in underdeveloped countries die from diarrhea. This, of course, is seldom seen in the hospitalized adult patient, but if left untreated, diarrhea may certainly progress to serious volume depletion and electrolyte imbalance. Some bacterial causes of diarrhea, if left untreated, may become *systemic*, life-threatening disorders.

■ BEDSIDE

Quick Look Test

Does the patient look well (comfortable), sick (uncomfortable or distressed), or critical (about to die)?

Most patients with acute diarrhea do not look unwell. However, if the diarrhea is due to an invasive organism (e.g., *Salmonella, Shigella*), the patient may look sick and complain of headaches, diffuse myalgias, chills, and fevers.

Airway and Vital Signs

What is the BP?

Resting hypotension suggests significant volume depletion. If the resting BP is normal, examine for postural changes. A postural rise in HR of > 15 beats/min, a fall in systolic BP of > 15 mm Hg, or any fall in diastolic BP indicates significant hypovolemia.

What is the HR?

Intravascular volume depletion usually results in tachycardia unless the patient has a coexisting disorder (e.g., autonomic dysfunction due to beta blockade, sick sinus syndrome [SSS], or autonomic neuropathy), which may prevent the generation of a tachycardia. However, in diarrheal diseases, a tachycardia may also be seen due to anxiety, pain, or fever. A relative bradycardia despite fever raises the suspicion of *Salmonella* infection.

What is the temperature?

A fever in the patient with diarrhea is nonspecific but suggests the presence of inflammation, as may be seen with infectious diarrhea, diverticulitis, inflammatory bowel disease, intestinal lymphoma, tuberculosis, and amebiasis. Some organisms (*Shigella* and *Salmonella* spp.) may cause systemic sepsis. However, remember that sepsis may occur in the absence of fever, especially in the elderly.

Selective Physical Examination I (Is the patient volume depleted? Is there evidence of systemic sepsis?)

Vitals	(See above)
CVS	Pulse volume, JVP (flat neck veins)
	Skin temperature, color

Management I

What immediate measures need to be taken to correct intravascular volume depletion?

1. Normalize the intravascular volume. This can be achieved quickly by administration of an IV fluid that will at least temporarily remain in the intravascular space, such as NS or Ringer's lactate. Give NS 250 to 500 ml IV over 1 to 2 hours, titrating the IV fluid to the patient's vital signs and JVP. Reassess the volume status after each bolus of IV fluid, aiming for a JVP of 2 to 3 cm H_2O above the sternal angle and concomitant normalization of HR and BP.

2. Check the chart for a recent electrolyte determination. If the patient has not had electrolytes checked within the last 24 hours, order serum electrolytes, urea, and creatinine levels now.

3. In the patient with fever $> 38.5°C$, two sets of blood cultures should be drawn. If the patient is also hypotensive, volume replacement should be instituted with NS, and consideration should be given to empiric antibiotic coverage (see Chapter 12, page 98).

4. A rectal examination should be performed, and stool samples sent for occult blood, culture, ova and parasite determination, *Clostridium difficile* toxin, and white blood cell (WBC) stain. If unusual organisms are suspected (e.g., in the acquired immunodeficiency syndrome [AIDS] patient), the laboratory should be alerted so appropriate culture technique and media can be used.

Selective Chart Review (Are potential causes of diarrhea apparent from the chart?)

Is the patient on any medications that may cause diarrhea?

Medications are the most common cause of diarrhea in the hospital. Frequent offenders include laxatives, stool softeners, magnesium-containing antacids, sorbitol-containing liquid dosage forms, digoxin, quinidine, colchicine, and xanthines. Laxatives and stool softeners should be discontinued. Magnesium-containing antacids may be withheld or switched to aluminum-containing preparations. Do not discontinue other medications without first asking your resident or attending physician. Remember, also, in the celiac patient, that some medications (e.g., Anacin, Dristan, Dyazide) contain gluten.

Has the patient received antibiotics recently?

Many antibiotics cause transient diarrhea through alteration of the intestinal flora. In addition, *pseudomembranous colitis* due to *C. difficile* enterotoxin may result in persistent diarrhea during or after antibiotic use. A stool sample for *C. difficile* toxin titer or stool for *C. difficile* culture should be collected, but the diagnosis can be made immediately with sigmoidoscopy and the findings of yellowish-white pseudomembranes. Treatment includes discontinuation of the offending antibiotic and administration of *metronidazole* 250 mg PO every 6 hours for at least 7 days. *Vancomycin* 125 to 250 mg PO every 6 hours for 7 days is an alternative therapy but is more expensive and no more effective than metronidazole.

Does the patient have AIDS?

Immunocompromised patients and patients with AIDS may develop diarrhea for many reasons. In addition to the "usual" causes of diarrhea, homosexual men should be tested for sexually transmitted anorectal conditions, including infection with *Treponema pallidum, Neisseria gonorrhoeae, Chlamydia* spp., and herpes simplex. Other nonvenereal agents include cytomegalovirus (CMV), *Mycobacterium avium-intracellulare,* and a variety of protozoa (*Cryptosporidium* spp., *Cyclospora* spp., *Entamoeba histolytica, Isospora belli, Enterocytozoon bieneusi*). If this is the first documented episode of diarrhea, stool samples should be sent for acid-fast stain, WBC stain, bacterial and mycobacterial culture, and ova and parasite determination. The test with the highest yield is microscopic examination including a search for ova and parasites. The correct transport medium must be used for specific pathogen cultures, and frequently laboratories require identification of the possible pathogens such as *Cryptosporidum, Yersinia, Aeromonas,* and *Escherichia coli* 0157. Diagnosis of anorectal infections may require proctoscopy or sigmoidoscopy with specimens taken for gonorrhea, herpes simplex viral culture, and dark-field examination for syphilis; this can be arranged in the morning.

Has the patient had recent surgery?

Postgastrectomy dumping of hypertonic boluses of stomach contents into the jejunum is associated with vasomotor symptoms of flushing, anxiety, palpitations, sweating, and dizziness, and there may be associated diarrhea. Resections of the ileum and right colon may result in diarrhea due to bile acid malabsorption.

Does the patient have known inflammatory bowel disease, celiac disease, lactase deficiency, or other conditions known to cause chronic diarrhea?

Has there been recent travel abroad?

E. coli enterotoxin is the most common cause of "traveler's diarrhea," although *Salmonella* spp., *Shigella* spp., and *Campylobacter jejuni* also may be responsible for acute, self-limiting traveler's diarrhea. Giardiasis, amebiasis, and tropical sprue may cause a more chronic picture.

Has the patient been admitted for the investigation of diarrhea?

In these cases, a plan of investigation usually is already outlined. If the patient is not volume depleted and is otherwise comfortable, no additional measures are required at night.

Is the patient receiving tube feedings?

Diarrhea often complicates enteral tube feedings, but in many cases it is due to factors other than the feeding formula itself, such as medications or underlying illnesses. Occasionally, diarrhea may develop because of the formula's composition (e.g., high fat, high osmolarity, presence of lactose), the manner in which it is delivered (bolus versus continuous infusion), or contamination of the formula.[1] In most cases, decisions regarding a change in formula or in manner or rate of delivery can wait until morning.

Selective Physical Examination II (Look for clues for specific causes of diarrhea)

Vitals	Repeat now
HEENT	Lymphadenopathy (lymphoma, Whipple's disease, AIDS)
ABD	Surgical scars (gastrectomy, cholecystectomy, intestinal resection)
	Hepatosplenomegaly (*Salmonella* infection)
	Epigastric tenderness (Zollinger-Ellison syndrome)
	RLQ mass or tenderness (Crohn's disease, ischemic colitis)
	LLQ mass or tenderness (diverticulitis, tumor, inflammatory bowel disease, ischemic colitis, fecal impaction)
Rectal	Rectal fissure (Crohn's disease)

	Hard mass (fecal impaction, tumor)
	Fresh blood or stool positive for occult blood (inflammatory bowel disease, infection, tumor)
MSS	Arthritis (inflammatory bowel disease, Whipple's disease)
Skin	Rose spots (*Salmonella* infection)
	Dermatitis herpetiformis (celiac disease)
	Pyoderma gangrenosum (Crohn's disease)
	Hyperpigmentation (Whipple's, Addison's, or celiac disease)
	Flushing (carcinoid)

Management II

It is unusual to be able to pinpoint the specific cause of diarrhea when seeing a patient for the first time at night. Occasionally a patient will tell you, "I'm sure it's my Crohn's disease acting up," or "I have lactose intolerance and the kitchen gave me yogurt for dinner," and in these cases, the patient most often turns out to be right. When the diagnosis is not obvious at night, your goals are to ensure that the patient is adequately hydrated, does not have a serious electrolyte imbalance, and does not have a systemic infection. Additional specialized investigations for diarrhea can, in most cases, wait until the morning to be arranged.

Remember, in many cases of infectious diarrhea, frequent loose stools are the body's way of expelling the offending organism or toxin. Do not compound the problem by inhibiting the body's ability to do this. Diarrhea is always best treated by addressing the underlying cause, and this may take a few days (and sometimes weeks) to identify. Unless the diarrhea is profuse or disabling, nonspecific antidiarrheal agents are best avoided. Explain this to the patient and to the nurses caring for him or her so everyone is clear about the treatment approach.

If the patient's diarrhea is severe and disabling, it is occasionally warranted to use *one* of the nonspecific antidiarrheal agents listed below. However, none of these agents should be prescribed before examining the patient (including rectal examination and possibly sigmoidoscopy) and deciding on an appropriate plan of investigation.

Loperamide (Imodium) 4 mg PO every 4 hours until diarrhea is controlled to a maximum dose of 16 mg in 24 hours. The drug is less effective if given on an as-needed (PRN) basis. Side effects include dry mouth, abdominal distention and cramping, occasionally nausea and vomiting, and rarely toxic megacolon. Other side effects include rash, drowsiness, dizziness, and tiredness.

Diphenoxylate hydrochloride (Lomotil) 5 mg PO three or four times a day until the diarrhea is controlled. It is as effective in acute nonspecific diarrhea as loperamide but has a slower onset of antidiarrheal action. Diphenoxylate is contraindicated in patients with hepatic failure or cirrhosis. Respiratory depression may occur when it is used in combination with phenothiazines, tricyclic antidepressants, or barbiturates. Toxic megacolon may result if ulcerative colitis is present.

Bismuth subsalicylate (Pepto-Bismol) 30 ml or 2 tablets (262 mg/tablet) PO every 30 minutes to a maximum of eight doses per day. Blackening of the tongue and stools is known to occur. It may inhibit the absorption of tetracycline. Salicylate overdose may be seen, especially if patient is also receiving aspirin.

Agents such as anticholinergics, kaolin, and pectin do not reduce fecal water loss in diarrheal illnesses and are best avoided.

References

1. Eisenberg PG: Causes of diarrhea in tube-fed patients: A comprehensive approach to diagnosis and management. Nutr Clin Pract 1993;8:3.
2. Hart CA, Batt RM, Saunders JR: Diarrhea caused by *Escherichia coli*. Ann Trop Paediatr 1993;13:121–131.

11

FALL-OUT-OF-BED

Patients always seem to be falling out of bed, but they fall while in other places, too. You will find the content of this chapter applicable to any fall occurring in the patient's room or elsewhere in the hospital.

■ PHONE CALL

Questions

1. **Was the fall witnessed?**
2. **Is there an obvious injury?**
3. **What are the vital signs?**
4. **Has there been a change in the level of consciousness?**
5. **Is the patient receiving anticoagulants or antiseizure medications?**
6. **What was the reason for admission?**

Orders

Ask the RN to call immediately if the level of consciousness changes before you are able to assess the patient.

Inform RN

"Will arrive at the bedside in . . . minutes."

When other sick patients are in need of assessment, they take priority over a patient who has had an uncomplicated fall. However, a change in the level of consciousness, a suspected fracture, or a coagulation disorder requires you to see the patient immediately.

■ ELEVATOR THOUGHTS
(Why does a patient fall?)

Cardiac   Postural hypotension (volume depletion, drugs, or autonomic failure)
Vasovagal attack
Dysrhythmia
MI

Neuro	Confusion and cognitive impairment (particularly in the elderly)
	Drugs (narcotics, sedatives, antidepressants, tranquilizers, antihypertension agents)
	Metabolic disorders (electrolyte abnormalities, renal failure, hepatic failure)
	Dementia (Parkinson's disease, Alzheimer's disease, multi-infarction, normal-pressure hydrocephalus) resulting in poor safety awareness
	Gait and balance disorders
	Visual impairment
	TIA, stroke
	Seizure
Environmental/ accidental	Disorientation at night
	Call bell inaccessible
	Restraints
	Improper bed height
	Wet floors
	Unsafe clothing (e.g., long hospital gowns or pajamas, tractionless slippers)
	Obstacles (e.g., bedrails, IV poles, clutter around bed)

There are many potential environmental hazards within the hospital setting. Elderly persons are particularly prone to accidental falls due to a combination of environmental hazards, poor vision, diminished muscular strength, and impaired righting reflexes.

■ MAJOR THREAT TO LIFE

- Head injury

Any patient who may have hit his or her head during a fall requires a complete neurologic examination immediately. Even seemingly minor trauma can result in a serious intracranial bleed in an anticoagulated patient. If a new neurologic problem is identified, an immediate computed tomography (CT) scan of the head can be helpful. The consideration of immediate reversal of anticoagulation should be discussed in consultation with the resident and hematologist (see Chapter 31, pages 342 to 343, for reversal of anticoagulation). If no neurologic deficit is identified at this time, observation through a frequent assessment of the neurovital signs is required.

■ BEDSIDE

Quick Look Test

Does the patient look well (comfortable), sick (uncomfortable or distressed), or critical (about to die)?

Most patients do not have life-threatening problems to account for falling. Usually, they look well and the vital signs are normal.

Airway and Vital Signs

What are the heart rate (HR) and rhythm?

Tachycardia, bradycardia, or irregular rhythm may indicate a dysrhythmia as the cause of the fall.

Are there postural (lying and standing) changes in blood pressure (BP) and HR?

A postural fall in BP together with a postural rise in HR ($>$ 15 beats/min) suggests volume depletion. A drop in BP without a change in HR suggests autonomic dysfunction. An initial drop in BP that corrects on standing also suggests autonomic dysfunction. Drugs are common causes of postural hypotension in elderly patients, particularly antihypertension agents, sedatives, and antidepressants.

Selective History

Ask the patient why he or she fell—after all, the patient may know the answer!

What was the patient doing just before the fall?

Coughing, micturating, or straining are examples of maneuvers that may result in vasovagal syncope. Question any witnesses who observed the fall. Did the patient trip or slip?

Were there any warning symptoms before the fall?

Lightheadedness and visual disturbances on standing may indicate postural hypotension. Palpitations suggest a dysrhythmia. A preceding aura would be rare in this situation but, if present, is highly suggestive of a seizure disorder.

Is there a history of previous falls?

Recurrent falls suggest an underlying disorder that has gone unrecognized. Although your main duty at night is to detect, document, and treat any injuries that have been sustained, a pattern of falling behavior may be an important clue to an unrecognized but treatable disorder.

Is the patient diabetic?

Hyperglycemia or hypoglycemia may cause confusion, and the patient may, as a consequence, fall. Order a Chemstrip or glucose meter reading. Check the diabetic record for the past 3 days.

Is the patient aware of any injury sustained during the fall?

Patients may fracture a wrist or hip as a result of falling. Elderly women are at particular risk because of osteoporosis.

Selective Physical Examination (Look for both cause and consequence of the fall)

Vitals	Repeat now. Only supine BP and HR are necessary, provided that both supine and standing measurements were already taken.
HEENT	Tongue or cheek lacerations (seizure)
	Hemotympanum (basal skull fracture)
CVS	Pulse rate and rhythm (dysrhythmia)
	Decreased JVP (volume depletion)
MSS	Palpate skull and face ⎫
	Palpate spine and ribs ⎪ Fractures, hematomas,
	Palpate long bones ⎬ and lacerations
	Check passive ROM of ⎪
	all four limbs ⎭
Neuro	Complete neurologic examination. Pay particular attention to the level of consciousness and to any asymmetric neurologic findings. New findings of asymmetry suggest structural brain disease.

Selective Chart Review (Search for the cause of the fall)

1. **What was the reason for admission?**
2. **Is there a past history of cardiac dysrhythmia, seizure disorder, autonomic neuropathy, disorientation at night, or diabetes mellitus?**
3. **What drugs is the patient receiving?**
   - Antihypertension agents
   - Diuretics (volume depletion)
   - Antidysrhythmic agents
   - Antiseizure medications
   - Narcotics
   - Sedatives, tranquilizers
   - Antidepressants
   - Insulin, oral hypoglycemic agents

4. Check the most recent laboratory results.

- □ Glucose
  □ Na } ↑ or ↓ may cause confusion
- □ ↑ K can cause atrioventricular (AV) blocks; ↓ K can cause weakness or tachydysrhythmias.
- □ ↑ Ca causes confusion; ↓ Ca may cause seizures.
- □ Urea, creatinine (uremia can result in confusion and seizures)
- □ Antiseizure drug levels (subtherapeutic levels may result in seizure breakthrough; toxic levels may be associated with ataxia)

Management

Provisional Diagnosis. Establish the reason for the fall (provisional diagnosis). The etiology is often multifactorial. For example, diuretic-induced nocturia forces an elderly patient, under the influence of nighttime sedation, to struggle to the bathroom in an unfamiliar, dimly lit hospital room.

Complications. Are there any complications resulting from the fall, giving rise to a second diagnosis? For example, the stroke victim may have unknowingly dislocated or subluxated his or her shoulder on the paralyzed side during the fall. The anticoagulated patient may develop a serious, delayed hemorrhage at any site of trauma. Reexamine these patients frequently.

Treat the Cause. Investigate and treat the suspected cause. A fall is a symptom, not a diagnosis!

Reversible Factors. Reversible factors must be corrected, especially volume depletion and inappropriate drug therapy in the elderly.

Nocturia. The majority of elderly patients who fall out of bed at night are on their way to the bathroom because of nocturia. Make sure the nocturia is not iatrogenic (e.g., an evening diuretic order or an unnecessary IV infusion).

Elderly Patient. If the patient is disoriented at night, ensure that the call bell is easily accessible, a nightlight is left on, and the evening's fluid intake is limited. The use of physical restraints (poseys and bed rails) may actually contribute to falls and should be discouraged.[1] It is best to leave the side rails down or lower the bed height.

Reference

1. Tinetti ME, Liu WL, Ginter SF: Mechanical restraint use and fall-related injuries among residents of skilled nursing facilities. Ann Intern Med 1992;116:369–374.

12

FEVER

It is unusual to spend an entire night on call without being called about a febrile patient. The majority of fevers seen in hospitalized patients are due to infections. Locating the source of a fever usually requires some detective work. Whether the cause of the fever requires specific immediate treatment will depend both on the clinical status of the patient and on the suspected diagnosis.

■ PHONE CALL

Questions

1. **How high is the temperature, and by what route was it taken?**
   (37°C oral = 37.5°C rectal or 36.5°C axillary)
2. **What are the other vital signs?**
3. **Are there any associated symptoms?**
   Pain may help localize a site of infection or inflammation. A headache, neckache, seizure, or change in sensorium, together with fever, suggests meningitis or encephalitis.
4. **Is this a "new" fever?**
5. **What was the reason for admission?**
6. **Is this a postoperative patient?**
   Postoperative fever is very common and may be due to atelectasis, pneumonia, pulmonary embolism, wound infection, infected intravenous (IV) sites, or urinary tract infection from a Foley catheter.

Orders

1. If febrile and hypotensive, give 500 ml of normal saline (NS) IV as rapidly as possible.
2. If febrile with meningitis symptoms (headache, neckache, seizure, or change in sensorium), order a lumbar puncture (LP) tray to the bedside now.

Inform RN

"Will arrive at bedside in . . . minutes."
An elevated temperature alone is seldom life threatening. How-

ever, fever in association with hypotension or meningitis symptoms requires you to see the patient immediately.

■ ELEVATOR THOUGHTS
(What causes fever?)

- *Infection* is by far the most common cause of fever in the hospitalized patient. Common sites of infection are the lung, urinary tract, wounds, and IV sites. Less common sites include central nervous system (CNS), abdominal, and pelvic infections. The *immunocompromised patient* is not only predisposed to infection but also more susceptible to serious complications of infection.
- Pulmonary embolism and deep vein thrombosis (DVT)
- Drug-induced fever
- Neoplasm
- Connective tissue diseases
- Postoperative atelectasis

■ MAJOR THREAT TO LIFE

- Septic shock
- Meningitis

Fever is most commonly a manifestation of infection in the hospitalized patient. Most infections can be brought under control by a combination of the body's natural defense mechanisms and judicious antibiotic use. Infection at any site, if progressive, may lead to septicemia with attendant *septic shock. Meningitis,* by virtue of its location, can result in permanent neurologic deficit or death if allowed to go untreated.

■ BEDSIDE

Quick Look Test

Does the patient look well (comfortable), sick (uncomfortable or distressed), or critical (about to die)?

Toxic signs, such as apprehension, agitation, or lethargy, suggest serious infection.

Airway and Vital Signs

What is the heart rate (HR)?

Tachycardia, proportionate to the temperature elevation, is an expected finding in the febrile patient. Normally, the

HR rises by 16 beats/min for each degree Celsius of temperature rise. A relative bradycardia in the febrile patient has been observed in *Legionella* pneumonia, *Mycoplasma pneumoniae* pneumonia, ascending cholangitis, typhoid fever, and *Plasmodium falciparum* malaria with profound hemolysis.

What is the blood pressure (BP)?

Fever in association with supine or postural hypotension indicates relative hypovolemia and can be the forerunner of septic shock. Ensure that an IV line is in place. Infuse NS or Ringer's lactate to correct the intravascular volume deficit.

Selective Physical Examination I

What is the volume status? Is the patient in septic shock? Are there signs of meningitis?

Vitals	Repeat now
HEENT	Photophobia, neck stiffness
CVS	Pulse volume, JVP, skin temperature, and color
Neuro	Change in sensorium
Special maneuvers	*Brudzinski's sign:* with the patient supine, passively flex the neck forward. Flexion of the patient's hips and knees in response to this maneuver constitutes a positive test result (see Fig. 14–3A)
	Kernig's sign: with the patient supine, flex one hip and knee to 90 degrees, then straighten the knee. Pain or resistance in the ipsilateral hamstrings constitutes a positive test result (see Fig. 14–3B)

Septic shock is a clinical diagnosis consisting of two states. Serious delays in treatment are made through failure to recognize the first state. Early in the development of septic shock, the patient may be warm, dry, and flushed because of peripheral vasodilation and increased cardiac output (*warm shock*). As septic shock progresses, the patient becomes hypotensive, and the skin becomes cool and clammy (*cold shock*) as a result of peripheral vasoconstriction.

Fever in the elderly patient, regardless of cause, can produce changes in sensorium ranging from lethargy to agitation. If a specific site of infection is not obvious, an LP should be performed to rule out meningitis (see pages 98 to 99).

Management I

What immediate measures need to be taken to prevent septic shock or to recognize meningitis?

Septic shock. If the patient is febrile and hypotensive, determine the volume status and give IV fluids (NS or Ringer's lactate) promptly until the volume status returns to normal. Aggressive volume repletion in a patient with a history of congestive heart failure (CHF) may compromise cardiac function. Do not overshoot the mark!

While IV fluid resuscitation is taking place, obtain samples for necessary cultures, usually including blood from two different sites, urine (for Gram's stain and culture), sputum, and any other potentially infected body fluid.

Septic shock is a major threat to life, and once culture samples are taken, antibiotics must be given to cover both Gram-positive and Gram-negative organisms. The choice of antibiotic will also depend on a knowledge of local antibiotic susceptibility patterns. Many institutions have protocols to guide empiric antibacterial therapy, particularly in neutropenic patients. A common empiric, broad-spectrum regimen includes a cephalosporin and an aminoglycoside, such as *ceftazidime* 1 to 2 g IV every 8 hours and *gentamicin* 2 to 3 mg/kg IV as a loading dose. Further maintenance doses of gentamicin should be 1.5 to 1.7 mg/kg IV given at an interval that is adjusted for creatinine clearance.

Some patients are allergic to penicillin. Ensure that the patient is *not* allergic before ordering penicillin or cephalosporin. Aminoglycosides are common causes of nephrotoxicity and ototoxicity. Select maintenance dosing intervals according to the patient's calculated creatinine clearance (see Appendix E, page 410). Follow the serum aminoglycoside concentrations, usually after the third or fourth dose, and the serum creatinine concentration.

If the volume status is normal and the patient is still hypotensive, transfer to the intensive care unit/cardiac care unit (ICU/CCU) for inotropic or vasopressor support. (Refer to Chapter 18 for further discussion of septic shock.)

A Foley catheter should be placed in a patient with septic shock to monitor urine output.

Meningitis. Fever plus headache, seizure, stiff neck, or change in sensorium is considered to be meningitis until proved otherwise.

An LP should be performed without delay to confirm the diagnosis and guide antimicrobial therapy. This procedure should not be undertaken if there are focal neurologic findings or signs of increased intracranial pressure such as papilledema (see Fig. 14–2), coma, irregular respirations, bradycardia, or decerebrate posture. Other contraindications include patients with a coagulopathy, in whom the risk of intrathecal hematoma formation may result in cord compression.

In bacterial meningitis, the cerebrospinal fluid (CSF) will usually show a pleocytosis ($> 10^9/L$), protein > 0.4 g/L, and glucose < 2 mmol/L. However, these findings may not be present early in the course. Gram's stain is positive in 80% of patients not previously treated with antibacterial agents. In patients who have been partially treated, detection of bacterial antigens with latex agglutination is helpful but unreliable in detecting group B meningococcal antigen.

If you are unable to visualize the fundi or if there is papilledema or focal neurologic signs (suggesting a mass lesion), give the first dose of antibiotics and arrange for an urgent computed tomography (CT) scan of the head to exclude a space-occupying lesion before performing the LP. An LP done in the presence of an intracranial space-occupying lesion can result in uncal herniation and brainstem compression (coning).

Selective Chart Review

If the patient is not in septic shock and does not have symptoms or signs of meningitis, perform a selective chart review—look for *localizing clues* (Table 12–1). Also check the chart for the following:

- Temperature pattern during hospital stay
- Recent white blood cell (WBC) count and differential
- Evidence of immunodeficiency (e.g., cancer chemotherapy, hematologic malignancy, HIV infection, CD4 lymphocyte count)
- Allergies to antibiotics
- Other possible reasons for fever (e.g., connective tissue disease, neoplasm)
- Antipyretics, antibiotics, or steroids that may modify the fever pattern

Selective Physical Examination II

Confirm localizing symptoms or signs already documented in chart review.

Vitals	Repeat now
HEENT	Fundi—papilledema (intracranial abscess), Roth's spots (infective endocarditis) (Fig. 12–1)
	Conjunctival or scleral petechiae (infective endocarditis)

Table 12–1 □ SELECTIVE CHART REVIEW—LOOKING FOR LOCALIZING CLUES

Localizing Clues	Diagnostic Considerations	Comments
Recent surgery	Atelectasis	Postoperative fever due to atelectasis is a diagnosis to be made after exclusion of infection
	Pneumonia	
	Pulmonary embolism	
	Infected surgical wound, biopsy site, or deeper infection of biopsy organ	Despite modern surgical techniques, *any* incision or puncture site may serve as a portal for bacteria
Blood transfusion	Tranfusion reaction	See Chapter 27
Headache, seizure, stiff neck, changes in sensorium	Meningitis	Delirium tremens can mimic meningitis in some patients; is the patient withdrawing from alcohol?
	Intracranial abscess	
	Encephalitis	
Sinus discomfort	Sinusitis	
Dental caries, toothache	Periodontal abscess	
Sore throat	Pharyngitis	
	Tonsillitis	
Dysphagia	Retropharyngeal abscess	Either of these diagnoses is a medical emergency; consult ENT or anesthesia immediately
	Epiglottitis	
SOB, cough, or chest pain	Pneumonia	
	Lung abscess	
	Pulmonary embolus	

Murmur, CHF, or peripheral embolic lesions	Infective endocarditis	
Pleuritic chest pain	Pneumonia	
	Empyema	
	Pulmonary embolus	
	Pericarditis	
Costovertebral angle (CVA) tenderness	Pyelonephritis	
	Perinephric abscess	
Foley catheter, dysuria, hematuria, or pyuria	Cystitis	Condom catheters and Foley catheters predispose patients to urinary tract infections
	Pyelonephritis	
Abdominal pain		If there are peritoneal signs, consider surgical consultation
RUQ	Subphrenic abscess	
	Hepatic abscess	
	Hepatitis	
	RLL pneumonia	
	Cholecystitis	
	Ascending cholangitis	Does the patient have Charcot's triad (fever, RUQ pain, plus jaundice)? If so, consider surgical consultation
RLQ	Appendicitis	
	Crohn's disease	
	Salpingitis	
LUQ	Splenic abscess	
	Subphrenic abscess	
	Infected pancreatic pseudocyst	
	LLL pneumonia	

Table continued on following page

Table 12–1 □ SELECTIVE CHART REVIEW—LOOKING FOR LOCALIZING CLUES *Continued*

Localizing Clues	Diagnostic Considerations	Comments
LLQ	Diverticular abscess Salpingitis	
Ascites	Peritonitis	Perform abdominal paracentesis to exclude spontaneous bacterial peritonitis in any ascitic patient who becomes unwell
Diarrhea	Enteritis Colitis	
Swollen red tender joint	Septic arthritis Gout or pseudogout	A monoarticular effusion or a disproportionately inflamed joint in polyarticular disease must be tapped to exclude infection
Prosthetic joint Vaginal discharge	Infected prosthesis Endometritis Salpingitis	
Red or tender IV site TPN line	Septic phlebitis Catheter sepsis	Fever may be the only symptom

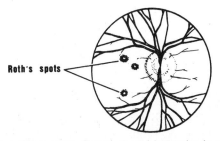

Figure 12–1 □ Roth's spots. Round or oval hemorrhagic retinal lesions with central pallor.

	Ears—red tympanic membranes (otitis media, a complication of the intubated patient)
	Sinuses—tenderness, inability to transilluminate (sinusitis)
	Oral cavity—dental caries, tender tooth on tongue blade percussion (periodontal abscess)
	Pharynx—erythema, pharyngeal exudate (pharyngitis, thrush)
	Neck—stiff (meningitis)
Resp	Crackles, friction rub, signs of consolidation (pneumonia, pulmonary embolism)
CVS	New murmurs (infective endocarditis)
ABD	Localized tenderness (see page 32)
Rectal	Tenderness or mass (rectal abscess)
MSS	Joint erythema or effusion (septic arthritis)
Skin	Decubitus ulcers (cellulitis)
	Osler's nodes and Janeway's lesions, petechiae (infective endocarditis)
	IV sites (phlebitis, cellulitis)
	All surgical wounds must be examined (that means taking off the dressings)
Pelvis	A pelvic examination should be done if a pelvic source of fever is possible

Management II

Any patient with an unexplained oral temperature > 38.5°C that has developed in hospital should have the following performed:

- Blood cultures immediately from two different sites
- Urinalysis (routine and microscopic) and urine culture immediately
- WBC count and differential

The performance of other, more *selective tests* depends on the *localizing clues* you have been able to elicit with your chart review, history, and physical examination.

- Throat swab for Gram's stain and culture
- Sputum for Gram's stain and culture
- Chest x-ray (CXR)
- LP
- Blood culture for infective endocarditis (refer to your institution's protocol)
- Cervical culture (also obtain specific medium for gonococcal isolation before performing the pelvic examination)
- Joint aspiration
- Swab decubitus ulcers or infected/draining wounds for Gram's stain and culture

Fluid from any source should be examined microscopically immediately to help in your choice of antibiotics.

Remove *suspected IV lines* and replace if necessary at a new site. Central total parenteral nutrition (TPN) lines that may be infected should be replaced in consultation with your resident or TPN service. Catheter tips should be sent to the laboratory for culture.

Remove a Foley catheter in a patient suspected of having *urinary tract infection.* A few days of incontinence in the patient is an annoyance for the nursing staff but will not harm the patient if there is no perineal skin breakdown. An exception to this occurs when a Foley catheter is placed to treat urinary retention because urinary stasis predisposes the patient to infection.

Broad-Spectrum Antibiotics

Three types of patients need broad-spectrum antibiotics now:

1. The patient with *fever and hypotension* requires broad-spectrum antibiotics (see page 98).
2. The patient (e.g., on chemotherapy) with *fever and neutropenia* ($< 500/mm^3$ or $< 1000/mm^3$ and falling) in whom a localizing site of infection is not apparent. A minimal workup includes the following:
   □ Blood cultures
   □ Urinalysis and urine culture
   □ Sputum for Gram's stain and culture
   □ CXR

   Anticipate this event in the immunocompromised patient and agree on an appropriate broad-spectrum antibiotic regimen with the hematologist or oncologist well ahead of time. One of the following regimens may be advised: (1) combination therapy with an aminoglycoside and an antipseudomonal beta-lactam (e.g., piperacillin), (2) double beta-lactam coverage for those with contraindications to aminoglycosides (i.e., a third-generation cephalosporin, such as cefoper-

azone or ceftazidime, plus piperacillin), or (3) imipenem.[1]
Your institution may have special protocols to follow.
3. A patient who is febrile, appears toxic and acutely ill, and is suspected of having an infection despite no evidence of clear-cut source also should receive broad-spectrum antibiotics.

Specific Antibiotics

Two types of patients need specific antibiotics now:
1. The patient with *fever and meningitis symptoms* requires antibiotics immediately after the LP is done. However, do not delay initial antibiotic treatment if a CT scan of the head must be done before the LP (see pages 98 to 99).
2. The patient with *fever and clear localizing clue* should be given specific antibiotics after collection of culture specimens. Antibiotic therapy should be considered an urgent requirement in the diabetic patient.

No Antibiotics Until a Specific Microbiological Diagnosis Is Made

A patient who does not look sick or critical, who is immunologically competent, and in whom the source of fever is not readily apparent (e.g., a patient admitted for workup of fever of unknown origin [FUO]) should not have antibiotics until a specific microbiological diagnosis is made.

Choice of Antibiotics

The common infecting organisms change much more slowly than the antibiotics synthesized to inhibit them. Specific antibiotic choices depend on knowledge of your institution's local microbial flora and their antibiotic susceptibilities. Current guidelines may be found in Appendix, pages 412–413).

Fever in the HIV-Positive Patient

Patients with HIV disease usually have a fever as a result of infection or lymphoma. In these patients, one should assume that fever is due to infection until proved otherwise. Occasionally, no specific cause of fever is found—in this case, the fever may be due to HIV infection itself, but this should be considered a diagnosis of exclusion.

Although HIV-positive patients are susceptible to any of the common infections, a number of opportunistic pathogens should be considered. The organ system involved in such a patient may suggest the offending organism (Table 12–2). More than in any other patient population, multiple infections are often present at the same time in the HIV-positive patient.

Table 12–2 □ COMMON INFECTING ORGANISMS RESPONSIBLE FOR FEVER IN PATIENTS WITH HIV DISEASE, BY SYSTEM INVOLVED

Organ System	Organism	Diagnostic Test
Lungs (cough, SOB)	*Pneumocystis carinii*	Induced sputum or bronchoscopy specimens for toluidine blue or silver stain
	Bacteria (*Pneumococcus, Haemophilus influenzae, Staphylococcus aureus*)	Sputum culture and Gram's stain, blood cultures
	Mycobacteria (*M. tuberculosis, M. avium-intracellulare*)	Sputum smears for AFB × 3; sputum and blood for mycobacterial culture
	Occasionally fungi (cryptococcosis, histoplasmosis, aspergillosis)	Sputum and blood for fungal culture
	Occasionally CMV	Definitive diagnosis requires lung biopsy, which is rarely indicated. CMV is often recovered on bronchoscopy specimens but does not indicate CMV pneumonia
CNS (meningitis)	*Cryptococcus neoformans*	Serum cryptococcal antigen; CSF: cryptococcal antigen, India ink stain, fungal culture
	Bacteria (*Pneumococcus, Meningococcus, Listeria*)	CSF: Gram's stain, culture, and bacterial antigens
	Mycobacterium (*M. tuberculosis*)	CSF: smears and culture for TB
	Treponema pallidum (syphilis)	Serum and CSF: VDRL, serum MHA-TP or FTA-ABS
	HIV	By exclusion

CNS (mass lesion)	*Toxoplasma gondii*	CT scan head (with contrast); serology (IgG ± IgM) usually positive but not diagnostic—if serology negative, argues against diagnosis. Brain biopsy may be required if no response to empiric treatment
	Occasionally tuberculoma, cryptococcoma, histoplasmoma	Brain biopsy
CNS (diffuse disease)	JC virus (progressive multifocal leuko-encephalopathy)	CT scan head ± brain biopsy
	Herpes simplex encephalitis	CT scan head ± brain biopsy
	CMV encephalitis	CT scan head ± brain biopsy
	HIV dementia complex	Clinical diagnosis plus exclusion of other causes
GI tract		
Esophagitis (dysphagia, odynophagia)	*Candida albicans*	Empiric antifungal treatment (ketoconazole, fluconazole, or itraconazole)—if no response, endoscopy brushings and biopsy; smears/cultures
	CMV	Endoscopy for biopsy and viral culture
	Herpes simplex	Endoscopy for biopsy and viral culture

Table continued on following page

Table 12–2 □ **COMMON INFECTING ORGANISMS RESPONSIBLE FOR FEVER IN PATIENTS WITH HIV DISEASE, BY SYSTEM INVOLVED** *Continued*

Organ System	Organism	Diagnostic Test
Diarrhea	Bacteria (*Salmonella, Shigella, Campylobacter, Yersinia, Clostridium difficile*)	Stool culture for bacterial pathogens, stool toxin assay and culture for *C. difficile*
	Parasites (*Giardia, Entamoeba histolytica, Cryptosporidium, Isospora belli, Enterocytozoon bieneusi*)	Stools for ova and parasites ×3; stools for cryptosporidia (modified AFB smear or fluorescent stain)
	CMV	Sigmoidoscopy ± colonoscopy and biopsy
	M. avium-intracellulare	Stool smear for AFB, culture ± endoscopy and biopsy, blood cultures for mycobacteria
Disseminated infection	Mycobacteria (*M. avium-intracellulare, M. tuberculosis*)	Blood, sputum, urine, stool for smears and mycobacterial culture
	CMV	Blood (buffy coat) and urine viral cultures; + biopsies
	Cryptococcosis	Blood, CSF, and urine fungal cultures; serum and CSF for cryptococcal antigen
	Histoplasmosis	Blood, sputum, and bone marrow biopsy for fungal culture; buffy coat smear for yeast forms in WBCs
	Herpes zoster	Tzanck smear, viral culture of skin lesions
	Coccidioidomycosis	Sputum, blood, and CSF for fungal culture; serology
	Bacillary angiomatosis (*Bartonella* sp.)	Biopsy of skin lesion, blood culture

■ REMEMBER

1. The immunocompromised patient is especially susceptible to infection and liable to complications. You should not hesitate to call for the help of the resident or attending physician.

2. The definition of FUO is a temperature $> 38.3°C$ for 3 weeks with no cause found despite thorough in-hospital investigation for 1 week.

3. Fever due to neoplasm, connective tissue disorder, or drug reaction is a diagnosis to be made *after* exclusion of fever due to infection.

4. Fever may result from the use of prescription or nonprescription drugs. Even such commonly used drugs as antibiotics can cause a "drug fever," which, when present, usually occurs within 7 days of beginning the offending drug.

   Antipsychotic medications may cause the *neuroleptic malignant syndrome*, characterized by fever, muscular rigidity, an altered sensorium, tachycardia, and elevations in creatine phosphokinase (CPK), white blood cell (WBC) count, and liver enzymes. The symptoms respond to discontinuation of the offending drug.

   Overdoses of some psychostimulants such as amphetamines and cocaine may acutely elevate the temperature, resulting in rhabdomyolysis and contributing to fatal cardiac dysrhythmias.[2] Prompt cooling, the use of antipyretics, and the judicious use of tranquilizers may be indicated in this setting.

5. Treating a fever due to infection with antipyretics is only treating a symptom. In fact, there is evidence that the ability to mount a febrile response is an adaptive mechanism that inhibits bacterial replication and enhances the ability of macrophages to kill bacteria.[3] It is also useful to observe the fever pattern, and if the fever is not very high ($> 40°C$) and the patient is not uncomfortable, it is not necessary to treat with aspirin or acetaminophen.

6. If antipyretics are ordered, ask the RN to indicate with an arrow the time of administration on the bedside temperature chart. In addition, assessment of therapeutic response is made easier by charting the antibiotics given (Fig. 12–2).

7. Steroids may elevate the WBC count and suppress fever response regardless of the cause. Defervescence with steroids should be interpreted cautiously.

8. Microorganisms love foreign bodies. Look for foreign bodies as sites of infection—IV lines, Foley catheters, ventriculoperitoneal (VP) shunts, prosthetic joints, peritoneal dialysis catheters, and porcine or mechanical heart valves.

9. Fever occurring while the patient is already on antibiotics may mean the following:

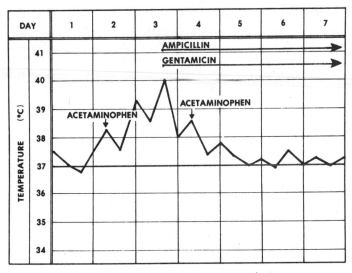

Figure 12–2 □ Bedside temperature chart.

    a. You are using an inappropriate antibiotic.
    b. You are giving an inadequate dose.
    c. You are not treating the right organism, or resistance or superinfection has developed.
    d. The antibiotic is not getting to the right place (e.g., thick-walled abscess requiring surgical drainage).
    e. The fever may not be due to an infection.
10. Delirium tremens is a serious cause of fever occasionally seen in patients withdrawing from alcohol. It is associated with confusion, including delusions and hallucinations, agitation, seizures, and signs of autonomic hyperactivity, such as fever, tachycardia, and sweating. This condition is sometimes fatal and requires high doses of benzodiazepines to stabilize the patient (see page 67).

References

1. Winston DJ: Beta-lactam antibiotic therapy in febrile granulocytopenic patients. Ann Intern Med 1991;115:849–859.
2. Callaway CW, Clark RF: Hyperthermia in psychostimulant overdose. Ann Emerg Med 1994;24:68–76.
3. Saper CB, Breder CD: The neurologic basis of fever. N Engl J Med 1994;330:1880–1886.

13

GASTROINTESTINAL BLEEDING

Gastrointestinal (GI) bleeding is common in hospitalized patients. Whether the bleeding is from minor gastric stress ulceration or from life-threatening exsanguination of aortoduodenal fistula, the initial principles of assessment and management are the same.

■ PHONE CALL

Questions

1. **Clarify the situation. Is the blood old or new, and from where is it coming?**

   Vomiting of bright red blood or "coffee grounds" and most cases of melena indicate an upper GI bleed. Bright red blood passed rectally (i.e., hematochezia) usually indicates a lower GI bleed but may be seen in upper GI bleeds when blood loss is sudden and massive.
2. **How much blood has been lost?**
3. **What are the vital signs?**

   This information helps determine the urgency of the situation.
4. **What was the admitting diagnosis?**

   Recurrent bleeding from duodenal ulcer or esophageal varices carries a high mortality rate.
5. **Is the patient receiving anticoagulants (heparin, warfarin) or thrombolytic therapy (streptokinase, tissue plasminogen activator)?**

   Anticoagulants or thrombolytic agents may require immediate discontinuation or reversal in an actively bleeding patient.

Orders

1. Large-bore intravenous (IV) line (size 16 if possible) immediately, if not already in place

   IV access is a priority in the bleeding patient. Two IV sites may be required if the patient is hemodynamically unstable.
2. Hemoglobin (Hb) stat

   Caution: The Hb level may be normal during an acute

bleed and drops only with correction of the intravascular volume by a shift of fluid from the extravascular space.

3. Crossmatch: Is there blood on hold? If not, order stat crossmatch of 2, 4, or 6 units of packed red blood cells (RBCs), depending on your estimation of blood loss.

4. If the admitting diagnosis is bleeding esophageal varices and the patient is hypotensive, order a Minnesota (or Sengstaken-Blakemore) tube to be at the bedside immediately. If not familiar with the use of this tube, call your resident for assistance now. Also, commence *octreotide* 50 μg bolus followed by 50 μg/hr IV infusion.

5. Ask the RN to take the patient's chart to the bedside.

Inform RN

"Will arrive at bedside in . . . minutes."

Hypotension or tachycardia requires you to see the patient immediately.

■ ELEVATOR THOUGHTS
(What causes gastrointestinal bleeding?)

1. Upper gastrointestinal bleed
   - Esophagitis
   - Esophageal varices
   - Mallory-Weiss syndrome (tear)
   - Gastric ulcer, gastritis
   - Duodenal ulcer, duodenitis
   - Neoplasm (esophageal Ca, gastric Ca)
2. Lower gastrointestinal bleed
   - Angiodysplasia
   - Diverticulosis
   - Neoplasm
   - Colitis (ulcerative, ischemic, infectious)
   - Mesenteric thrombosis
   - Meckel's diverticulum
   - Hemorrhoids

GI bleeding in the human immunodeficiency virus (HIV)-positive patient may result from any of the conditions listed, which are unrelated to the HIV-positive state. However, additional etiologies should be considered—upper GI bleeding may result from Kaposi's sarcoma, gastric lymphoma, cytomegalovirus (CMV) infection of the esophagus or duodenum, or herpes simplex infection of the esophagus. Lower GI bleeding also may result from Kaposi's sarcoma or from colitis caused by CMV, bacterial pathogens (including atypical mycobacteria), or herpes simplex.

■ MAJOR THREAT TO LIFE

- Hypovolemic shock

The major concern with GI bleeding is the progressive loss of intravascular volume in the patient whose bleeding lesion is not identified and managed correctly. If allowed to progress, even minor intermittent or continuous bleeding eventually may result in hypovolemic shock, with hypoperfusion of vital organs.

Initially, lost blood volume may be corrected by infusion of normal saline (NS) or Ringer's lactate, but if bleeding continues, the replacement of lost RBCs will also be required in the form of packed RBC transfusion. Hence, your initial assessment should be directed at the patient's volume status to determine whether a significant amount of intravascular volume has been lost.

■ BEDSIDE

Quick Look Test

Does the patient look well (comfortable), sick (uncomfortable or distressed), or critical (about to die?)
    The patient in hypovolemic shock due to blood loss appears pale and apprehensive and may have other symptoms and signs, including cold and clammy skin, due to stimulation of the sympathetic nervous system.

Airway and Vital Signs

Are there any postural changes in blood pressure (BP) or heart rate (HR)?
    First, check for changes with the patient in the lying and sitting (with legs dangling) positions. If there are no changes, the BP and HR should then be checked with the patient standing. A rise in HR > 15 beats/min, a fall in systolic BP > 15 mm Hg, or any fall in diastolic BP indicates significant hypovolemia. *Caution:* A resting tachycardia alone may indicate decreased intravascular volume. If the resting systolic BP is < 90 mm Hg, order a second large-bore IV line immediately.

Selective Physical Examination I

What is the patient's volume status? Is the patient in shock?
    Vitals   Repeat now
    CVS   Pulse volume, JVP
               Skin temperature and color
    Neuro   Mental status
Shock is a clinical diagnosis as follows: systolic BP < 90 mm

Hg with evidence of inadequate tissue perfusion, such as skin (cold and clammy) and central nervous system (CNS) (agitation or confusion). In fact, the kidney is a sensitive indicator of shock (i.e., urine output < 20 ml/hr). The urine output of a patient who is hypovolemic ordinarily correlates with the renal blood flow, which, in turn, is dependent on cardiac output and is an extremely important measurement. However, placement of a Foley catheter should not take priority over resuscitation measures.

Management I

What immediate measures need to be taken to correct or prevent shock from occurring?

Replenish the intravascular volume by giving IV fluids. The best immediate choice is a crystalloid (NS or Ringer's lactate), which will at least temporarily stay in the intravascular space. Albumin or banked plasma can be given but is expensive, carries a risk of hepatitis, and is not readily available.

Blood has been lost from the intravascular space, and ideally blood is what needs to be replaced. If there is no blood on hold for the patient, a stat crossmatch will usually take 50 minutes. If blood is on hold, it should be available at the bedside in 30 minutes. In an emergency, O-negative blood may be given, although this practice is usually reserved for the acute trauma victim. Transfusion-associated hepatitis can be minimized by transfusing only when necessary. *Rule of thumb:* Maintain a hemoglobin (Hb) level of 90 to 100 g/L.

Order the appropriate IV rate, which will depend on the patient's volume status. *Shock* will require running IV fluid wide open through at least two large-bore IV sites. Elevating the IV bag, squeezing the IV bag, or using IV pressure cuffs may help increase the rate of delivery of the solution. *Moderate volume depletion* can be treated with 500 to 1000 ml of NS given as rapidly as possible, with serial measurements of volume status and assessment of cardiac status. If blood is not at the bedside within 30 minutes, delegate someone to find out why there is a delay.

Aggressive volume repletion in a patient with a history of congestive heart failure (CHF) may compromise cardiac function. Do not overshoot the mark!

What can you do at this time to stop the source of bleeding?

Treat the underlying cause. Treating hypovolemia is treating a symptom.

Upper GI bleed (hematemesis and most cases of melena). Many clinicians begin a parenteral acid-suppressing agent even though studies have not confirmed an influence on complications such as rebleeding, need for surgery, or death within the first 48 to 72 hours.[1, 2] Parenteral H_2-blocking drugs used include *cimetidine* (Tagamet) 300 mg IV every 6 hours, *ranitidine* (Zantac) 50 mg IV every 8 hours, and *famotidine* (Pepcid) 20 mg IV every 8 hours. These agents may be just as effective orally. *Nizatidine* (Axid) is another H_2 blocker available only in the oral form at a dose of 150 mg PO every 12 hours. *Omeprazole* (Losec) 20 mg PO daily is the most potent antisecretory agent currently available, but it is more expensive than the H_2 blockers. Antacids are contraindicated if endoscopy or surgery is anticipated. They obscure the field in endoscopy and increase the risk of aspiration in surgery.

Lower GI bleed (usually bright red blood per rectum and, occasionally, melena). No other treatment is immediately required until the specific site of bleeding is identified, but continue to monitor the volume status.

Abnormal coagulation. If the prothrombin time (PT) or activated partial thromboplastin time (aPTT) is prolonged or if the patient is thrombocytopenic, fresh frozen plasma (2 units) and platelet infusion (6 to 8 units), respectively, may be required. If the patient has recently received thrombolytic therapy, additional agents, such as *antagosan* (Trasylol), may be required but should be initiated only after consultation with your resident or attending physician.

Selective Chart Review

What was the reason for admission?

Has the cause of this GI bleed already been identified during this admission?

Is the patient on any medication that may worsen the situation?

NSAIDs	Counteract the protective effect of prostaglandins on gastric mucosa and may result in gastric erosions or peptic ulcers.
Steroids	Increased frequency of ulcer disease in patients on steroids. Most disease processes for which the patient is receiving steroids will not allow their immediate discontinuation.
Heparin	Prevents clot formation by enhancing the action of antithrombin III.
Warfarin	Prevents activation of vitamin K–dependent clotting factors.

| Streptokinase | Converts free plasminogen to plasmin, which then causes lysis of fibrin. |
| Tissue plasminogen activator | Binds specifically to fibrin, becoming active, and then converts plasminogen to plasmin on the tissue surface. |

Laboratory Data

Most recent Hb value

PT, aPTT, platelets. Are there any platelet or coagulation abnormalities that may predispose the patient to bleeding?

Bleeding time (if a platelet disorder is suspected)

Urea, creatinine levels. (Uremia prolongs bleeding time.) Remember, in prerenal failure, urea level may be more markedly elevated than creatinine level. This difference may be further accentuated in a GI bleed by absorption of urea from the breakdown of blood in the GI tract.

Selective Physical Examination II

Where is the site of bleeding?

Vitals	Repeat now
HEENT	Nosebleed
ABD	Epigastric tenderness (peptic ulcer disease)
	RLQ tenderness or mass (cecal cancer)
	LLQ tenderness (sigmoid cancer, diverticulitis, or ischemic colitis)
Rectal	Bright red blood, melena, hemorrhoids, or mass (rectal cancer)

Also, look for signs of chronic liver disease (hepatosplenomegaly, ascites, parotid gland hypertrophy, spider angiomata, gynecomastia, palmar erythema, testicular atrophy, dilated abdominal veins), which may suggest the presence of esophageal varices.

Management II

Once hypovolemia is corrected, ongoing management includes maintaining adequate intravascular volume while trying to determine the specific site of bleeding.

What procedures are available to determine the site of bleeding?

Esophagogastroduodenoscopy

Tagged RBC scan

Angiography

Sigmoidoscopy

Colonoscopy

In a patient with an *upper GI bleed* that has stopped and who is stable hemodynamically, elective endoscopy can be performed within the next 24 hours. Urgent endoscopy may be required if bleeding continues or the patient is hemodynamically unstable.

Some conditions can be temporarily stabilized at the time of endoscopy. *Esophageal varices* can be treated with sclerotherapy or banding, *octreotide* (50 μg bolus, then 50 μg/hr IV infusion), or a Minnesota (or Sengstaken-Blakemore) tube (Fig. 13–1). In most cases, the presence of bleeding varices should be documented endoscopically before initiating any treatment. Sclerotherapy or banding are the preferred emergency treatments. Sclerotherapy

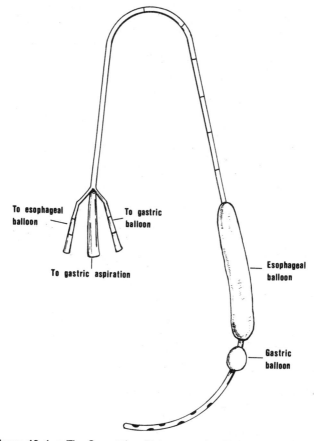

Figure 13–1 □ The Sengstaken-Blakemore tube. The Minnesota tube is similar; it has an additional port for esophageal aspiration.

plus *octreotide* (25 μg/hr IV × 5 days) is more effective than sclerotherapy alone in controlling variceal bleeding in patients with cirrhosis.[3] A Minnesota tube is a temporizing measure reserved for a life-threatening bleed. *Gastric* or *duodenal ulcers* with a visible vessel at the base may be treated with electrocoagulation, heater probe therapy, or direct injection (epinephrine, ethanol, or polidocanol).

Patients with *lower GI bleeds* who are hemodynamically stable should be scheduled for colonoscopy. If unstable, an urgent tagged RBC scan should be arranged and, if possible, be followed by angiography. Tagged RBC scans and mesenteric angiography are most sensitive if performed while there is still active bleeding but should not take priority over resuscitation measures.

Angiographic diagnosis and management of upper GI bleeds are rarely necessary owing to recent improvements in endoscopic therapy. Intra-arterial infusion of vasoconstrictors or selective arterial embolization may be helpful if severe or persistent bleeding occurs in a patient at high risk for surgery, or in centers where endoscopic therapy is unavailable.

When is early surgical consultation appropriate?
- Exsanguinating hemorrhage
- Continued bleeding with transfusion requirements > 5 units/day
- A second bleed from an ulcer, requiring transfusion during the same hospital stay
- Ulcer with a visible vessel at the base on endoscopy

Order an ECG and cardiac enzyme tests if there are any risk factors for coronary artery disease. A hypotensive episode in a patient with atherosclerosis may result in myocardial infarction.

■ REMEMBER

1. Keep the patient NPO for endoscopy or possible surgery.
2. Insertion of an NG tube to look for bright red blood may help identify an upper GI source of bleeding. However, negative NG returns do not rule out an upper GI bleed. Do not leave the NG tube in to monitor bleeding. The patient's volume status is the best indicator of further blood loss, and an NG tube may cause mucosal artifacts, hampering interpretation of endoscopic findings.
3. Bismuth compounds (e.g., Pepto-Bismol) and iron supplements can turn stools black. True melena is pitch black, sticky, and tarlike, with an odor that is hard to forget.
4. An aortoduodenal fistula can appear as a sentinel (minor) bleed that can be followed by rapid exsanguination. Con-

sider this possibility in any patient with abdominal vascular surgery or in any patient with a midline abdominal scar who is unable to give a history.

5. Never attribute a GI bleed to hemorrhoids before thorough exclusion of other sources of bleeding.

References

1. Zuckerman G, Welch R, Douglas A, et al: Controlled trial of medical therapy for active upper gastrointestinal bleeding and prevention of rebleeding. Am J Med 1984;76:361–366.
2. Daneshmend TK, Hawkey CJ, Langman MJS, et al: Omeprazole versus placebo for acute upper gastrointestinal bleeding: Randomized double blind controlled trial. BMJ 1992;304:143–147.
3. Besson I, Ingrand P, Person B, et al: Sclerotherapy with or without octreotide for acute variceal bleeding. N Engl J Med 1995;333:555–560.

14

HEADACHE

Patients in the hospital often complain of headache. You must decide whether the headache is chronic and of no urgent concern or is a symptom of a more serious problem.

■ PHONE CALL

Questions

1. **How severe is the headache?**
   Most headaches are mild and not of major concern unless associated with other symptoms.
2. **Was the onset sudden or gradual?**
   The sudden onset of a severe headache is suggestive of a subarachnoid hemorrhage.
3. **What are the vital signs?**
4. **Has there been a change in the level of consciousness?**
5. **Is there a past history of chronic or recurrent headaches?**
6. **What was the reason for admission?**

Orders

1. Ask the RN to measure the patient's temperature if it has not been recorded within the past hour.
   Bacterial meningitis may present with only fever and headache.
2. If you are confident that the headache represents a chronic or previously diagnosed, recurrent problem, the patient can be given medication that has relieved the headache in the past or a nonnarcotic analgesic agent (e.g., acetaminophen). Ask the RN to call back in 2 hours if the headache has not been relieved by the medication.

Inform RN

"Will arrive at the bedside in . . . minutes."

Headaches associated with a fever, vomiting, or a decreased level of consciousness and severe headaches of acute onset require you to see the patient immediately. Assessment of chronic recurrent headaches at the bedside is necessary if the headache is more severe than usual or if the character of the pain is different.

■ ELEVATOR THOUGHTS
(What causes headaches?)

Chronic (Recurrent) Headaches

1. Muscle contraction
   a. Psychogenic—depression, anxiety, stress (tension headaches)
   b. Cervical osteoarthritis
   c. Temporomandibular joint disease
2. Vascular
   a. Migraine
   b. Cluster
3. Drugs
   a. Nitrates
   b. Calcium channel blockers
   c. Nonsteroidal anti-inflammatory drugs (NSAIDs)

Acute Headaches

1. Infectious
   a. Meningitis
   b. Encephalitis
2. Posttrauma
   a. Concussion
   b. Cerebral contusion
   c. Subdural or epidural hematoma
3. Vascular
   a. Subarachnoid hemorrhage
   b. Intracerebral hemorrhage
4. Increased intracranial pressure
   a. Space-occupying lesions
   b. Malignant hypertension
   c. Benign intracranial hypertension
5. Local causes
   a. Temporal arteritis
   b. Acute angle-closure glaucoma

■ MAJOR THREAT TO LIFE

- Subarachnoid hemorrhage
- Bacterial meningitis
- Herniation (transtentorial, cerebellar, central)

Subarachnoid hemorrhage is associated with a very high mortality rate if not recognized and treated to prevent rebleeding. *Bacterial meningitis* must be recognized early if antibiotic treatment is to be successful. Any intracranial mass lesion (e.g., tumor, blood, pus) may result in *herniation* (Fig. 14–1).

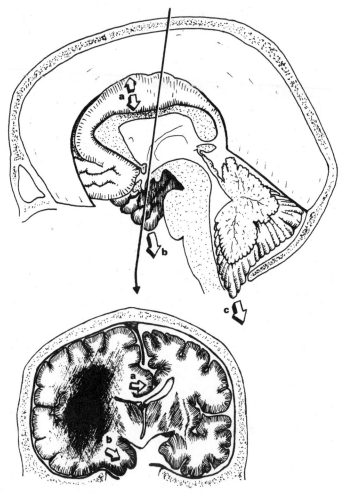

Figure 14–1 □ CNS herniation. a, Cingulate herniation; b, uncal herniation; c, cerebellar herniation.

■ BEDSIDE

Quick Look Test

Does the patient look well (comfortable), sick (uncomfortable or distressed), or critical (about to die)?

Most patients with chronic headaches look well. Those with

subarachnoid hemorrhage, meningitis, or severe migraines look sick.

Airway and Vital Signs

What is the temperature?
Fever associated with a headache requires you to decide soon whether a lumbar puncture (LP) should be performed.

What is the blood pressure (BP)?
Malignant hypertension (hypertension with papilledema) is usually associated with a systolic BP > 190 mm Hg and a diastolic BP > 120 mm Hg. Headache usually is not a symptom of hypertension unless there has been a recent increase in pressure and the diastolic BP is > 120 mm Hg.

What is the heart rate (HR)?
Hypertension in association with bradycardia may be a manifestation of increasing intracranial pressure.

Selective Physical Examination I (Does the patient have increased intracranial pressure or meningitis?)

HEENT	Nuchal rigidity (meningitis or subarachnoid hemorrhage)
	Papilledema (increased intracranial pressure)—see Figure 14–2 for the fundoscopic features of papilledema. An early sign of increased intracranial pressure is absence of venous pulsations.
Neuro	Mental status
	Pupil symmetry
	Asymmetric pupils associated with a rapidly decreasing level of consciousness represent a life-threatening situation. Ask for a neurosurgery consult immediately for assessment and treatment of probable uncal herniation.
	Kernig's sign and Brudzinski's sign (meningitis or subarachnoid hemorrhage) (Fig. 14–3).
	A full neurologic examination is required if there is nuchal rigidity, pupillary asymmetry, or papilledema.
Skin	Maculopapular rash, petechiae, or purpura may be seen in bacterial meningitis.

Management I

If there is papilledema, then there is very likely to be increased intracranial pressure. In the context of "headache," this should

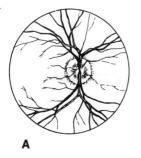
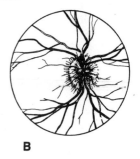

A   **B**

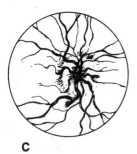
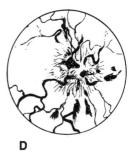

C   **D**

Figure 14–2 □ Disc changes seen in papilledema. *A*, Normal. *B*, Early papilledema. *C*, Moderate papilledema with early hemorrhage. *D*, Severe papilledema with extensive hemorrhage.

suggest a mass lesion (tumor, pus, or blood) but may also be seen with less localized processes such as subarachnoid hemorrhage or meningitis. An immediate computed tomography (CT) scan of the head will help differentiate among these possibilities. An LP is contraindicated because of the risk of brain herniation.

If *fever* is present in addition to papilledema, then empiric antibiotic coverage should be implemented even before the CT scan, as follows.

Suspected Bacterial Meningitis

- Adult, community-acquired infection (most often *Streptococcus pneumoniae, Neisseria meningitidis, Listeria monocytogenes,* streptococcci)—*penicillin G* 2 million units intravenously (IV) over 30 minutes every 2 hours. In areas with a high incidence of penicillin-resistant *S. pneumoniae,* a third-generation cephalosporin (e.g., *cefotaxime* 2 g IV every 6 hours or *ceftriaxone* 2 g IV every 12 hours) may be preferred.

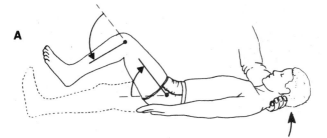

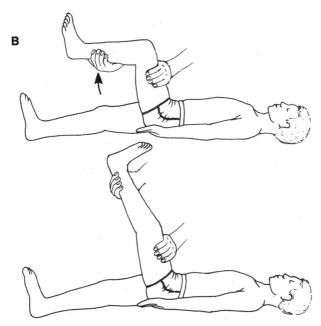

Figure 14–3 □ *A*, Brudzinski's sign. The test result is positive when the patient actively flexes his or her hips and knees in response to passive neck flexion by the examiner. *B*, Kernig's sign. The test result is positive when pain or resistance is elicited by passive knee extension, from the 90-degree hip/knee flexion position.

- Immunosuppressed, alcoholic, or > 60 years old (Gram-negative bacilli)—a third-generation cephalosporin (*cefotaxime* 2 g IV every 6 hours or *ceftriaxone* 2 g IV every 12 hours) plus penicillin or ampicillin

- Postcraniotomy, head trauma, or cerebrospinal fluid (CSF) shunt—*vancomycin* 1 g IV every 12 to 16 hours and a third-generation cephalosporin

Suspected Subdural Empyema or Brain Abscess

- Secondary to frontoethmoid sinusitis, otitis media, mastoiditis, or lung abscess—*cloxacillin* plus a third-generation cephalosporin plus *metronidazole* (60% to 90% of subdural empyemas are caused by extension of a sinusitis or an otitis media)
- After trauma—*cloxacillin* or *nafcillin* plus a third-generation cephalosporin

In addition to beginning antibiotics, a patient with a subdural empyema or a brain abscess should be referred for neurosurgical assessment. Also, prophylactic antiepileptic therapy should be administered routinely as follows: *phenytoin* (Dilantin) loading dose 18 mg/kg IV at a rate no faster than 25 to 50 mg/min IV followed by a maintenance dosage of 100 mg IV every 8 hours or 300 mg PO daily. Steroid treatment, surgery, or both may be required to relieve increased intracranial pressure due to cerebral edema.

If there is fever, nuchal rigidity, and no papilledema, then the likelihood of meningitis is high. In this case, perform an LP, to be followed immediately by IV antibiotics, as recommended above. If there is a delay of ≥ 1 hour in performing the LP, antibiotic therapy should be initiated first—the initial dose will have little effect on the evaluation of the CSF, which is obtained later.

If there is nuchal rigidity, no fever, and no papilledema, then a subarachnoid hemorrhage should be considered. In this case, a noncontrast CT of the brain should be performed before the LP. If a subarachnoid hemorrhage is present, the CT scan will show subarachnoid blood in most cases. If the CT brain scan is normal and a subarachnoid hemorrhage is still suspected, an LP should be performed looking for xanthochromia. Confirmation of a subarachnoid hemorrhage requires immediate neurosurgical consultation.

If there is no papilledema, no fever, and no nuchal rigidity, a more detailed history and chart review may be performed.

Selective History and Chart Review

Was the onset of the headache sudden or insidious?
   The abrupt onset of severe headache suggests a vascular cause, with the most serious being subarachnoid or intracerebral hemorrhage.

How severe is the headache?
Most muscle contraction headaches are mild and not incapac-

itating. However, when migraine headaches are associated with severe pain, the patient may look sick.

Is the headache improved or worsened in the supine position?
Most muscle contraction headaches are improved by lying down. Headaches made worse by lying down suggest increasing intracranial pressure, and an intracranial mass should be considered.

Were there any prodromal symptoms?
Nausea and vomiting are associated with increased intracranial pressure but may also occur with migraine or acute angle-closure glaucoma. Photophobia and neck stiffness are associated with meningitis. The classic visual aura (scintillations, migratory scotomata, and blurred vision) that precedes a migraine headache is helpful in making the diagnosis, but the absence of an aura does not rule out migraine headache.

Is there a past history of chronic, recurring headaches?
Migraine and muscle contraction headaches follow a pattern. Ask the patient whether this headache is the same as his or her "usual headache." The patient will probably make the diagnosis for you!

Is there a history of recent head trauma?
An epidural hematoma may occur after even a relatively minor head injury, particularly in teenagers or young adults. Subdural hematomas can appear insidiously 6 to 8 weeks after seemingly minor trauma and are not uncommonly seen in the alcoholic patient.

Does the patient have joint disease in the neck or upper back?
Muscle contraction headaches in the elderly often are caused by cervical osteoarthritis. These headaches characteristically start in the neck region and radiate to the temple or forehead.

Does the patient have clicking or popping when opening or closing the jaw?
These symptoms are a clue to the presence of temporomandibular joint dysfunction. In addition, the pain may be located predominantly in the ear or face.

Has an ophthalmologist or another physician (MD) dilated the patient's pupils within the past 24 hours?
Acute angle-closure glaucoma can be precipitated by pupillary dilatation. The patient complains of a severe unilateral headache located over the brow and may experience nausea, vomiting, and abdominal pain.

Is there any decrease or loss in vision? Is there a history of jaw claudication?

Temporal arteritis is a systemic illness (fever, malaise, weight loss, anorexia, weakness, myalgia) seen in patients > 50 years of age. If this condition is suspected, order a stat erythrocyte sedimentation rate (ESR). Visual loss in temporal arteritis is a medical emergency and should be managed in consultation with a neurologist or rheumatologist (for treatment, see page 130).

What drugs is the patient receiving?

Drugs such as nitrates, calcium channel blockers, and NSAIDs can cause headaches. Any head trauma or unusual headache occurring in a patient receiving anticoagulants or thrombolytic therapy should raise the suspicion of an intracranial hemorrhage. In this case, a CT scan of the head should be performed and consideration given to reversal of the anticoagulant or thrombolytic agent.

Selective Physical Examination II

Vitals	Repeat now
HEENT	Red eye (acute angle-closure glaucoma)
	Hemotympanum or blood in the ear canal (basal skull fracture)
	Tender, enlarged temporal arteries (temporal arteritis)
	Retinal hemorrhages (hypertension)
	Lid ptosis, dilated pupil, eye deviated down and out (posterior communicating cerebral artery aneurysm)
	Tenderness on palpation or failure of transillumination of the frontal and maxillary sinuses (sinusitis or subdural empyema)
	Inability to fully open the jaw (temporomandibular joint dysfunction)
	Cranial bruit (arteriovenous malformation)
Neuro	Complete neurologic examination

What is the level of consciousness?

Drowsiness, yawning, and inattentiveness associated with headache all are ominous signs. In a patient with a small subarachnoid hemorrhage, these may be the only signs.

Is there any asymmetry of pupils, visual fields, eye movements, limbs, tone, reflexes, or plantar responses?

Asymmetry suggests structural brain disease.

If this is a new finding, a CT scan of the head will be required.

MSS   Palpate skull and face looking for fractures, hematomas, and lacerations

Evidence of recent head trauma suggests the possibility of a subdural or an epidural hematoma.

Management II

Muscle Contraction Headaches. Chronic muscle contraction headaches may temporarily be treated with nonnarcotic analgesics. These are the most common types of headaches you will see in the hospital. A long-term treatment plan, if not already established, may be discussed in the morning.

Mild Migraine Headaches. Mild migraine headaches can be treated adequately with analgesics such as *aspirin* 650 to 1300 mg PO every 4 hours for two doses, *ibuprofen* 400 to 800 mg PO every 6 hours for two doses, or *naproxen sodium* 275 to 550 mg PO every 2 to 6 hours.[1] Patients with allergies to these medications may be given acetaminophen 650 to 1300 mg PO every 4 hours for two doses or *codeine* 30 to 60 mg PO or IM every 3 to 4 hours as needed (PRN).

Severe Migraine Headaches. Severe migraine headaches are best treated immediately during the prodromal stage, but it is unlikely you will be called until the headache is well established. Ask the patient what he or she usually takes for the migraine headache. It will probably be the most effective agent you can prescribe immediately.

Serotonin receptor agonists, such as *dihydroergotamine* or *sumatriptan succinate* (Imitrex), are first-line therapy for most severe migraines. *Dihydroergotamine* 0.5 to 1.0 mg IM, SC, or IV may be given and repeated in 1 hour if ineffective. Alternatively, *sumatriptan* 50 to 100 mg PO or 6 mg SC may be given.

Sumatriptan should not be given within 24 hours of the administration of dihydroergotamine.[2]

These agents are contraindicated in uncontrolled hypertension, unstable coronary artery disease, coronary spasm, or pregnancy and in the presence of hemiplegic migraine. Side effects of sumatriptan include chest or throat tightness, tingling in the head or limbs, and nausea. Dihydroergotamine is less likely to induce chest pain but more likely to cause nausea.

In patients with severe migraines in whom vasoconstrictors are contraindicated, one of the following dopamine antagonists may be tried:

Metoclopramide 10 mg IV

Chlorpromazine 0.1 mg/kg IV over 20 minutes. Repeat after 15

minutes to a maximum dose of 37.5 mg (pretreatment with 5 ml/kg normal saline IV may prevent the hypotensive effects of chlorpromazine).
Prochlorperazine 5 to 10 mg IV or IM or 25 mg PR

Cluster Headaches. Cluster headaches are difficult to treat. Most last less than 45 minutes, and oral treatment has minimal effect. If a cluster headache develops in hospital and is severe, a parenteral narcotic, such as *codeine* 30 to 60 mg IM or *meperidine* (Demerol) 50 to 100 mg IM, may be tried. Alternatively, *dihydroergotamine* or *sumatriptan* in the same doses recommended for migraine headaches may be effective.

Postconcussion Headaches. Postconcussion headaches (provided intracranial hemorrhage has been ruled out by a CT scan of the head) should be treated with an analgesic agent that is unlikely to cause sedation, such as *acetaminophen* or *codeine*. Aspirin is contraindicated in the posttrauma patient because the inhibition of platelet aggregation may predispose the patient to bleeding complications.

Hemorrhages and Space-Occupying Lesions. Patients with subdural, epidural, and subarachnoid hemorrhages and space-occupying lesions (brain abscess, tumor) causing raised intracranial pressure should be referred to a neurosurgeon as soon as possible. While awaiting neurosurgical consultation, *nimodipine* 60 mg PO every 4 hours may improve outcome in patients with subarachnoid hemorrhage.[3]

Malignant Hypertension. Malignant hypertension (hypertension and papilledema) should be managed by careful reduction of BP (see Chapter 16, page 161).

Benign Intracranial Hypertension. Benign intracranial hypertension (pseudotumor cerebri) is a syndrome of unknown etiology, with increased intracranial pressure (headache and papilledema) and no evidence of a mass lesion or hydrocephalus. Refer the patient to a neurologist in the morning for further investigation and management.

Temporal Arteritis. Temporal arteritis should be treated immediately to prevent irreversible blindness. *Prednisone* 60 mg PO daily can be started immediately when this diagnosis is suspected and supported by an ESR of > 60 mm/hr (Westergren's method). Confirmation by temporal artery biopsy should be arranged within the next 3 days.

Glaucoma. A patient with acute angle-closure glaucoma should be referred to an ophthalmologist immediately.

References

1. Pryse-Phillips W, Dodick D, Edmeads J, et al: Guidelines for the diagnosis and management of migraine in clinical practice. Can Med Assoc J 1997;156:1273–1287.
2. Kubacka RT: Practical approaches to the management of migraine. Am Pharm 1994;34:34–44.
3. Pickard JD, Murray GD, Illingworth R, et al: Effect of oral nimodipine on cerebral infarction and outcome after subarachnoid hemorrhage: British Aneurysm Nimodipine Trial. Br Med J 1989;298:636–642.

Headache
Migranes : [Maxeran (Metochlopramide) 10mg IM/IV/PO
                                        q6h prn (max 4/day)
          [Aspirin 650mg   →Side effects
                                        - 10% Extrapyramidal signs

15

HEART RATE AND RHYTHM DISORDERS

There are only three abnormalities in heart rate (HR) or rhythm that you will be called to assess at night—too fast, too slow, and irregular. Remember that the main purpose of the HR is to keep cardiac output high enough to perfuse the following three vital organs: (1) the heart, (2) the brain, and (3) the kidney. Your task is to find out why the heart is beating too quickly, too slowly, or irregularly before it results in hypoperfusion of the patient's vital organs. Begin by asking whether the HR is too fast or too slow. (Rapid HRs are discussed subsequently, slow HRs are addressed on page 149 of this chapter.) Next, decide whether the rhythm is regular or irregular.

RAPID HEART RATES

■ PHONE CALL

Questions

1. **What is the HR?**
2. **Is the rhythm regular or irregular?**
3. **Is this a new problem since admission?**
4. **What is the blood pressure (BP)?**
   Remember that hypotension may be a *cause* of tachycardia (i.e., compensatory) or a *result* of tachycardia that does not allow adequate diastolic filling of the left ventricle to maintain cardiac output.
5. **Is the patient having chest pain or shortness of breath (SOB)?**
   Dysrhythmias are common in patients with underlying coronary artery diseases. A rapid HR may be the result of myocardial ischemia or congestive heart failure (CHF) or may precipitate ischemia or CHF in such a patient.
6. **What is the respiratory rate?**
   Any illness causing hypoxia may result in tachycardia.
7. **What is the temperature?**
   Tachycardia, proportional to the temperature elevation, is an expected finding in a febrile patient. However, you must still examine the patient to ensure that there is no other cause for the rapid HR.

Orders

1. If the patient is experiencing tachycardia and *hypotension,* order a large-bore (size 16 if possible) intravenous (IV) line immediately.
2. If the patient is having *chest pain,* ask the RN to put the cardiac arrest cart in the room and attach the patient to the electrocardiogram (ECG) monitor.
3. Order a stat 12-lead ECG and rhythm strip.

Inform RN

"Will arrive at bedside in . . . minutes."

A rapid HR in association with chest pain (angina), SOB (CHF), or hypotension requires you to see the patient immediately.

■ ELEVATOR THOUGHTS (What causes rapid heart rates?)

Rapid irregular HR	Atrial fibrillation
	Atrial flutter with variable block
	Multifocal atrial tachycardia
	Sinus tachycardia with premature atrial contractions (PACs) or premature ventricular contractions (PVCs)
Rapid regular HR	Sinus tachycardia
	Atrial flutter
	"Supraventricular tachycardias (SVTs)"
	Reentrant
	Atrioventricular (AV) nodal reentry
	Accessory pathways (e.g., Wolff-Parkinson-White [WPW] syndrome, concealed pathways)
	Nonreentrant
	Unifocal atrial tachycardia
	Junctional tachycardia
	Ventricular tachycardia

As electrophysiologic studies have enhanced our knowledge, the classification of SVTs has become more mechanistic but sometimes less practical. Although sinus tachycardia, atrial fibrillation, and atrial flutter are tachycardias with a supraventricular origin, their mechanisms are sufficiently distinct from the other SVTs that they often are classified separately. The term *supraventricular tachycardia* is commonly reserved for (usually narrow-complex) tachycardia that is not clearly sinus, atrial fibrillation, or atrial flutter. Do not be distressed because you cannot differentiate an SVT due to AV nodal reentry from one resulting from orthodromic reentry using a concealed bypass tract! The precise mechanism of an SVT often is not apparent on the surface ECG, and in most cases the initial management is the same.

■ MAJOR THREAT TO LIFE

- *Hypotension,* leading to shock
- *Angina,* progressing to myocardial infarction
- *CHF,* leading to hypoxia

It is useful to recall the determinants of BP as expressed in the following two formulas:

$$BP = \text{cardiac output (CO)} \times \text{total peripheral resistance (TPR)}$$

$$CO = HR \times \text{stroke volume (SV)}$$

As demonstrated by the first equation, any decrease in CO will result in a decrease in BP, unless it is accompanied by a compensatory increase in TPR. Although in most instances a rapid HR serves to increase CO, many of the rapid HRs do not allow adequate time for diastolic filling of the ventricles, resulting in a low SV and, hence, a decreased CO. The low CO may result in *hypotension,* in *angina* in the patient with underlying coronary artery disease, or in CHF in the patient with inadequate left ventricular reserve.

■ BEDSIDE

Quick Look Test

Does the patient look well (comfortable), sick (uncomfortable or distressed), or critical (about to die)?

Patients with tachycardia sufficiently severe to cause hypotension usually look sick or critical. However, a patient with SVT or ventricular tachycardia may look deceptively well if adequate BP is maintained.

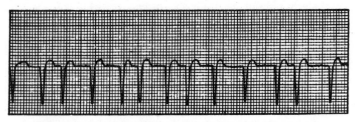

Figure 15–1 □ Atrial fibrillation with rapid ventricular response.

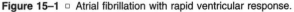

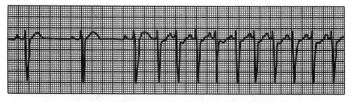

Figure 15–2 □ Supraventricular tachycardia.

Airway and Vital Signs

What is the HR? Is it regular or irregular?
Read the ECG and rhythm strip.

What is the BP?
If hypotensive (systolic BP < 90 mm Hg), you must decide the following quickly:

- Whether the tachycardia is a result of the hypotension (i.e., a compensatory tachycardia)

OR

- Whether the hypotension is a result of the tachycardia (i.e., inadequate diastolic filling leading to low CO with low BP). Three rapid heart rhythms occasionally can cause hypotension due to decreased diastolic filling, resulting in hypoperfusion of vital organs. These rhythms are atrial fibrillation with rapid ventricular response, SVT, and ventricular tachycardia (Figs. 15–1 through 15–3). If the patient is hypotensive, it is important to immediately recognize these three rhythms because prompt treatment is required to restore adequate cardiac output.

Management I

If the patient is *hypotensive* and has atrial fibrillation with rapid ventricular response, SVT, or ventricular tachycardia, emergency cardioversion may be required.

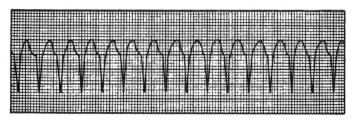

Figure 15–3 □ Ventricular tachycardia.

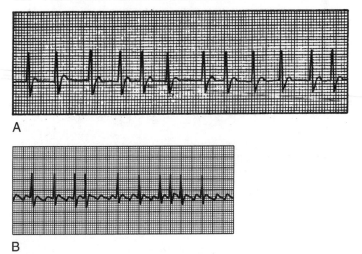

Figure 15–4 □ *A*, Rapid irregular rhythms. Atrial fibrillation. *B*, Rapid irregular rhythms. Atrial flutter with variable block.

- Ask the RN to immediately call for your resident and an anesthetist.
- Ask the RN to bring the cardiac arrest cart into the room. Attach the patient to the ECG monitor.
- Give the patient 100% O_2 by mask (28% if chronic obstructive pulmonary disease [COPD]).
- Ask the RN to draw *midazolam* 5 mg IV into a syringe.
- Ensure that an IV line is in place.
- If the patient has an SVT, also ask the RN to draw *adenosine* 6 mg IV into a syringe. IV adenosine may terminate some SVTs and save you from having to electrically cardiovert the hypotensive patient.

If the patient is *hypotensive* and none of these three rhythms are present, the tachycardia is most likely *secondary* to hypotension.

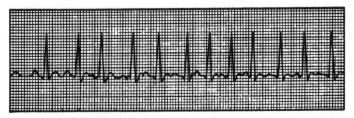

Figure 15–5 □ Rapid irregular rhythms. Multifocal atrial tachycardia.

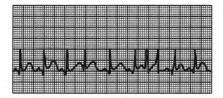

Figure 15–6 ▫ Rapid irregular rhythms. Sinus tachycardia with PACs.

You must perform a selective physical examination to decide which of the four major causes of hypotension is resulting in compensatory tachycardia: (1) cardiogenic causes, (2) hypovolemic causes, (3) sepsis, or (4) anaphylaxis. (Refer to Chapter 18 for investigation and management of hypotension.)

Fortunately, most of the patients you will see with rapid HRs will not be hypotensive. In these cases, you may relax for a minute. Look at the ECG and rhythm strip and decide which rapid rhythm the patient is experiencing.

Rapid Irregular Rhythms
- Atrial fibrillation (Fig. 15–4A)
- Atrial flutter with variable block (Fig. 15–4B)
- Multifocal atrial tachycardia (Fig. 15–5)
- Sinus tachycardia with PACs (Fig. 15–6)
- Sinus tachycardia with PVCs (Fig. 15–7)

Rapid Regular Rhythms
- Sinus tachycardia (Fig. 15–8)
- Atrial flutter (Fig. 15–9)
- SVT: e.g., unifocal atrial tachycardia (Fig. 15–10)
- SVT: e.g., AV nodal reentry or orthodromic WPW tachycardia (Fig. 15–11)
- Ventricular tachycardia (Fig. 15–12)

Note: A wide-complex regular tachycardia such as that shown in Figure 15–3 may in fact represent either ventricular tachycardia or SVT with aberrancy. Most cases of wide-complex tachycardia

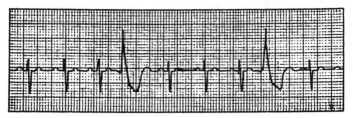

Figure 15–7 ▫ Rapid irregular rhythms. Sinus tachycardia with PVCs.

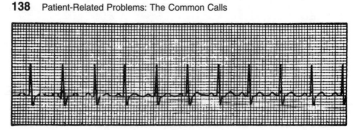

Figure 15–8 □ Rapid regular rhythms. Sinus tachycardia.

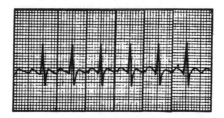

Figure 15–9 □ Rapid regular rhythms. Atrial flutter.

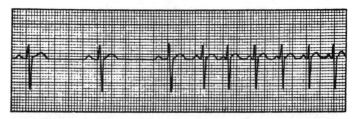

Figure 15–10 □ Rapid regular rhythms. SVT. Ectopic atrial tachycardia.

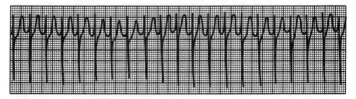

Figure 15–11 □ Rapid regular rhythms. SVT. AV nodal reentry or WPW tachycardia.

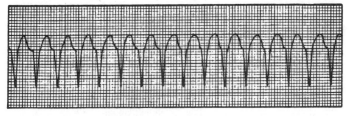

Figure 15–12 □ Rapid regular rhythms. Ventricular tachycardia.

in hospitalized patients are ventricular tachycardia, particularly if occurring in a patient with known or suspected coronary artery disease or cardiomyopathy. Do not assume that a wide-complex tachycardia is SVT with aberrancy just because the rhythm is well tolerated by the patient or the patient is young. If you are uncertain, call your resident for help. A trial of *adenosine* 6 mg IV may help differentiate between these two dysrhythmias. Verapamil can be dangerous in this situation and may result in cardiovascular collapse in a patient with ventricular tachycardia. If uncertainty remains, IV *procainamide* may be effective in treating both dysrhythmias.

Management of Rapid Irregular Rhythms

Management of Atrial Fibrillation. If the patient is *unstable*—is hypotensive, has chest pain (angina), or has SOB (CHF)—and if atrial fibrillation is of recent onset (< 2 days), the treatment of choice is cardioversion, beginning with 100 J.

Atrial fibrillation with ventricular rates of > 100/min and without evidence of hemodynamic compromise (no hypotension, angina, or CHF) can be treated with oral or IV digoxin. If the patient is not already receiving digoxin, give *digoxin* 0.25 mg PO or IV every 4 hours for four doses. Then, give 0.25 mg PO daily thereafter in a patient with normal renal function, and reassess the HR response. Because digoxin is predominantly excreted by glomerular filtration, smaller maintenance doses are required in the presence of renal dysfunction.

In a patient already receiving digoxin, additional doses should be given with caution and careful observation.

Digoxin overdose is a common cause of morbidity in both community and hospital settings. Common side effects include dysrhythmias, heart blocks, anorexia, nausea, vomiting, and neuropsychiatric symptoms, such as hallucinations. It is unusual for these side effects to develop acutely when digoxin is prescribed in the regimen previously outlined. The subsequent development of these side effects can be minimized by adjusting maintenance

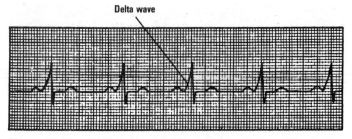

Delta wave

Figure 15–13 □ Wolff-Parkinson-White syndrome. This condition is characterized by a regular rhythm, a PR interval < 0.12 second, a QRS complex > 0.11 second, and a delta wave (i.e., slurred beginning of the QRS).

digoxin doses according to renal function. The risk of digoxin-induced ventricular dysrhythmias can be reduced by avoiding hypokalemia.

Atrial fibrillation with ventricular rates of < 100/min in the untreated patient suggests underlying AV nodal dysfunction. These patients do not require immediate treatment unless hemo-dynamically compromised (e.g., hypotension, angina, or CHF).

SELECTIVE HISTORY AND CHART REVIEW. Once the ventricular rate is controlled, perform a selective history and chart review looking for the following causes of atrial fibrillation:

- Coronary artery disease
- Hypertension
- Hyperthyroidism (check T_4, TSH)
- Pulmonary embolism (check for risk factors, see page 275)
- Mitral or tricuspid valve disease (stenosis or regurgitation)
- Cardiomyopathy
- Congenital heart disease (e.g., atrial septal defect)
- Pericarditis, recent cardiac surgery
- Recent alcohol ingestion (holiday heart syndrome)
- WPW syndrome (Fig. 15–13)
- Sick sinus syndrome (SSS)
- Hypoxia
- Idiopathic (lone fibrillator)

SELECTIVE PHYSICAL EXAMINATION. Look for specific causes of atrial fibrillation. Note that this process takes place after you have already begun to treat the patient.

Vitals	Repeat now
HEENT	Exophthalmos, lid lag, lid retraction (hyperthyroidism)
Resp	Tachypnea, cyanosis, wheezing, pleural effusion (pulmonary embolus)

CVS	Murmur of mitral regurgitation or mitral stenosis (mitral valve disease)
Ext	Swelling, erythema, calf tenderness (DVT)
	Tremor, hyperactive deep tendon reflexes (hyperthyroidism)

Management of Multifocal Atrial Tachycardia. This rhythm does not always require specific management. One should treat the underlying cause, which is usually pulmonary disease and usually already being treated. Check for the following underlying causes.

- Pulmonary disease (especially COPD)
- Hypoxia, hypercapnia
- Hypokalemia
- CHF
- Drugs: theophylline toxicity
- Caffeine, tobacco, alcohol use

Multifocal atrial tachycardia can be a forerunner of atrial fibrillation. If no remediable causes can be found, *verapamil* 80 mg PO three times daily or *diltiazem* 30 to 60 mg PO four times daily may provide rate control and diminish the frequency of ectopics.

Management of Sinus Tachycardia with PACs. Treatment is the same as that for multifocal atrial tachycardia. Again, PACs may be forerunners of multifocal atrial tachycardia or of atrial fibrillation, but PACs do not need to be treated unless atrial fibrillation develops.

Management of Sinus Tachycardia with PVCs. Look carefully at the ECG and rhythm strip and decide whether the PVCs are "malignant." The following features suggest a more ominous arrhythmia: *R on T phenomenon* (Fig. 15–14), *multifocal PVCs* (Fig. 15–15), *couplets or salvos* (≥ 3 PVCs in a row) (Fig. 15–16), and > 5 PVCs/min (Fig. 15–17).

Unless you can be certain that (1) the patient has not had a myocardial infarction (MI), (2) the patient is hemodynamically stable, and (3) the patient has had PVCs chronically, the patient with very frequent PVCs or runs of nonsustained ventricular

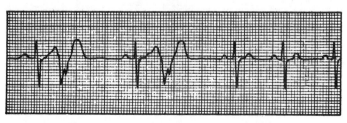

Figure 15–14 □ PVCs. R on T phenomenon.

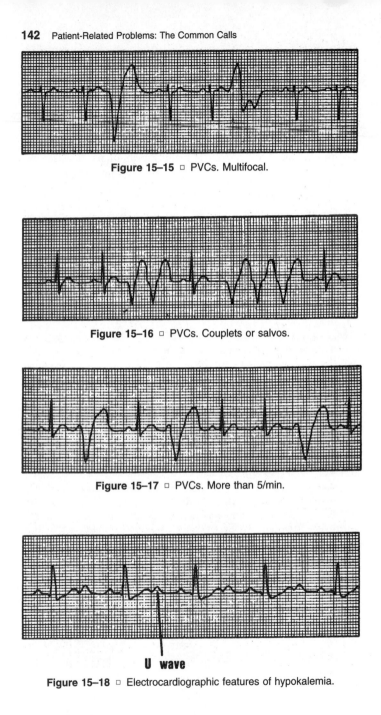

Figure 15–15 □ PVCs. Multifocal.

Figure 15–16 □ PVCs. Couplets or salvos.

Figure 15–17 □ PVCs. More than 5/min.

U wave

Figure 15–18 □ Electrocardiographic features of hypokalemia.

tachycardia should be transferred to a telemetry ward or the intensive care unit/cardiac care unit (ICU/CCU) for further investigation and continuous ECG monitoring.

Look for the following common causes of PVCs in the hospital.

- *Myocardial ischemia* (symptoms or signs of angina or MI). This is the most important cause of PVCs to identify, if present. PVCs are not generally associated with an increased risk of death unless they occur in the setting of myocardial ischemia or MI.

- *Hypokalemia.* Look for a recent serum potassium value in the chart, and order a repeat measurement if a recent one is not available. Check the 12-lead ECG for evidence of hypokalemia (Fig. 15–18). Determine whether the patient is on diuretics that may cause hypokalemia (refer to Chapter 33 for treatment).

- *Hypoxia.* Obtain arterial blood gas (ABG) measurements if hypoxia is suspected clinically.

- *Acid-base imbalance.* Check the chart for a recent HCO_3^- determination. Obtain ABGs if acidosis or alkalosis is suspected.

- *Cardiomyopathy.* Patients with cardiomyopathy sufficiently severe to cause PVCs almost always have a cardiologist and an established diagnosis of cardiomyopathy before you see them. Consult the patient's cardiologist for guidance in treating cardiomyopathy-related PVCs.

- *Mitral valve prolapse.* Mitral valve prolapse (MVP) may be associated with PVCs. Listen carefully for a systolic click and murmur. Diagnosis can usually await confirmation by echocardiography in the morning.

- *Drugs.* Drugs such as digoxin and other antiarrhythmic agents may actually *cause* PVCs.

- *Hyperthyroidism.* Look for signs of hypermetabolism, such as diaphoresis, tremor, heat intolerance, diarrhea, and ocular manifestations of hyperthyroidism, including lid lag, lid retraction, and exophthalmos. Order a serum T_4 and TSH if hyperthyroidism is suspected.

Try to identify whether any of the preceding eight factors are responsible for the PVCs, and correct them if possible. Hypokalemia, hypoxia, and acid-base disturbances usually can be identified and corrected in the patient's room. However, if there is suspicion of myocardial ischemia, cardiomyopathy, digoxin toxicity, or hyperthyroidism, the patient should be transferred to a telemetry ward or the ICU/CCU for continuous ECG monitoring and initiation of antiarrhythmic agents if indicated.

After the PVCs have been treated, the patient may still be left with *sinus tachycardia*. Investigation and management of the underlying sinus tachycardia should be undertaken as subsequently outlined.

Management of Rapid Regular Rhythms

Management of Sinus Tachycardia. There is no specific drug for the treatment of sinus tachycardia. The key is to find the *underlying cause* of this dysrhythmia. The most common causes in hospitalized patients of persistent sinus tachycardia are as follows:

- *Hypovolemia*
- *Hypotension* (cardiogenic, hypovolemic, sepsis, anaphylaxis) (Refer to Chapter 18 for investigation and management of hypotension.)
- *Hypoxia* of any cause (CHF, pulmonary embolism, pneumonia, bronchospasm [COPD, asthma]) (Refer to Chapter 24 for investigation and management of shortness of breath [SOB].)
- *Fever*
- *Anxiety or pain*
- *Hyperthyroidism*
- *Drugs*

The treatment for sinus tachycardia is *always* treatment of the underlying causes.

Management of SVT: Atrial Flutter. The treatment of atrial flutter is similar to that of atrial fibrillation. If *unstable,* the patient may require synchronized cardioversion; if *stable,* the patient may be treated with verapamil, diltiazem, or digoxin IV (see pages 146 to 147). Often, atrial flutter requires higher doses of digoxin than atrial fibrillation to slow the ventricular rate. Ironically, treatment of atrial flutter sometimes produces atrial fibrillation. Look for causes in the chart that may predispose the patient to atrial flutter; for the most part, these are the same diseases that can cause atrial fibrillation (see page 140).

Management of SVT: AV Nodal Reentry and Ectopic Atrial Tachycardias. You will undoubtedly be anxious if called to see a patient with paroxysmal atrial tachycardia (PAT) who is unstable because you know that may require *electrical cardioversion,* a technique with which you may not be familiar. Stay calm; there is still much you can do. If the patient is *unstable,* that is, hypotensive or has chest pain (angina) or SOB (CHF), prepare for immediate cardioversion as follows:

- Ask the RN to immediately call your resident and an anesthetist
- Ask the RN to bring the cardiac arrest cart into the room. Attach the patient to the ECG monitor. Set the defibrillator to 25 J, in the *Synchronize* mode.
- Give the patient 100% O_2 by mask (28% for COPD).
- Ask the RN to draw *midazolam* 5 mg IV into a syringe. Double check that an IV line is in place.
- Ask the RN to draw *adenosine* 6 mg IV into a syringe. Adeno-

sine has a very brief half-life, may be given to an unstable patient, and may terminate an SVT such as AV nodal reentry without the need for cardioversion. This **should not be given,** however, without the guidance of your resident.

- While waiting for your resident to arrive, try nonelectrical means to convert the rhythm, such as the Valsalva maneuver or carotid sinus massage (see the next section).

If the patient is hemodynamically stable, you may try one or more of the following measures to break the tachycardia.

- *Valsalva maneuver.* Ask the patient to hold his or her breath and to "bear down as if you are going to have a bowel movement." This maneuver increases vagal tone and may terminate an SVT.

- *Carotid sinus massage.* This maneuver is an effective form of vagal stimulation and may thereby terminate some SVTs. It should always be performed with IV atropine available and with continuous ECG monitoring, both for safety (some patients have developed asystole) and for documentation of results.

- Listen over the carotid arteries for bruits, and if they are present, do not perform carotid sinus massage. If no bruit is heard, proceed as follows. Turn the patient's head to the left. Locate the carotid sinus just anterior to the sternocleidomastoid muscle at the level of the top of the thyroid cartilage (Fig. 15–19). Feel the carotid pulsation at this point, and apply steady pressure to the carotid artery with two fingers for 10 to 15 seconds. Try the right side, and if not effective, try the left side. Simultaneous bilateral massage of the carotid sinus should never be done because you will effectively cut off cerebral blood flow!

  Carotid sinus massage has resulted, on several occasions, in cerebral embolization of an atherosclerotic plaque from carotid artery compression. Although this is a rare complication, it can be minimized by first listening over the carotid artery for a bruit. If a bruit is heard, forego carotid sinus massage on that side.

- *Adenosine.* Adenosine may be given at 6 mg as a rapid IV bolus followed by a saline flush. If ineffective, increase to 12 mg IV push. A third dose of 18 mg IV push may be given if the first two lower doses were ineffective but well tolerated. Because of the very short half-life of adenosine, the three incremental doses may be administered at intervals of 60 seconds, if required. IV adenosine should be used with caution in patients with asthma and COPD. Lower doses may be required in patients on dipyridamole and in patients who have undergone cardiac transplantation because of supersensitivity to the drug. Common side effects are transient and include facial flushing, dyspnea, and chest pressure. Some

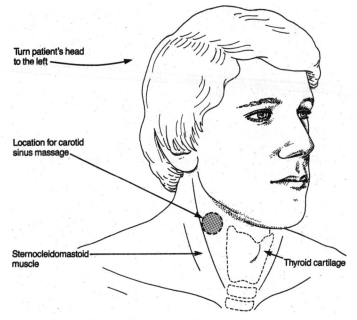

Figure 15–19 □ Carotid sinus massage.

SVTs, particularly unifocal atrial tachycardia, may not be responsive to adenosine, in which case IV verapamil may be effective.

- *Verapamil.* Begin with 2.5 to 5.0 mg IV over 2 minutes. If there has been no effect, the dose may be repeated in 5 to 10 minutes. Verapamil increases atrioventricular (AV) conduction time and may slow ventricular rate. Its advantage over IV digoxin is its more rapid onset of action (1 to 2 minutes for verapamil, 5 to 30 minutes for digoxin).

  Verapamil may cause hypotension if injected too rapidly. It is essential to give the dose slowly over 2 minutes. Verapamil is also a negative inotropic agent and may precipitate pulmonary edema in the patient with a predisposition to CHF. Pretreatment or post-treatment with *calcium chloride* (500 to 1000 mg IV over 5–10 minutes) may minimize the hypotensive effects of verapamil.

- *Diltiazem.* 0.25 mg/kg IV (usual initial dose, 15 to 20 mg) given slowly over 2 minutes will terminate many reentrant SVTs. A second dose of 0.35 mg/kg may be given 15 minutes later if the initial dose is ineffective.

Common side effects of IV diltiazem include bradycardias and hypotension.

- *Digoxin.* Provided that the SVT is not due to digoxin toxicity (i.e., PAT with block), you may use *digoxin* 0.25 to 0.5 mg IV, followed by 0.125 to 0.25 mg every 4 to 6 hours until a full loading dose of 1 mg is given instead of verapamil. Then, a daily maintenance dose of 0.125 to 0.25 mg PO daily may be given if the patient has normal renal function.

  Digoxin slows AV nodal conduction and may terminate SVT. The common side effects of digoxin (dysrhythmias, heart blocks, GI upsets, neuropsychiatric symptoms) are seldom seen acutely when digoxin is prescribed in the regimen as outlined.

- If the patient is known to have **WPW syndrome** and is having SVT, *procainamide* is the drug of choice.

If hemodynamically stable and the aforementioned measures have not worked, the patient should be transferred immediately to the ICU/CCU for semielective cardioversion.

Unlike atrial fibrillation and flutter, the reentrant SVTs are not usually secondary to acquired structural cardiac disease or to other illnesses. Of the nonreentrant SVTs, unifocal atrial tachycardia (particularly with 2:1 or 3:1 block) may be a manifestation of *digoxin toxicity,* and junctional tachycardia may be seen with *digoxin toxicity* or after *acute MI* or *aortic or mitral valve surgery.*

Management of Sustained Ventricular Tachycardia. If the patient has no BP or pulse, call for a cardiac arrest cart and proceed with resuscitation as described on page 370.

If the patient is *unstable* (hypotensive, angina, CHF, or impaired mentation), do the following.

- Call for the cardiac arrest cart, your resident, and an anesthetist, and order a 12-lead ECG immediately.
- Attach the patient to the ECG monitor.
- Make sure that an IV line is in place.
- Give the patient 100% O_2 by mask (28% for COPDs).
- Prepare for *synchronized electrical cardioversion* at 100 J.

If the patient is *stable* (not hypotensive, no angina, CHF, or impaired mentation), do the following.

- Call for the cardiac arrest cart, your resident, and an anesthetist, and order a 12-lead ECG immediately.
- Attach the patient to the ECG monitor.
- Make sure that an IV line is in place.
- Give the patient 100% O_2 by mask (28% for COPDs).
- Order *lidocaine* 1 mg/kg IV to be given by syringe as rapidly as possible. At the same time, begin a maintenance infusion of lidocaine at a rate of 1 to 4 mg/min. In elderly patients and in patients with liver disease, CHF, or hypotension, give half the maintenance dose. In 5 to 15 minutes after the initial

loading dose, give a second bolus of lidocaine, 0.5 mg/kg IV. Lidocaine may cause drowsiness, confusion, slurred speech, and seizures, especially in the elderly and in patients with heart failure or liver disease. Once your patient has been transferred to the ICU/CCU, the staff there will need to watch carefully for these signs of lidocaine toxicity.

- Alternatively, *procainamide* 750 to 1000 mg IV given at a rate of 50 mg/min may also be tried. Although it is often more effective than lidocaine in breaking ventricular tachycardia, the patient will need to be monitored carefully for hypotension.

- If chemical cardioversion with lidocaine or procainamide is unsuccessful, then electrical cardioversion is usually required. The patient should be continuously monitored, your resident and an anesthetist should be called to the bedside, the patient should be sedated, and *synchronized electrical cardioversion*, beginning at 50 J, should be given.

Ventricular tachycardia with hemodynamic compromise or without prompt response to lidocaine or procainamide requires cardioversion. A patient with an episode of ventricular tachycardia should be transferred to the ICU/CCU for continuous ECG monitoring.

After immediate resuscitation, look for the following precipitating or potentiating causes of ventricular tachycardia.

- Myocardial ischemia or MI
- Hypoxia
- Electrolyte imbalance (hypokalemia, hypomagnesemia, hypocalcemia)
- Hypovolemia
- Valvular heart disease (MVP)
- Acidemia
- Cardiomyopathy, CHF
- Drugs
  Digoxin
  Quinidine
  Procainamide
  Disopyramide
  Phenothiazines
  Tricyclic antidepressants
  Sotalol
  Amiodarone
  Cisapride

These drugs may prolong the QT interval to produce a characteristic type of ventricular tachycardia known as torsades de pointes, which resembles a corkscrew pattern in the ECG rhythm strip, with complexes rotating above and below the baseline (Fig. 15–20). The drugs listed should be discontinued if such a rhythm develops. *Magnesium sulfate* 1 to 2 g IV is often effective in terminating this type of ventricular tachycardia.

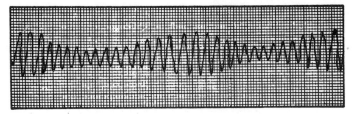

Figure 15–20 □ Torsades de pointes.

SLOW HEART RATES

■ PHONE CALL

Questions

1. **What is the HR?**
2. **What is the BP?**
3. **Is the patient on digoxin, a beta blocker, a calcium channel blocker, or other antiarrhythmic drug?**

   Drugs such as digoxin, beta blockers, diltiazem, and verapamil possess both sinus and AV nodal suppressant properties and may result in profound sinus bradycardias or heart blocks. Other antiarrhythmics such as sotalol or amiodarone possess beta-blocking properties and may also cause bradycardias.

Orders

1. If the patient is hypotensive (systolic BP < 90 mm Hg), order an IV line to be started immediately and ask the RN to place the patient in the Trendelenburg position (foot of the bed up). IV access is essential to deliver medications to increase the heart rate. Placement of the patient in Trendelenburg position achieves an autotransfusion of 200 to 300 ml of blood.
2. If the heart rate is < 40/min, ask the RN to have a premixed syringe of *atropine* 1 mg ready at the bedside.
3. Obtain a stat ECG and rhythm strip.
4. Ask the RN to bring the cardiac arrest cart into the room and to attach the patient to the ECG monitor.

Inform RN

"Will arrive at bedside in . . . minutes."

"Bradycardia + hypotension" or any HR < 50/min requires you to see the patient immediately.

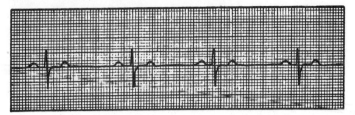

Figure 15–21 □ Slow heart rate. Sinus bradycardia.

■ ELEVATOR THOUGHTS (What causes slow HRs?)

Sinus Bradycardia (Fig. 15–21)

Drugs	Beta blockers
	Calcium channel blockers
	Digoxin
	Other antiarrhythmic agents (amiodarone, sotalol)
Cardiac	SSS
	Acute MI (usually of inferior wall)
	Vasovagal attack
Misc	Hypothyroidism
	Healthy young athletes
	Increased intracranial pressure in association with hypertension

Second-Degree Atrioventricular Block: Type I (Wenckebach) (Fig. 15–22) and Type II (Fig. 15–23)

Drugs	Beta blockers
	Digoxin
	Calcium channel blockers
	Other antiarrhythmic agents (amiodarone, sotalol)
Cardiac	Acute MI
	SSS

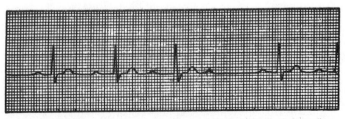

Figure 15–22 □ Slow heart rate. Second-degree AV block (type I).

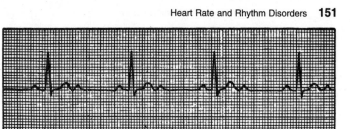

Figure 15–23 □ Slow heart rate. Second-degree AV block (type II).

Third-Degree Atrioventricular Block
(Fig. 15–24)

Drugs	Beta blockers
	Calcium channel blockers
	Digoxin
	Other antiarrhythmic agents (amiodarone, sotalol)
Cardiac	Acute MI
	SSS

Atrial Fibrillation with Slow Ventricular Rate
(Fig. 15–25)

Drugs	Digoxin
	Beta blockers
	Calcium channel blockers
	Other antiarrhythmic agents (amiodarone, sotalol)
Cardiac	SSS

Notice that no matter which bradycardia is present, the most common causes are drug related and cardiac.

■ MAJOR THREAT TO LIFE

- Hypotension
- MI

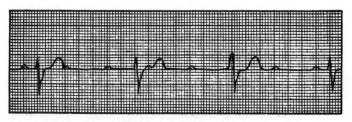

Figure 15–24 □ Slow heart rate. Third-degree AV block.

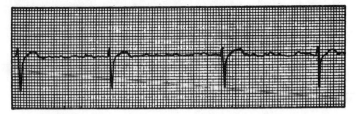

Figure 15–25 □ Atrial fibrillation with slow ventricular rate.

Two major threats to life exist in the patient with bradycardia, as follows. First, if the HR is sufficiently low, it will result in hypotension due to inadequate CO, resulting in hypoperfusion of vital organs. Second, if the bradycardia is due to MI, the patient will be prone to even more ominous dysrhythmias, such as ventricular tachycardia or fibrillation or asystole.

■ BEDSIDE

Quick Look Test

Does the patient look well (comfortable), sick (uncomfortable or distressed), or critical (about to die?)

If the patient looks sick or critical, ask the RN to bring the cardiac arrest cart to the bedside and attach the patient to the ECG monitor. This may give instant diagnosis of the patient's rhythm, allow continuous monitoring, and provide instant feedback on the effects of your interventions.

Airway and Vital Signs

What is the HR?

Read the ECG to identify which slow rhythm is occurring.

What is the BP?

Most causes of hypotension are accompanied by a compensatory reflex *tachycardia*. If hypotension exists with any of the bradycardias, proceed as follows.

- Notify your resident as soon as possible.
- Elevate the legs. This is a temporary measure serving to shift blood volume from the legs to the central circulation. At the same time begin 250 to 500 ml IV NS bolus.
- *Atropine* 0.5 mg IV as rapidly as possible. If no response after 5 minutes, give an additional 0.5 mg atropine IV every 5 minutes up to a total dose of 2.0 mg IV. If still no improvement, begin an IV *isoproterenol* (Isuprel) infusion

by adding 2 mg of isoproterenol to 500 ml of D5W, running at 1 to 10 μg/min (15 to 150 ml/hr). Any patient receiving an isoproterenol infusion should be transferred to the ICU/CCU for further monitoring and possible pacemaker placement.

Selective History and Chart Review

Look for the cause of bradycardia.

Drugs	Beta blockers
	Calcium channel blockers
	Digoxin
	Other antiarrhythmic agents (amiodarone, sotalol)
Cardiac ischemia	Does the patient have a history of angina or previous MI?
	Has there been any hint (chest pain, SOB, nausea, or vomiting) of a cardiac ischemic event's having occurred within the past few days?
	Does the patient have other evidence of atherosclerosis (previous stroke, transient ischemic attacks [TIAs], peripheral vascular disease) that may be a clue to the concomitant presence of coronary artery disease?
	Does the patient have current risk factors (hypertension, diabetes mellitus, smoking, hypercholesterolemia, family history of coronary artery disease) that may suggest that this is the first episode of cardiac ischemia?
	If there is any evidence that the bradycardia is due to an acute myocardial infarction, the patient should go to the ICU/CCU for ECG monitoring.
Vasovagal attack	Is there a history of pain, straining, or other Valsalva-like maneuver immediately before the occurrence of the bradycardia?

Selective Physical Examination

Look for a cause of bradycardia.

Vitals	Bradypnea (hypothyroidism)
	Hypothermia (hypothyroidism)
	Hypertension (risk factor for coronary artery disease)

HEENT	Coarse facial features (hypothyroidism)
	Loss of lateral third of eyebrows (hypothyroidism)
	Periorbital xanthomas (coronary artery disease)
	Fundi with hypertensive or diabetic changes (coronary artery disease)
	Carotid bruits (cerebrovascular disease with concomitant coronary artery disease)
CVS	New S_3, S_4, or mitral regurgitant murmur (nonspecific but common findings in acute MI)
ABD	Renal, aortic, or femoral bruits (concomitant coronary artery disease)
Ext	Poor peripheral pulses (peripheral vascular disease with concomitant coronary artery disease)
Neuro	Delayed return phase of deep tendon reflexes (hypothyroidism)

Management

Sinus Bradycardia

- No immediate treatment is required if the patient is not hypotensive.
- If the patient is on digoxin with an HR < 60/min, further digoxin doses should be held until the HR is > 60/min.
- If the patient is on medications that depress conduction, no immediate treatment is required as long as the patient is not hypotensive. However, with very slow HRs (< 40/min), one should hold subsequent doses of these medications until the HR is > 60/min. Further maintenance doses can be determined in consultation with the attending physician.

Second-Degree Atrioventricular Block (Type I and Type II) and Third-Degree Block

- Patients with either second- or third-degree AV block should be temporarily taken off any drugs that are known to prolong AV conduction and transferred to a bed where continuous ECG monitoring is available.

Atrial Fibrillation with Slow Ventricular Response

- This dysrhythmia does not require treatment unless the patient is hypotensive or has symptoms (syncope, confusion, angina, CHF) suggestive of vital organ hypoperfusion. Definitive treatment includes discontinuation of drugs that depress conduction and, in some cases, requires transfer to the ICU/CCU for pacemaker placement.

■ REMEMBER

1. Abrupt discontinuation of some beta blockers may result in rebound hypertension, angina, or MI. Observe the patient closely over the next several days. When the HR rises to > 60/min, the beta blocker may be reinstituted at a lower dosage. If treated in this manner, rebound hypertension or cardiac ischemia is seldom a problem.

2. Occasionally, digoxin overdose results in life-threatening dysrhythmias that are unresponsive to conventional measures. In these instances, *digoxin-specific antibodies* may be effective in reversing the toxic effects of digoxin.

16

HIGH BLOOD PRESSURE

Calls concerning high blood pressure (BP) are frequent at night. They rarely require the use of drugs that rapidly reduce the pressure. The level of the BP itself is of less importance than the rate of the rise and the setting in which the high BP is occurring.

■ PHONE CALL

Questions

1. **Why is the patient in the hospital?**
2. **Is the patient pregnant?**
   Hypertension in the pregnant patient may indicate the development of preeclampsia or eclampsia and should be assessed immediately.
3. **Is the patient taking antidepressant drugs?**
   Hypertension occurring in a patient receiving monoamine oxidase (MAO) inhibitors or tricyclic antidepressants suggests the possibility of a catecholamine crisis due to food or drug interaction.
4. **Is the patient in the emergency department?**
   Hypertension in young individuals appearing in the emergency department may be caused by catecholamine hypertension due to cocaine or amphetamine abuse.
5. **How high is the BP, and what has the BP been previously?**
6. **Does the patient have symptoms suggestive of a hypertensive emergency?**
   a. Back and chest pain (aortic dissection)
   b. Chest pain (myocardial ischemia)
   c. Shortness of breath (pulmonary edema)
   d. Headache, neck stiffness (subarachnoid hemorrhage)
   e. Headache, vomiting, confusion, seizures (hypertensive encephalopathy)
7. **What antihypertensive medication has the patient been taking?**

Orders

If the patient has any symptoms of a hypertensive emergency, order intravenous (IV) 5% dextrose in water (D5W) to keep the vein open (TKVO) immediately.

Inform RN

"Will be at bedside in . . . minutes."

Situations requiring immediate assessment and possibly prompt lowering of BP include the following:

Eclampsia

Aortic dissection

Pulmonary edema resistant to other emergency treatment (see Chapter 24, pages 273 to 274)

Myocardial ischemia

Catecholamine crisis

Hypertensive encephalopathy

Uncontrolled bleeding anywhere, including worsening vision secondary to retinal hemorrhage

■ ELEVATOR THOUGHTS

The diagnosis of *preeclampsia* can be made in the obstetric patient with hypertension, edema, and proteinuria. This syndrome usually occurs in the third trimester of pregnancy, at which stage hypertension is defined as BP $\geq 140/85$ mm Hg for > 4 to 6 hours or as an increase of 30 mm Hg in systolic BP, 15 mm Hg in diastolic BP, or more, compared with the pregestational values.

Aortic dissection is potentiated by high shearing forces determined by the rate of rise of the intraventricular pressure as well as the systolic pressure.

Elevation of afterload (increased systemic vascular resistance and elevated BP) may be a readily correctable detrimental factor in *myocardial ischemia* and *pulmonary edema.*

Catecholamine crises can be caused by the following:

Drug overdoses	Cocaine and amphetamines
Drug interactions	MAO inhibitors and indirect-acting catechols (wine, cheese, ephedrine)
	Tricyclics and direct-acting catechols (epinephrine, pseudoephedrine, norepinephrine)
Drug withdrawal	Abrupt withdrawal from antihypertensive agents, such as beta blockers, centrally acting alpha agonists, and angiotensin-converting enzyme (ACE) inhibitors, may result in a rebound hypertensive crisis
Pheochromocytoma	May produce a hypertensive crisis through overproduction of epinephrine or norepinephrine
Burns	Some patients with second- or third-degree burns will develop a transient hy-

pertensive crisis, usually resolving within 2 weeks, due to high circulating levels of catecholamines, renin, and angiotensin II

Hypertensive encephalopathy is a rare complication of hypertension and even more unusual in hospitalized patients. Vomiting developing over several days, and headache, lethargy, and confusion are suggestive symptoms. Focal neurologic deficits are uncommon in the early course of encephalopathy.

BP fluctuates in normal individuals and more so in hypertensive individuals. Excitement, fear, and anxiety from unrelated medical conditions or procedures can cause marked transient increases in BP. BP measurements require care with regard to proper cuff size and proper cuff placement and should be repeated to confirm the readings.

■ MAJOR THREAT TO LIFE

The major immediate threat to life is a marked increase in blood pressure with the following:
- Eclampsia
- Aortic dissection
- Pulmonary edema
- Myocardial infarction (MI)
- Hypertensive encephalopathy

■ BEDSIDE

Quick Look Test

Does the patient look well (comfortable), sick (uncomfortable or distressed), or critical (about to die)?
   Unless the patient is having seizures (eclampsia, hypertensive encephalopathy) or is markedly short of breath (SOB) (pulmonary edema), the severity of the situation cannot be assessed by the initial appearance. The patient may have hypertensive encephalopathy yet look deceptively well.

Airway and Vital Signs

What is the BP?
   Retake the BP in both arms.
   Accompanying arteriosclerosis may unilaterally reduce brachial artery flow and may give an artifactually low BP reading. A lower pressure in one arm may be a clue to

aortic dissection. Too small a cuff on an obese patient or a patient with rigid arteriosclerotic peripheral vessels may give readings that are factitiously high in relation to the intra-arterial pressure.

What is the HR?

Bradycardia and hypertension in a patient not receiving beta blockers may indicate increasing intracranial pressure.

Tachycardia and hypertension can be seen in catecholamine crisis.

Selective History

Can the patient further elucidate the duration of hypertension?

Ask the patient about any symptoms suggestive of a hypertensive emergency.

- Headache (an occipital headache or a neckache, lethargy, or visual blurring suggests hypertensive encephalopathy)
- Chest pain (myocardial ischemia)
- SOB (pulmonary edema)
- Back or chest pain (aortic dissection)
- Unilateral weakness or sensory symptoms suggest a cerebrovascular accident. Such an episode in a previously hypertensive patient may be associated with a transient increase in BP.

Selective Physical Examination

Does the patient have evidence of a hypertensive emergency?

HEENT	Assess the fundi for hypertensive changes (generalized or focal arteriolar narrowing, flame-shaped hemorrhages near the disc, dot-and-blot hemorrhages, exudates)
	Papilledema is an ominous finding in patients with hypertension and is seen in malignant hypertension and hypertensive encephalopathy (Fig. 16–1); hypertensive encephalopathy can occur without papilledema, but retinal hemorrhages and exudates are almost always present
Resp	Crackles, pleural effusion (CHF)
CVS	Elevated JVP, S_3 (CHF)
Neuro	Confusion, delirium, agitation, or lethargy (hypertensive encephalopathy)
	Localized deficits (stroke)

Management

Most often, the elevated BP will be an isolated finding in an asymptomatic patient known to have hypertension. Although

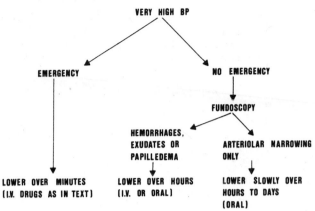

VERY HIGH BP

EMERGENCY

NO EMERGENCY

FUNDOSCOPY

HEMORRHAGES,
EXUDATES OR
PAPILLEDEMA

ARTERIOLAR NARROWING
ONLY

LOWER OVER MINUTES
(I.V. DRUGS AS IN TEXT)

LOWER OVER HOURS
(I.V. OR ORAL)

LOWER SLOWLY OVER
HOURS TO DAYS
(ORAL)

Figure 16–1 □ Approach to management of very high blood pressure.

long-term control of hypertension in such patients is of proved benefit, acute lowering of BP is not. Remember there is a risk of overshooting the mark in acute reduction of BP in patients with longstanding high BP and reduced ability to autoregulate cerebral blood flow. Do not treat the BP reading. Treat the condition associated with it!

True emergencies require special management. These include the following:

- Hypertensive encephalopathy
- Malignant hypertension (marked elevation of diastolic BP with fundal hemorrhages and exudates and usually some compromise in renal function)
- Eclampsia
- Subarachnoid or cerebral hemorrhage
- Aortic dissection
- Hypertension and pulmonary edema or myocardial ischemia
- Catecholamine crisis

Call your resident now for help if you are unfamiliar with the management of these conditions.

Hypertensive Encephalopathy. This is almost always accompanied by retinal exudates and hemorrhages and often by papilledema. Focal neurologic deficits are unusual early on and suggest that the elevated pressure is most likely associated with a stroke. Remember particularly the risk of lowering pressure too quickly in patients with atherothrombotic cerebrovascular disease; you can precipitate a stroke!

1. Transfer the patient to the intensive care unit/cardiac care

unit (ICU/CCU) for electrocardiographic (ECG) monitoring and intra-arterial BP monitoring.

2. Because transfer to the ICU/CCU often takes > 30 minutes, you may temporarily achieve BP control by giving the patient a single oral tablet of one of the following:

   a. *Nifedipine* 5 to 10 mg PO for one dose. Patients with longstanding hypertension are at risk from abrupt reduction in BP, which may compromise coronary and cerebral blood flow. In the presence of atherosclerosis, this circumstance can result in MI or stroke. The risk can be reduced if nifedipine is given orally as the intact capsule in an initial dose of 5 to 10 mg. The effect of this dose usually is apparent within 30 minutes, and a repeat dose of 5 to 10 mg may be given if insufficient BP lowering has been achieved. Few situations require the more rapid (by 5 to 10 minutes) but less predictable response that occurs after biting and swallowing the capsule. The sublingual route should not be used because nifedipine is not absorbed by the oral mucosa. Aim for diastolic BP levels of around 100 mm Hg.

   b. *Captopril* 25 mg PO

   c. *Labetolol* 200 mg PO

   d. *Atenolol* 25 mg PO or *nadolol* 20 mg PO

3. *Labetalol* is a combined alpha- and beta-blocking agent that may be given IV without intra-arterial monitoring. It may be given in repeated incremental doses, beginning at 20 mg IV every 10 to 15 minutes (e.g., 20 mg, 20 mg, 40 mg, 40 mg) to a maximum of 300 mg. Alternatively, a labetalol infusion beginning at 2 mg/min and titrating to a BP response may be given. Labetalol is not as useful in lowering BP if the patient is already on a beta blocker.

4. A *nitroprusside infusion* may be required. In most medical situations, IV nitroprusside cannot be given to patients in general medical units because of the requirement for intra-arterial BP monitoring. However, you may expedite treatment by informing the ICU/CCU staff in advance when patients will be requiring IV nitroprusside infusions. The usual dose is 0.5 to 10.0 μg/kg/min.

5. Once BP control is achieved through parenteral means, the patient should be started on an appropriate oral regimen to maintain satisfactory BP control.

Malignant Hypertension. Unless accompanied by another feature (e.g., encephalopathy, pulmonary edema), you have more time to gain control of the BP. Control may be achieved by using a combination of orally effective antihypertensive drugs. Review the patient's current antihypertensive treatment. Increase to the maximum effective dose or add other agents. More aggressive approaches can wait until morning.

Preeclampsia and Eclampsia. Treatment in these patients is complicated by the risk to the fetus and to the mother from both the disorder and the treatment. The treatment of choice near term is magnesium sulfate until delivery of the baby can be effected. Treatment should be initiated only in consultation with the patient's obstetrician. *Magnesium sulfate* is given as an IV infusion: mix 16 g of magnesium sulfate in 1 L of D5W and give a loading dose of 250 ml (4 g) IV over 20 minutes. The maintenance dose is 1 to 2 g (62.5 to 125 ml)/hr or more, as required. Order a serum magnesium level every 4 hours, aiming for serum magnesium level of 6 to 8 mmol/L.

Note that magnesium sulfate does not lower BP. Local practice may include other drug selections, such as *labetalol, hydralazine,* or *nitroprusside.* Diuretics should be avoided because these patients are usually already volume depleted, with an activated renin-angiotensin system.

Subarachnoid or Cerebral Hemorrhage. Although there is no proof that lowering of pressure alters outcome, many neurologists will administer drugs to control elevated pressures in these situations. Unless you are familiar with the local practice, a neurologist should be consulted.

Aortic Dissection

1. Transfer the patient to the ICU/CCU immediately for intra-arterial BP monitoring and control of BP with parenteral drugs.
2. *Nitroprusside* 0.5 to 10.0 μg/kg/min is useful in the management of aortic dissection but should not be used without an accompanying beta blocker, which will reduce the rate of rise of intraventricular pressure and, hence, the shearing force. These beta blockers should be given parenterally, and high doses may be required as follows:
   a. *Propranolol* 0.5 mg IV followed by 1 mg IV every 5 minutes until the pulse pressure is reduced to 60 mm Hg or to a total dose of 0.15 mg/kg in any 4-hour period, with a maintenance dosage of every 4 to 6 hours, or
   b. *Esmolol* 500 μg/kg/min for 1 to 4 minutes and then 50 to 300 μg/kg/min by maintenance infusion. The only advantage of esmolol is its short half-life, thus providing a rapid onset and offset of action.
3. *Labetalol* alone may be used for aortic dissection in the same regimen as for hypertensive encephalopathy (see page 161).

Hypertension and Pulmonary Edema or Myocardial Ischemia

1. In addition to BP control, pulmonary edema should be treated with the measures outlined in Chapter 24, pages 273 to 274.
2. Transfer the patient to the ICU/CCU for continuous ECG and intra-arterial BP monitoring.
3. Notify the ICU/CCU staff that the patient will require an IV *nitroglycerin infusion.* Experimental evidence suggests that IV nitroglycerin is preferable to IV nitroprusside for the control of BP in a patient with myocardial ischemia because nitroprusside may cause a coronary steal phenomenon, resulting in extension of the ischemic zone. It is therefore preferable to attempt control of the BP in a cardiac patient with IV nitroglycerin and, if unsuccessful, nitroprusside.
4. If the patient is hypertensive and tachycardic and has myocardial ischemia but no evidence of pulmonary edema, beta blockade is helpful in addition to IV nitroglycerin. Any of the following agents may be used acutely:
   a. *Propranolol* 0.5 mg IV followed by 1 mg IV every 5 minutes until the pulse pressure is reduced to 60 mm Hg or to a total dose of 0.15 mg/kg in any 4-hour period, with a maintenance dosage of every 4 to 6 hours, or
   b. *Esmolol* 500 μg/kg/min for 1 to 4 minutes and then 50 to 300 μg/kg/min by maintenance infusion, or
   c. *Metoprolol* 5 to 15 mg IV, or
   d. *Atenolol* 5 mg IV

Catecholamine Crisis. *Pheochromocytoma* is the classic condition (pallor, palpitations, and perspiration) associated with intermittent and alarmingly high BPs. Other conditions associated with similar, sudden, and severe increase in BP include *cocaine* and *amphetamine* abuse, major second- or third-degree *burns*, abrupt antihypertensive *drug withdrawal*, and food (cheese), drug (ephedrine), and drink (wine) interactions with *MAO inhibitors* (antidepressants). Currently used MAO inhibitors include tranylcypromine sulfate (Parnate), phenelzine sulfate (Nardil), and isocarboxazid (Marplan). If sudden increases in pressure are observed in patients on these drugs, the most likely cause is an interaction with a substance that is releasing the stores of catecholamines, which are overabundant because of inhibition of one of the catecholamine-metabolizing enzymes (MAO).

1. Transfer the patient to the ICU/CCU for ECG and intra-arterial BP monitoring.
2. Notify the ICU/CCU staff that the patient will require special parenteral antihypertensive drugs.
3. In cases of known or suspected ***pheochromocytoma***, *phentolamine mesylate*, a direct alpha blocker, may be given IV for

marked elevation of BP. This drug causes a decrease in peripheral resistance and an increase in venous capacity due to a direct action on vascular smooth muscle. This effect may be accompanied by cardiac stimulation with tachycardia that is more than can be explained as a reflex response to peripheral vasodilation. In an emergency, 2.5 to 5 mg may be given intravenously. However, if time permits and for continuous control, phentolamine mesylate should be given at an initial dosage of 5 to 10 µg/kg/min by continuous IV infusion. Alternatively, *labetalol* or *nitroprusside* may be used in the same dosages as described previously.

4. In *cocaine-induced hypertension, labetalol, phentolamine,* or *nitroprusside* may be used in the same dosages as described previously. Propranolol and beta-blockers other than labetalol should be avoided because of the risk of resulting in unopposed alpha stimulation.[1]

5. In *amphetamine-induced hypertension, chlorpromazine* 1 mg/kg IM can reverse hypertension and hyperactivity.

6. In catecholamine crisis associated with *MAO inhibitors,* phentolamine, labetalol, or nitroprusside may each be effective.

Reference

1. Lange RA, Cigarroa RG, Flores ED, et al: Potentiation of cocaine-induced coronary vasoconstriction by beta-adrenergic blockade. Ann Intern Med 1990;112:897–903.

17

HYPNOTICS, LAXATIVES, ANALGESICS, AND ANTIPYRETICS

Telephone calls regarding the reordering of hypnotic, laxative, analgesic, and antipyretic medications are frequent. The majority of these requests can be managed over the telephone.

HYPNOTICS

■ PHONE CALL

Questions

1. **Why is a hypnotic being requested?**
   The majority of requests for nighttime sedation are due to insomnia. Sleeping pills should not be prescribed for restless or agitated patients who have not been examined.
2. **Has the patient received hypnotics before?**
3. **What are the vital signs?**
4. **What was the reason for admission?**
5. **Does the patient have any of the following conditions in which hypnotics are contraindicated?**
   a. Depression: an antidepressant is the drug of choice if insomnia is a manifestation of depression
   b. Confusion
   c. Hepatic or respiratory insufficiency
   d. Sleep apnea
   e. Myasthenia gravis
6. **Is the patient receiving other centrally active drugs that may interact, such as alcohol, antidepressants, antihistamines, and narcotics?**
7. **Does the patient have any drug allergies?**
   The major contraindication to a specific hypnotic is a known allergy to the drug.

Orders

A benzodiazepine is the drug of choice for short-term treatment of insomnia. Sedative effects are comparable among all benzodiazepines; only the onset and duration of the effects differ. Table 17–1 lists the drug doses of various benzodiazepines.

Table 17–1 □ CHARACTERISTICS OF SOME BENZODIAZEPINES

Drug	Usual Adult Dose (mg)	Time of Peak Effect (hr)	Biological Half-life (hr)
Premedication			
Midazolam (Versed)	0.035–0.1/kg IV		
Hypnotic			
Temazepam (Restoril)	30 PO hs	0.8–1.4	8–10
Nitrazepam (Mogadon)	5–10 PO hs	2	26
Flurazepam (Dalmane)	15–30 PO hs	1	50–100
Antianxiety			
Oxazepam (Serax)	30–120/d	1–4	4–13
Bromazepam (Lectopam)	6–30/d	1–4	12
Alprazolam (Xanax)	0.5–1.5/d	1–2	6–20
Lorazepam (Ativan)	2/d	1–6	12–15
Chlordiazepoxide (Librium)	15–75/d	2–4	20–24
Clorazepam (Traxene)	30/d	1–2	48
Ketazolam (Loftran)	15–30/d	?	50
Diazepam (Valium)	4–40/d	2	50–100

Inform RN

"Will arrive at the bedside in . . . minutes."

Agitated, restless patients should be assessed before hypnotics are prescribed.

■ REMEMBER

1. The biological half-lives of benzodiazepines vary from 4 hours for oxazepam to 50 to 100 hours for diazepam (Valium). Accumulation can occur if the second and subsequent doses of drugs are given before the previous dose has been metabolized and excreted. Diazepam and flurazepam (Dalmane) have active metabolites; the half-lives (see Table 17–1) include the active metabolites. When the drugs are prescribed once or twice, the half-life of the drug is of no great concern because diffusion out of the brain rather than the rate of elimination from the body is the major factor respon-

sible for the duration of effect. However, with repeated use of benzodiazepines, the drug half-life must be taken into account because the rates of metabolism then become more important in determining the duration of effects. Flurazepam given repeatedly will cause a daytime hangover, whereas oxazepam (Serax) will not. However, the shortest-acting drugs may be associated with early morning insomnia and rebound daytime anxiety.

2. Benzodiazepines should not be prescribed on a continuous nightly basis but should be discontinued temporarily once one or two nights of acceptable sleep have been achieved. The use of benzodiazepines for less than 14 consecutive nights helps to prevent the development of drug tolerance and dependence.

3. Be aware of the adverse effects of any drug you prescribe. The *adverse effects of benzodiazepines* are central nervous system (CNS) depression (tiredness, drowsiness, detached feeling), headache, dizziness, ataxia, confusion, disorientation in the elderly, and psychological dependence.

4. Barbiturates and nonbarbiturate hypnotics other than benzodiazepines usually carry more risks than advantages as hypnotics and should be avoided.

LAXATIVES

Constipation is frequently aggravated or caused by drugs (e.g., iron supplements, calcium entry blockers, aluminum-containing antacids) or medical conditions (e.g., hypothyroidism, diabetes mellitus, Parkinson's disease, diverticular disease). Hospitalized patients commonly require laxatives, particularly after acute myocardial infarction to limit straining, during the administration of narcotics, during prolonged bedrest, and during evacuation of the bowels before abdominal surgery and some gastrointestinal (GI) diagnostic procedures. The solutions used in *enemas* have either hypertonic properties to stimulate rectal peristalsis or surfactant properties to achieve softening of impacted feces.

■ PHONE CALL

Questions

1. Why is a laxative being requested?

The frequency of bowel movements is highly variable in the normal population, ranging from twice daily to once every 3 days. Make certain you know what this patient's normal bowel pattern is before prescribing a laxative.

2. **Has the patient received laxatives before? If so, which ones have been tried so far?**
3. **What are the vital signs?**
4. **What was the reason for admission?**
5. **When was a rectal examination last performed?**

   Fecal impaction, which requires a rectal examination for diagnosis (and sometimes for treatment), is a relative contraindication to oral laxative use.

6. **Does the patient have nausea, vomiting, or abdominal pain?**

   These symptoms suggest an acute GI disorder.

Orders

Table 17–2 lists the drug doses of selective laxatives, and Table 17–3 lists the drug doses of enemas. Bowel movements can be increased in frequency by liquefying the stool. Both bulk and osmotic laxatives increase the water content in the intestine. An increase in the frequency of bowel movements can also be induced by stool softeners and colon-irritating drugs that increase peristalsis.

Inform RN

"Will arrive at the bedside in . . . minutes."

The only time you need to assess a patient when a laxative has been requested is when the patient has associated nausea, vomiting, or abdominal pain or when fecal impaction is suspected. (See Chapter 5 for the assessment and management of abdominal pain.)

■ REMEMBER

1. When a patient is constipated (unless there is fecal impaction), an oral laxative is the treatment of choice. If the oral laxative fails, a stronger-acting laxative can be used; if this is not effective, a suppository is prescribed. Finally, enemas can be used as follows: first, a hypertonic enema solution (e.g., Fleet) and, if unsuccessful, an oil-retention enema may then be tried.
2. When there is fecal impaction, an oil-based enema is the treatment of choice.
3. Soapsuds enemas are primarily used for preoperative bowel cleansing. They are quite uncomfortable because of the large

Table 17-2 □ SOME CHARACTERISTICS OF LAXATIVES

Drug	Dose	Comments
Bulk Forming		
Psyllium hydrophilic mucilloid (Metamucil and others)	3–6.5 g PO once to TID	Cellulose binds drugs (e.g., digoxin) Not useful for acute constipation
Surface Active		
Docusate (dioctyl sodium sulfosuccinate, Colace)	100 mg PO TID 50 mg/90 ml enema fluid	See page 435
Lubricant		
Mineral oil	Emulsion 15 ml BID	Impairs the absorption of fat-soluble vitamins
Osmotic		
Lactulose	15–30 ml PO	Onset in 30 min
Glycerin	2.67 g suppository	Do not use Mg preparations in renal impairment
Milk of magnesia	15–30 ml PO	
Magnesium citrate oral solution	15 g/300 ml solution, or 7–21 ml of a 70% solution	
Stimulant		
Anthraquinones (cascara, senna)	Variable	Onset in 6 hr; urine may be brown
Diphenylmethanes (e.g., bisacodyl)	5–15 mg PO or 10 mg PR	See page 430
Castor oil	15–60 ml	May give profound evacuation

Table 17–3 □ EXAMPLES OF ENEMAS

Sodium Phosphate and Sodium Biphosphate (Fleet Enema)

Onset: Immediate

Caution: Do not use when nausea, vomiting, or abdominal pain is present.

Usual adult dose: 60–120 ml (6 g sodium phosphate and 16 g sodium biphosphate/100 ml). (Available in a disposable plastic container.)

Use: Acute evacuation of the bowel prior to diagnostic procedures; acute constipation.

Bisacodyl (Fleet Bisacodyl)

Onset: Immediate

Caution: Do not use when nausea, vomiting, or abdominal pain is present. Avoid in pregnancy and MI. May worsen orthostatic hypotension, weakness, and incoordination in the elderly.

Usual adult dose: 37.5 ml (10 mg/30 ml). (Available in disposable plastic containers.)

Use: Acute evacuation of the bowel prior to diagnostic procedures; acute constipation.

Mineral Oil (Fleet Mineral Oil Enema)

Onset: Immediate

Caution: Do not use when nausea, vomiting, or abdominal pain is present.

Usual adult dose: 60–120 ml. (Available in disposable plastic containers.)

Use: Impacted feces.

Microlax (Na citrate 450 mg, Na alkylsulfoacetate 45 mg, sorbic acid 5 mg)

Onset: 5–15 min

Caution: Do not use when nausea, vomiting, or abdominal pain is present.

Usual adult dose: 5 ml.

Use: Fecal impaction when hard stool is present in the rectum. Not useful if rectum is empty.

---

volumes used and are rarely required in the treatment of constipation.

ANALGESICS

Most hospital pharmacies do not allow narcotic medication orders to stand indefinitely. Narcotic medications need to be reordered every 3 to 5 days, depending on the individual medical institution. Consequently, if the housestaff fail to reorder these medications during the day, you may be called to do so at night.

■ PHONE CALL

Questions

1. Why is an analgesic being requested?
The majority of requests are for reordering of medications.

2. How severe is the pain?
This question will help to determine whether a nonnarcotic analgesic may be sufficient.

3. Is this a new problem?
The new onset of undiagnosed pain requires you to assess the patient, at the bedside, before ordering an analgesic medication.

4. What are the vital signs?
The onset of fever in association with pain suggests a localized infectious process.

5. What was the reason for admission?

6. Does the patient have any drug allergies?

Orders

Tables 17–4 and 17–5 provide the drug dosages of selected analgesics.

Inform RN

"Will arrive at bedside in . . . minutes."

Any undiagnosed pain, new onset of severe pain, or change in character of previous pain requires you to assess the patient at the bedside before ordering an analgesic.

■ REMEMBER

If reversal of a narcotic overdose is required, the following are recommended.

1. *Reversal of postoperative narcotic depression.* Give *naloxone* (Narcan) 0.2 to 2.0 mg IV every 5 minutes until the desired improved level of consciousness is achieved (maximum total dose, 10 mg). Doses every 1 to 2 hours may be required to maintain reversal of CNS depression.

2. *Reversal of suspected narcotic overdose.* If the patient is comatose, intubation for airway protection should be undertaken before reversal. Abrupt reversal may induce nausea and vomiting with the attendant risk of aspiration pneumonia. Give *naloxone* 0.2 mg IV, SC, or IM every 5 minutes for several doses. If the initial dosages are ineffective, the dose may be increased incrementally to a maximum total dose of 10 mg.

Table 17–4 □ CHARACTERISTICS OF SOME COMMONLY USED ANALGESICS IN MILD TO MODERATE PAIN

Drug	Usual Adult Dose (mg)	Comments
Acetaminophen* (Paracetamol, Tylenol)	650–975 q4h PO	As effective an analgesic as NSAIDs with no anti-inflammatory effects
Aspirin (acetylsalicylic acid)	650–975 q4h PO	
Diflunisal (Dolobid)	1000, then 500 q12h PO	Salicylate derivative
Ibuprofen (Motrin and many others)	400 q4–6h PO	NSAID
Naproxen (Naprosyn)	250 q8h PO	NSAID
Fenoprofen (Nalfon)	300 q6–8h PO	NSAID
Diclofenac sodium (Voltaren)	25–50 q8h PO	NSAID
Indomethacin (Indocin)	25 q6–8h PO	NSAID
Codeine*	30–60 PO/SC/IM q4–6h	More effective than propoxyphene and less addicting than oxycodone
Propoxyphene (Darvon)	100 q4–6h PO	Equipotent to 650 mg acetylsalcylic acid

*Acetaminophen and codeine are available in a variety of commercial preparations, usually containing 300 mg of acetaminophen and 8–60 mg of codeine phosphate.

Table 17–5 □ CHARACTERISTICS OF SOME NARCOTIC DRUGS

| Drug | Usual Adult Dose | | Comments |
	Oral (mg)	*SC/IM (mg)*	**Comments**
Morphine sulfate preparations			
MSIR (immediate release)	5–30 q4–6h*		Available in oral solution or tablet form.
MS Contin (sustained release)	15–120 q12h		Because it is difficult to titrate sustained-release doses, it is best to initiate morphine treatment with an immediate-release preparation.
Morphine injection		5–15 q4–6h*	
Anileridine (Leritine)	25–50 q4–6h*	25–50 q4–6h*	
Hydromorphone (Dilaudid)	2–4 q4h*	2 q4h*	
Meperidine (Demerol)	50–150 q4h*	50–150 q4h*	

*The duration of action tends to be longer with oral than with parenteral administration.

3. *Adverse effects of abrupt narcotic reversal.* Nausea and vomiting, if provoked in the patient with an unprotected airway, may result in aspiration pneumonia. Hypertension and tachycardia can occur during narcotic reversal and may result in congestive heart failure in the patient with poor left ventricular function.

ANTIPYRETICS

Antipyretics should not be prescribed in the adult patient with fever unless the cause of the fever is known or the patient is symptomatic from the fever itself. (Refer to Chapter 12 for the approach to the febrile patient. See Table 17–4 for the dosages and side effects of acetaminophen and aspirin.)

18

HYPOTENSION AND SHOCK

Hypotension is a common call at night. Do not panic. Remember that hypotension does not become shock until there is evidence of inadequate tissue perfusion. An adequate blood pressure (BP) is required to perfuse three vital organs—the *brain*, *heart*, and *kidneys*. Some patients normally have systolic BPs in the range of 85 to 100 mm Hg. The BP is usually adequate as long as the patient is not confused, disoriented, or unconscious; is not having angina; and is passing urine. However, a BP of 105/70 mm Hg may result in serious hypoperfusion in a patient who is normally hypertensive.

■ PHONE CALL

Questions

1. **What is the BP?**
2. **What is the heart rate (HR)?**
3. **What is the temperature?**
   "Fever + hypotension" suggests impending septic shock.
4. **Is the patient conscious?**
5. **Is the patient having chest pain?**
6. **Is there evidence of bleeding?**
7. **Has the patient been given intravenous (IV) contrast material or an antibiotic within the last 6 hours?**
   If you are called to see a hypotensive patient in the x-ray department or a patient who has recently returned to the room after undergoing an x-ray procedure involving the administration of IV contrast material, your primary thought should be that the patient may be having an anaphylactic reaction.
8. **What was the admitting diagnosis?**

Orders

1. If the information provided over the telephone supports the possibility of impending or established shock, order the following.
   a. Two large-bore (no. 16, if possible) IV lines immediately, if not already in place. IV access is a high priority in the hypotensive patient.
   b. Place the patient in reverse Trendelenburg position (i.e.,

head of the bed down and foot of the bed up). Although hypotension should be assessed immediately, if you are unable to get to the bedside for 10 to 15 minutes, also ask the nurse to give 500 ml normal saline (NS) IV as rapidly as possible.

   c. Have an arterial blood gas (ABG) tray at the bedside. Identification and correction of hypoxia and acidemia are essential in the management of shock.

   d. Administer oxygen at a rate of 4 to 10 L by face mask while awaiting the results of the ABG.

2. If there is a suspicion of *anaphylaxis*, ask the RN to have available a premixed syringe of IV epinephrine from the cardiac arrest cart.

3. If the admitting diagnosis is *gastrointestinal (GI) bleed* or if there is visible evidence of blood loss

   a. Ensure that there is blood on hold for the patient. If not, order a stat cross-match for 2, 4, or 6 units of packed red blood cells (RBCs), depending on your estimate of blood loss.

   b. Order a hemoglobin (Hb) stat. *Caution*: The Hb may be normal during an acute hemorrhage and drop only with correction of the intravascular volume by a shift of fluid from the interstitial and intracellular spaces, or by fluid therapy. (Refer to Chapter 13 for further investigation and management of GI bleeds.)

4. If an arrhythmia or ischemic myocardial event is suspected, order a stat electrocardiogram (ECG) and rhythm strip. These may help you identify a rapid heart rhythm or an acute myocardial infarction (MI), which may be responsible for hypotension.

Inform RN

"Will arrive at bedside in . . . minutes."
Hypotension requires you to see the patient immediately.

■ ELEVATOR THOUGHTS (What causes hypotension or shock?)

- Cardiogenic causes
- Hypovolemia
- Sepsis
- Anaphylaxis

Two formulas, as follow, are useful to remember when considering the causes of hypotension.

BP = cardiac output (CO) × total peripheral resistance (TPR)

$$CO = HR \times \text{stroke volume (SV)}$$

From these formulas, it can be seen that hypotension results from a fall in either CO or TPR. *Cardiogenic causes* result from a fall in CO due to either a fall in HR (e.g., heart block) or a fall in SV (e.g., acute MI, cardiac tamponade, massive pulmonary embolism, superior vena cava obstruction, or tension pneumothorax). *Hypovolemia* reduces stroke volume, and hence CO falls. *Sepsis* and *anaphylaxis* cause hypotension by lowering TPR.

■ MAJOR THREAT TO LIFE

- Shock

    Remember that hypotension does not become shock until there is evidence of inadequate tissue perfusion. As you will see, shock is a relatively easy diagnosis to make. Your goal is to identify and correct the cause of hypotension before it results in hypoperfusion of vital organs.

■ BEDSIDE

Quick Look Test

Does the patient look well (comfortable), sick (uncomfortable or distressed), or critical (about to die)?

A patient with hypotension but adequate tissue perfusion usually looks well. However, once perfusion of vital organs becomes compromised, the patient will look sick or critical.

Airway and Vital Signs

Is the airway clear?

If the patient is obtunded and cannot protect his or her airway, endotracheal intubation will be required. Ask the RN to notify the intensive care unit/cardiac care unit (ICU/CCU) immediately. Roll the patient onto the left side to avoid aspiration until intubation is achieved.

Is the patient breathing?

Assess respiration by checking the respiratory rate, the position of the trachea and chest expansion and performing auscultation. All patients in shock should receive high-flow oxygen. If acute respiratory distress and marked respiratory effort accompany shock, intubation and ventilation may be necessary.

Assess the circulation.

1. If hypotension is not severe, examine for postural changes.

A postural rise on standing in HR of > 15 beats/min, a fall in systolic BP of > 15 mm Hg, or any fall in diastolic BP indicates significant hypovolemia.

2. Measure the HR. Most causes of hypotension are accompanied by a compensatory reflex sinus tachycardia. If the patient is experiencing bradycardia or if you suspect a rhythm other than sinus tachycardia, refer to the discussion of bradycardia (below) for further evaluation and management.

3. Is the patient in *shock*? This should take < 20 seconds to determine.

Vitals	Repeat now
CVS	Pulse volume, JVP
	Skin temperature and color
	Capillary refill (normal < 2 seconds)
Neuro	Mental status

Shock is a clinical diagnosis: systolic BP < 90 mm Hg with evidence of inadequate tissue perfusion, such as inadequate perfusion of the skin (cold, clammy, and cyanotic) and of the central nervous system (CNS) (agitation, confusion, lethargy, and coma). In fact, the kidney is a sensitive indicator of shock (urine output < 20 ml/hr), but the immediate placement of a Foley catheter should not take priority over resuscitation measures.

What is the temperature?

An elevated temperature or hypothermia (< 36°C) suggests sepsis. However, remember that sepsis may appear in some patients, especially the elderly, with a normal temperature. Hence, the absence of fever does not rule out the possibility of septic shock.

Look at the ECG and take the pulse.

Bradycardia. If the resting HR is < 50 beats/min in the presence of hypotension, suspect one of three things, as follows.

1. *Vasovagal attack.* If this is the case, the patient is usually normotensive by the time you arrive. Look for retrospective evidence of straining, Valsalva's maneuver, pain, or some other stimulus to vagal outflow. If vasovagal attack is suspected and there is persistent bradycardia despite leg elevation, give *atropine* 0.5 mg IV. If not effective, the same dose may be repeated every 15 minutes up to a total dose of 2 mg IV.

2. *Autonomic dysfunction.* The patient may be on a beta blocker or calcium channel blocker and has been administered too much, resulting in hypotension, or the patient may be hypotensive for some other reason but is

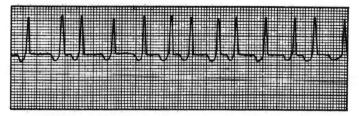

Figure 18–1 □ Atrial fibrillation with rapid ventricular response.

unable to generate a tachycardia because of beta blockade, calcium channel blockade, underlying sick sinus
syndrome, or autonomic neuropathy. If the systolic BP
is < 90 mm Hg, administer *atropine* 0.5 mg IV. If not
effective, the same dose may be repeated every 5 minutes up to a total dose of 2 mg IV.

3. *Heart block.* The patient may have a heart block (e.g.,
after acute MI). Obtain a stat ECG to document the
dysrhythmia. If systolic BP is < 90 mm Hg, administer
atropine 0.5 mg IV. If not effective, the same dose may
be repeated every 5 minutes up to a total dose of 2 mg
IV. Refer to Chapter 15 for further investigation and
management of heart block.

Tachycardia. A compensatory sinus tachycardia is an expected appropriate response in the hypotensive patient.
Ensure by looking at the ECG that the patient does not
have one of the following three rapid heart rhythms, which
may themselves cause hypotension due to inadequate diastolic filling with or without loss of the atrial kick.

1. Atrial fibrillation with rapid ventricular response (Fig.
18–1)
2. Supraventricular tachycardia (Fig. 18–2)
3. Ventricular tachycardia (Fig. 18–3)

If any one of these three rhythms is present in the hypoten-

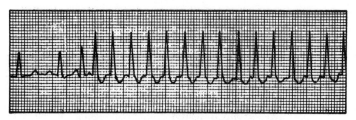

Figure 18–2 □ Supraventricular tachycardia.

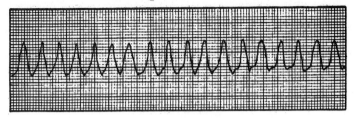

Figure 18–3 □ Ventricular tachycardia.

sive patient, emergency electrical cardioversion may be required.

- Ask the RN to notify your resident and an anesthetist immediately.
- Ask the RN to bring the cardiac arrest cart into the room.
- Attach the patient to the ECG monitor.
- Ask the RN to draw up *midazolam* (Versed) 5 mg IV in a syringe.
- Ensure that an IV line is in place. (Refer to Chapter 15, page 135, for further treatment of rapid heart rates associated with hypotension.)
- If the patient has a supraventricular tachycardia, also ask the RN to draw *adenosine* 6 mg IV into a syringe. IV adenosine may terminate some supraventricular tachycardias (SVTs) and save you from having to electrically cardiovert the hypotensive patient.

Selective Physical Examination

Determine the cause of hypotension or shock by *assessing the volume status.*

Only cardiogenic shock will result in a clinical picture of volume overload. Hypovolemic, septic, or anaphylactic shock will result in a clinical picture of volume depletion.

Vitals	Repeat now
HEENT	Elevated JVP (CHF), flat neck veins (volume depletion)
Resp	Stridor (anaphylaxis)
	Crackles, pleural effusions (CHF)
	Wheezes (anaphylaxis, CHF)
CVS	Cardiac apex displaced laterally, S_3 (CHF)
ABD	Hepatomegaly with positive HJR (CHF)
Ext	Presacral or ankle edema (CHF)
Skin	Urticaria (anaphylaxis)
Rectal	Melena or hematochezia (GI bleed)

Remember that *wheezing* may be seen in both CHF and anaphylaxis. The administration of epinephrine may save the life of someone with anaphylaxis but may kill someone with CHF. Anaphylactic shock comes on relatively suddenly, and nearly always an inciting factor (e.g., IV contrast material, penicillin) can be identified. Usually, other clues, such as angioedema or urticaria, are present.

Management

What immediate measures need to be taken to correct or prevent shock from occurring?

Normalize the intravascular volume. In the case of *cardiogenic shock* due to suspected MI, stop the IV NS bolus (ordered over the telephone) and replace with 5% dextrose in water (D5W) to keep the vein open (TKVO). Proper management also will require preload and afterload reduction and further investigation, as outlined in Chapter 24.

All other forms of shock will require volume expansion. This can be achieved quickly through elevation of the legs (i.e., reverse Trendelenburg) and the administration of repeated small volumes (200 to 300 ml over 15 to 30 minutes) of an IV fluid that will at least temporarily remain in the intravascular space, such as NS or Ringer's lactate. Reassess volume status after each bolus of IV fluid, aiming for a JVP of 2 to 3 cm H_2O above the sternal angle and concomitant normalization of HR, BP, and tissue perfusion.

If the patient is in *anaphylactic shock*, treat rapidly as follows.

1. IV NS wide open until normotensive
2. *Epinephrine* 0.3 mg (3 ml of 1:10,000 solution) IV immediately or 0.3 mg (0.3 ml of a 1:1000 solution) SC immediately, with repeat doses every 10 to 15 minutes if indicated; because the skin is usually hypoperfused during shock, it is better to administer epinephrine IV rather than SC
3. *Salbutamol* 2.5 mg/3 ml NS by nebulizer
4. *Diphenhydramine* 50 mg IV
5. *Hydrocortisone* 250 mg IV bolus, followed by 100 mg IV every 6 hours

Correct hypoxia and acidemia. If the patient is in shock, obtain ABGs and administer oxygen. If the arterial pH is < 7.2 in the absence of respiratory acidosis, order $NaHCO_3$ 0.5 to 1 amp (44.6 mmol) IV. Monitor the effects of your treatment by repeat ABGs every 30 minutes until the patient is stabilized.

While restoring the intravascular volume, determine the specific cause of hypotension or shock.

Cardiogenic shock. This is commonly a result of acute MI.

Order stat ECG, portable chest x-ray (CXR), and cardiac enzyme tests. However, any of the CHF etiologic factors listed on page 274 may be operative.

Be certain that the patient is in CHF! Patients with four other conditions can experience hypotension and elevated JVP, as follows.

1. *Cardiac tamponade* may cause elevated JVP, arterial hypotension, and soft heart sounds (Beck's triad). Suspect this as the diagnosis if there is a pulsus paradoxus of > 10 mm Hg during relaxed respirations (see page 269).

2. A massive *pulmonary embolus* can cause hypotension, elevated JVP, and cyanosis and may be accompanied by additional evidence of acute right ventricular overload (e.g., positive HJR, right ventricular [RV] heave, loud P_2, right-sided S_3, murmur of tricuspid insufficiency). If pulmonary embolism is suspected, call your resident immediately, and treat as outlined in Chapter 24, pages 277 to 279.

3. *Superior vena cava obstruction* may cause hypotension and elevated JVP that does not vary with respiration. Additional features may include headache, facial plethora, conjunctival injection, and dilatation of collateral veins on the upper thorax and neck.

4. *Tension pneumothorax* can also cause hypotension and elevated JVP due to positive intrathoracic pressure that decreases venous return to the heart. Look for severe dyspnea, unilateral hyperresonance, and decreased air entry, with tracheal shift *away* from the involved side. If a tension pneumothorax is suspected, do not wait for x-ray confirmation. Call for your resident and get a 14- to 16-gauge needle ready to aspirate the pleural space at the second intercostal space in the midclavicular line on the affected side. This is a medical emergency!

Hypovolemia. If there is suspicion that a *GI bleed* or another *acute blood loss* (e.g., ruptured abdominal aortic aneurysm) is responsible for hypotension, consult a surgeon immediately.

Excess fluid losses via sweating, vomiting, diarrhea, and polyuria and *third space losses* (e.g., pancreatitis, peritonitis) will respond to simple intravascular volume expansion with NS or Ringer's lactate and correction of the underlying problem.

Drugs are common causes of hypotension, resulting from relative hypovolemia with or without bradycardias due to their effects on the heart and peripheral circulation. Common offenders are morphine, meperidine, quinidine, nitroglycerin, beta blockers, calcium channel blockers, angiotensin-converting enzyme (ACE) inhibitors, and antihypertensive agents. In these instances, hypotension is seldom accompanied by evidence of inadequate tissue perfusion and usually can be avoided by reducing the dose or altering the schedule of administration of the drug.

Reverse Trendelenburg position or a small volume (300 to 500 ml) of NS or Ringer's lactate usually suffices to support the BP until the effect of most drugs wears off. The hypotension of narcotics (morphine, meperidine) can be reversed by *naloxone hydrochloride* 0.2 to 2.0 mg (maximum total dose, 10 mg) IV, SC, or IM every 5 minutes until the desired degree of reversal is seen.

Sepsis. Occasionally, intravascular volume repletion and appropriate antibiotics are sufficient to resolve hypotension associated with septic shock. Continuing hypotension despite intravascular volume repletion, however, requires ICU/CCU admission for vasopressor support.

Anaphylactic shock. This must be recognized and treated immediately to prevent fatal laryngeal edema. Treat as described on page 180.

■ REMEMBER

1. Consider *toxic shock syndrome* in any hypotensive premenopausal female. Ask about tampon use, or if the patient is obtunded, perform a pelvic examination and remove the tampon, if present.

2. The skin is not a vital organ but gives valuable evidence of tissue perfusion. Remember that during the early stage of septic shock, the skin may be warm and dry due to abnormal peripheral vasodilation.

3. Adequate BP is required to perfuse the three vital organs—*brain, heart,* and *kidney.* After you have successfully rescued your patient from an episode of hypotension, look out for hypotensive sequelae during the next few days. Not surprisingly, the common sequelae involve these three vital organs.

   a. *Brain* — thrombotic stroke in a patient with underlying cerebrovascular disease

   b. *Heart* — MI in a patient with preexisting atherosclerosis

   c. *Kidney* — acute tubular necrosis; monitor urine output and check urea and creatinine levels in a few days

4. Centrilobular hepatic necrosis (manifested by jaundice and elevated liver enzymes) and bowel ischemia or infarction also may be seen as sequelae of hypotension in the critically ill patient.

19

LEG PAIN

The easiest approach to leg pain at night is to identify which part of the leg hurts. Most leg pain originates from the muscle, joints, bone, or vascular supply to the legs; however, there also are several referred causes of leg pain.

■ PHONE CALL

Questions

1. **Which part of the leg hurts? Is the leg swollen or discolored?**
2. **What are the vital signs?**
3. **Was the pain sudden in onset, or is it chronic?**
4. **What was the reason for admission?**
5. **Has there been a recent leg injury or fracture? Does the patient have a leg cast on?**
   Leg pain after a leg injury, fracture, or casting raises the possibility of a compartment syndrome.

Orders

None.

Inform RN

"Will arrive at the bedside in . . . minutes."

An acute pulseless limb, fever, or severe leg pain of any etiology requires you to see the patient immediately. Increasing leg pain 24 to 48 hours after casting also requires you to see the patient immediately.

■ ELEVATOR THOUGHTS
(What causes leg pain?)

Bone and Joint Disease

1. Lumbar disc disease (sciatica)
2. Arthritis
   a. Septic (*Staphylococcus aureus, Neisseria gonorrhoeae, Streptococcus pneumoniae, Haemophilus influenzae,* and gram-negative bacilli)

    b. Inflammatory (gout, pseudogout, rheumatoid arthritis [RA], systemic lupus erythematosus [SLE])
    c. Degenerative (osteoarthritis)
  3. Osteomyelitis
  4. Ruptured Baker's cyst
  5. Skeletal tumors

Vascular Disease

  1. Arterial disease
    a. Acute arterial insufficiency (e.g., thromboembolism, cholesterol embolism)
    b. Arteriosclerosis obliterans (chronic arterial insufficiency)
    c. Thromboangiitis obliterans (Buerger's disease)
  2. Venous disease
    a. Deep venous thrombosis (DVT)
    b. Superficial thrombophlebitis

Muscle, Soft Tissue, or Nerve Pain

  1. Fasciitis, pyomyositis, myonecrosis
  2. Compartment syndrome
  3. Cellulitis
  4. Neuropathies (diabetes)
  5. Reflex sympathetic dystrophy syndrome
  6. Erythema nodosum
  7. Nodular liquefying panniculitis
  8. Benign nocturnal leg cramps

■ MAJOR THREAT TO LIFE

- Loss of limb from arterial insufficiency
- Pulmonary embolism from a DVT
- Septic arthritis
- Fasciitis, pyomyositis, myonecrosis
- Compartment syndrome

Acute arterial occlusion of the lower extremity, if left untreated, may result in gangrene in as little as 6 hours. A *DVT* may result in severe respiratory insufficiency or death if pulmonary embolism occurs. Although *septic arthritis* is not likely to result in loss of life overnight, its prompt recognition and management are essential to avoid permanent joint damage. Anaerobic infections resulting in *fasciitis, pyomyositis,* or *myonecrosis* may lead to septic shock. An unrecognized *compartment syndrome* can result in permanent ischemic muscle contractures within hours.

■ BEDSIDE

Although the list of possible diagnoses of leg pain is long, only the five major threats to life require emergency treatment at night. You should perform a systematic inspection, looking for evidence of each of these in the patient with leg pain.

Quick Look Test

Does the patient look well (comfortable), sick (uncomfortable or distressed), or critical (about to die)?
Most patients with significant leg pain lie still, appear apprehensive, and are reluctant to move the affected extremity.

Airway and Vital Signs

Leg pain should not compromise the vital signs; however, abnormalities in the vital signs may provide clues to the cause of leg pain.

What is the heart rate (HR)? Is it regular or irregular?
Pain from any cause may result in tachycardia. However, an irregularly irregular rhythm suggests atrial fibrillation, raising the possibility of an embolic event.

What is the blood pressure (BP)?
Pain or anxiety from any cause may raise the BP.

What is the temperature?
Fever suggests infection or inflammation, as may be seen with DVT, septic arthritis, fasciitis, pyomyositis, or myonecrosis.

ACUTE ARTERIAL INSUFFICIENCY

Selective History

Was the pain sudden in onset, suggesting an arterial embolism?

Is there a history of underlying cardiac disease (e.g., atrial fibrillation, mitral stenosis, ventricular aneurysm, prosthetic heart valve) that might predispose to arterial embolization?

Is there a history of intermittent claudication, which suggests long-standing chronic arterial insufficiency?

Is the patient receiving heparin?
Heparin-induced thrombocytopenia (platelet count ≤ 150,000/mm³) may result in acute intravascular thrombosis

due to platelet aggregation by heparin-dependent IgG antibodies. When present, this usually occurs after about 5 days of heparin therapy, but it may be seen earlier in patients with a prior history of receiving heparin.

Selective Physical Examination

Look for the four Ps.
1. Pain
2. Pallor
3. Pulselessness
4. Paresthesias

The following suggest a major arterial embolism.

Skin	Pallor
	Focal areas of gangrene
	Bilateral brawny discoloration (arteriosclerosis obliterans)
	Diminished temperature, especially if unilateral
CVS	Check the femoral, popliteal, and pedal pulses
	In an acute or a chronic arterial occlusion, pulses will be absent distal to the site of occlusion
Neuro	Paresthesias, diminished light touch in a stocking distribution

An *acute arterial embolism* tends to cause unilateral pain, pallor, paresthesias, and pulselessness (the four Ps), whereas *chronic arterial insufficiency* due to arteriosclerosis obliterans usually involves both lower limbs to a variable extent, with bilateral diminished pulses, trophic skin changes, loss of limb hair, and dependent rubor. Do not be fooled, however—although the presentation of arteriosclerosis obliterans is almost always chronic and progressive, fresh thrombosis on top of a fixed atherosclerotic plaque may completely obstruct arterial flow, resulting in an acute on chronic presentation.

Management

Acute arterial insufficiency is a surgical emergency. If you suspect that an arterial embolism has occluded a major artery
1. Immediately notify your resident and a vascular surgeon.
2. Draw a stat blood sample for a complete blood cell count (CBC) and activated partial thromboplastin time (aPTT).
3. If there are no contraindications, begin heparin 100 U/kg IV bolus, followed by a maintenance infusion of 1000 to 1600 U/hr, with the lower range selected for patients with a higher risk of bleeding. (See pages 278 to 279 for precautions in the use of heparin.)
4. If limb viability is threatened, the patient may require emergency thrombectomy or bypass. If limb viability is not a

concern, direct intra-arterial streptokinase may achieve lysis of a thrombus, but this should be initiated **only** under the guidance of a vascular surgeon.

Acute arterial insufficiency due to *heparin-induced thrombocytopenia* is a complex situation; notify your resident and a hematologist for help. Most cases require immediate discontinuation of heparin. If continued intravenous (IV) anticoagulation is necessary (i.e., for the original indication that heparin was prescribed), ancrod (Arvin) may be substituted for heparin. Ancrod is a thrombin-like enzyme obtained from the venom of the Malayan pit viper and achieves anticoagulation through defibrinogenation.

Chronic arterial insufficiency due to arteriosclerosis obliterans is not usually an emergency unless an acute thrombosis occurs on top of a long-standing fixed plaque. In this case, direct intra-arterial streptokinase or urokinase may result in clot lysis, but this should be administered only under the guidance of a vascular surgeon. The more common scenario is the complaint of rest pain in a patient with chronic intermittent claudication. If there is no immediate concern regarding limb viability, rest pain can be treated with nonnarcotic analgesics, such as *acetaminophen* 325 to 650 mg PO every 4 hours as needed, and placement of the affected extremity in the dependent position. More definitive therapy, including lumbar sympathectomy or direct arterial surgery, is seldom required on an emergency basis.

DEEP VENOUS THROMBOSIS

Selective History

Look for predisposing causes.
- Stasis
  - Prolonged bedrest
  - Immobilized limb
  - Congestive heart failure (CHF)
  - Pregnancy (particularly post partum)
- Vein injury
  - Trauma (especially hip fractures)
  - Surgery (especially abdominal, pelvic, and orthopedic procedures)
- Hypercoagulability
  - Malignancy
  - Inflammatory bowel disease
  - Nephrotic syndrome
  - Polycythemia vera
  - Antiphospholipid syndrome

- Deficiencies of antithrombin III, protein C or S
- Factor V Leiden mutation
- Older age (> 50 years)
- Recent abdominal, orthopedic, or neurologic surgery
- Recent general anesthesia

Selective Physical Examination

Look for the following signs involving the calf or thigh:
- Tenderness
- Erythema
- Edema: Subtle degrees of swelling may be appreciated by measuring and comparing the circumferences of both calves or thighs at several different levels.
- Warmth
- Distention of the overlying superficial veins
- *Homan's sign:* With the patient supine, flex the knee and then sharply dorsiflex the ankle. Pain in the calf during ankle dorsiflexion is supportive evidence of a calf DVT; its absence in no way excludes the diagnosis.

Management

A DVT should be recognized and treated immediately to prevent embolization and pulmonary infarction. If your suspicion of a DVT is high, you are obligated to begin anticoagulation without further confirmation of the diagnosis at this point. Heparin will inhibit further growth and promote resolution of the thrombus. However, before ordering heparin, ensure that the patient has no history of bleeding disorders, peptic ulcer, and intracranial disease, such as recent stroke, subarachnoid hemorrhage, tumor, and recent surgery. All are contraindications to anticoagulation. These patients will require confirmation of DVT by an imaging modality and, if DVT is documented, consultation for consideration of interruption of the inferior vena cava by the insertion of a transvenous caval device or, occasionally, inferior vena cava ligation.

Draw a blood sample for CBC, aPTT, PT, and platelet count immediately. If there are no contraindications, begin *heparin* 100 U/kg IV bolus (usual dose 5000 to 10,000 U IV) and follow with a maintenance infusion of 1000 to 1600 U/hr, with the lower range selected for patients with a higher risk of bleeding.

Heparin should be delivered by infusion pump, with maintenance dosing ordered as in the following example: heparin 25,000 U/500 ml 5% dextrose in water (D5W) to run at 20 ml/hr = 1000 U/hr. It is dangerous to put large doses of heparin in small-volume IV bags because runaway IV lines filled with heparin can result in serious overdose.

Heparin and warfarin are dangerous drugs because of their potential for causing bleeding disorders. Write and double check your heparin orders carefully. Also, measure platelet counts once or twice a week to detect reversible heparin-induced thrombocytopenia, which may occur at any time while a patient is on heparin.

Low-molecular-weight heparin (LMWH) is a safe and effective alternative to IV unfractionated heparin in the treatment of selected patients with DVTs.[1, 2] Several formulations of LMWH exist, with different distributions of molecular weight resulting in differences in their inhibitory activities against factor Xa and thrombin, the extent of plasma protein binding, and their plasma half-lives. You should familiarize yourself with the LMWH formulation used in your hospital. Also, be careful to note that the dose of LMWH used in the *treatment* of DVT is considerably higher than that used for *prophylaxis* of DVT. One formulation used for the *treatment* of DVT is *tinzaparin* 175 U/kg SC daily.

After starting heparin, the diagnosis should be confirmed in the morning by real-time B-mode or Duplex ultrasonography, which is the most sensitive noninvasive test to confirm a symptomatic DVT.[3] If this test is not available, impedance plethysmography, nuclear venography, and contrast venography are other options.

In patients receiving IV unfractionated heparin, monitor the aPTT every 4 to 6 hours and adjust the heparin maintenance dose until the aPTT is in the therapeutic range (1.5 to 2.5 × normal). After this, daily aPTT measurements are sufficient. Initial measurements of aPTT are made only to ensure adequate anticoagulation. Because of the more predictable anticoagulant response of LMWHs, patients receiving this medication do not require monitoring of the aPTT.

Continue heparin for approximately 5 days. Add *warfarin* (Coumadin) on the first day, beginning at 10 mg PO and titrating the dose to achieve a prothrombin time (PT) with an international normalized ratio (INR) of 2.0 to 3.0 (this corresponds to a PT of 1.3 to 1.5 × control, using rabbit brain thromboplastin; if you are unsure of the method used by your laboratory, call them and ask). Attainment of a therapeutic INR will usually take 5 days, at which time the heparin can be discontinued.

Numerous drugs interfere with warfarin metabolism to increase or decrease the PT. Before prescribing any drug to a patient on warfarin, look up its effect on warfarin metabolism and monitor PTs carefully if an interaction is anticipated.

Write an order that the patient should receive no aspirin-containing drugs, sulfinpyrazone, dipyridamole, or thrombolytic agents and no IM injections while on anticoagulation.

Ask your patient daily about signs of bleeding or bruising. Instruct your patient that prolonged pressure after venipuncture will be required to prevent local bruising while on anticoagulation.

SEPTIC ARTHRITIS

Selective History

In septic arthritis, the patient most often points to the painful joint involved. Your job is to determine whether the joint in question is infected. Two rules can be helpful. (1) If a single joint is swollen, red, and tender, it should be considered septic until proved otherwise. (2) In a patient with multiple joint involvement (as may be seen with RA or other inflammatory arthritides), if a single joint is inflamed out of proportion to the other joints involved, the joint in question should be considered possibly infected.

Look for predisposing factors:

Has there been a penetrating wound?

Has there been recent arthroscopy or intra-articular injection of steroids?

Does the patient have a joint prosthesis or other foreign body in the involved joint?

Has there been bacteremia (e.g., endocarditis)?

Selective Physical Examination

Fever may be present. The knee joint is most commonly affected. The joint is swollen, tender, restricted in range, and erythematous. These signs may be less marked, however, in the elderly patient or the patient on steroids.

Septic arthritis of the hip is often missed because of the deep location of the hip joint—swelling may not be detected easily. Conditions involving the hip joint are sometimes manifested only by referred pain to the groin, buttocks, lateral thigh, or anterior aspect of the knee. The affected extremity is usually held in adduction, flexion, and internal rotation.

Management

Septic arthritis is a medical emergency. Any suspected septic joint should be aspirated without delay. You will need your resident's help or the assistance of a rheumatologist to perform joint aspiration. The diagnosis of septic arthritis is made by demonstrating microorganisms on Gram's stain of synovial fluid. Prompt treatment with appropriate antibiotics is required, should not await confirmation by culture, and should be directed by the results of the Gram's stain. When microorganisms are not seen on the synovial fluid sample, empirical antibiotics should be administered. A good choice is a penicillinase-resistant penicillin and gentamicin until culture and sensitivity results are available.

Synovial fluid should be sent for
- White blood cell (WBC) count and differential
- Glucose determination
- Gram's stain
- Aerobic and anaerobic cultures
- Gonococcal culture
- Tuberculosis (TB) stain and culture

Blood samples should be sent for
- Simultaneous serum glucose determination
- Blood cultures for aerobes and anaerobes
- Gonococcal culture

In septic arthritis, the synovial fluid is usually cloudy or purulent, with WBC $\geq 10,000/mm^3$ with $\geq 90\%$ neutrophils. Synovial glucose is $\leq 50\%$ of a simultaneously drawn serum glucose.

FASCIITIS, PYOMYOSITIS, AND MYONECROSIS

This group of infections is usually caused by anaerobes, most often involving *Clostridium* sp.

Selective History

These infections usually result as a complication of **surgery** or **deep traumatic wounds**. The diagnosis may be more elusive in cases that arise spontaneously without a history of obvious injury. **Heroin addicts** are predisposed to a localized form of pyomyositis that may involve the thigh.

Selective Physical Examination

Look for
- Pus and/or gas formation in soft tissues
- Subcutaneous crepitance
- Local swelling and edema over a wound site, sometimes with a "frothy" wound exudate
- Dark patches of cutaneous gangrene are a late finding.
- Patients with clostridial myonecrosis may develop systemic toxemia with tachycardia, hypotension, renal failure, and feel-

ings of impending doom followed by toxic delirium and coma.

Management

These infections are surgical emergencies. If you think the patient has fasciitis, pyomyositis, or myonecrosis, consult a surgeon immediately. Systemic antibiotics (usually high-dose penicillin) are also indicated in the treatment of these clostridial infections.

COMPARTMENT SYNDROME

Some muscle groups in the leg are surrounded by well-fitted fascial sheaths, leaving no space for swelling should an injury occur. An increase in pressure within these sheaths may interfere with the circulation to the nerves and muscles within the compartment, resulting in a compartment syndrome.

Selective History

Look for predisposing causes.
- Recent fractures of the tibia and fibula
- Overly tight pressure bandages or casts
- Blunt leg trauma
- Prolonged, unaccustomed, vigorous exertion
- Anticoagulant medication
  Patients receiving heparin or warfarin are at risk for developing compartment syndrome due to bleeding within the enclosed fascial sheath, sometimes after relatively minor trauma.[4]

Selective Physical Examination

The anterior compartment of the leg is affected most commonly. It contains the anterior tibial muscle, the extensor hallucis longus, and the extensor digitorum longus muscles.
Look for
- Pain and tenderness over the involved compartment
- Overlying skin possibly erythematous, glossy, and edematous
- Sensory loss on the dorsum of the foot between the first and second toes
- Increasing pain on passive stretching of the involved muscle groups
- Weakness of dorsiflexion of the ankles and toes (footdrop)
Caution: Do not be fooled by the pulses! The pedal pulses are

rarely obliterated by the compartment swelling and may be easy to feel despite progressive muscle and nerve damage within the compartment.

If the patient has had a tibial fracture and has been casted, it may be difficult to properly examine the affected extremity. Any such patient who develops increasing pain 24 to 48 hours after casting should be suspected of having a compartment syndrome and should have the cast removed so the leg can be properly examined.

Management

Once the diagnosis of compartment syndrome is confirmed, a *decompressing fasciotomy* must be performed immediately by a surgeon. A delay of > 12 hours may lead to irreversible muscle necrosis and contracture formation. Conservative measures are only temporizing and may involve ice packs and elevation. Pressure dressings should be removed.

LESS URGENT CONDITIONS

If the five major threats to life have been excluded, a more leisurely approach to the diagnosis can be taken, looking for other, less urgent conditions.

Selective Physical Examination II

Skin	Localized skin and subcutaneous erythema, swelling, and warmth (cellulitis)
	Painful subcutaneous red nodules (erythema nodosum, nodular liquefying panniculitis)
	Tender superficial vein with surrounding erythema and edema (superficial thrombophlebitis)
	"Blue toe syndrome" or levido reticularis (cholesterol emboli)
	Focal areas of gangrene from cholesterol emboli (usually from the thoracic or abdominal aorta) may give one or more toes a bluish discoloration. Levido reticularis refers to cyanotic mottling of the skin in a fishnet-like pattern.
	Erythema, swelling, dysesthesias, increased hair growth of one foot (reflex sympathetic dystrophy syndrome)
MSS	Posterior knee joint swelling (Baker's cyst)
	Joint inflammation (RA, SLE, gout, pseudogout)
	Hip palpation and ROM (hip joint pathology may

cause leg pain with little or no evidence of inflammation)

Neuro   If no visible abnormality is found, a complete neurologic examination is required to look for lumbar disc disease (sciatica) or peripheral neuropathy (e.g., diabetes)

Benign nocturnal leg cramps often occur in the absence of physical findings.

Management of Selective Non–Life-Threatening Conditions

Acute Gout. Acute gout results from the sudden release of monosodium urate crystals from the cartilage and synovial membranes into the joint space. The diagnosis is made by synovial fluid aspiration and demonstration of negatively birefringent monosodium urate crystals with the use of polarizing microscopy.

At night, your main goal is to terminate the acute attack as quickly as possible. This can be done by administering *indomethacin* (Indocin) 100 mg PO, followed by 50 mg PO every 6 hours until pain relief occurs. *Colchicine* is a good alternative choice and may be administered as 1 mg PO initially, followed by 0.5 mg PO every 2 hours until either the pain improves, abdominal discomfort or diarrhea occurs, or a total of 8 mg is given. Intraarticular *triamcinolone hexacetonide* (15 to 30 mg) or *methylprednisolone acetate (Depo-Medrol)* (20 to 40 mg) is occasionally required.

Pseudogout. Pseudogout is a result of release of calcium pyrophosphate dihydrate crystals from the joint cartilage into the joint space. Diagnosis is made by joint aspiration and demonstration of weakly positive birefringent rods when viewed under polarized light. Acute inflammation usually responds to *indomethacin* (Indocin) 25 to 50 mg PO three times daily for 10 to 14 days, aspiration of fluid, and steroid injection.

Lumbar Disk Disease. Lumbar disk disease initially can be treated conservatively with bedrest, analgesics, and muscle relaxants.

Thromboangiitis Obliterans (Buerger's Disease). The only known effective treatment for this condition is complete abstinence from tobacco.

Erythema Nodosum. Erythema nodosum should be considered a symptom of some other underlying disorder, including drugs (oral contraceptives, penicillin, sulfonamides, bromides), inflammatory bowel disease, TB, fungal infections, and sarcoidosis. Treatment is that of the underlying condition.

Nodular Liquefying Panniculitis. The appearance of these nodules can be differentiated from erythema nodosum by their mobility with palpation. They are seen in association with acute pancreatitis or pancreatic neoplasms. Treatment is that of the underlying condition.

Reflex Sympathetic Dystrophy Syndrome. This disorder is often precipitated by a myocardial infarction (MI), stroke, or local trauma occurring weeks to months before characteristic redness, swelling (usually of the entire foot), and burning pain occur. Increased sweating and hair growth of the involved extremity also may occur. The condition may respond to analgesic agents and physical therapy. Occasionally, surgical sympathectomy or a short course of steroids is required.

Baker's Cyst. A Baker's cyst is caused by extension of inflamed synovial tissue into the popliteal space, resulting in pain and swelling behind the knee. A well-known complication is rupture of the synovial sac into the adjacent tissues. This may mimic a calf DVT with tenderness, swelling, and a positive Homan's sign. The diagnosis can be confirmed with a popliteal ultrasonogram or arthrogram. Treatment involves drainage of the cyst or intra-articular steroid injection. Occasionally, surgical synovectomy is required.

Superficial Thrombophlebitis. This condition presents with a tender lower extremity vein with surrounding edema and erythema. Often fever is present. Superficial venous thrombosis seldom propagates into the deep venous system, and anticoagulation therapy is not recommended. Treatment involves local measures, such as leg elevation, heat, and nonsteroidal anti-inflammatory drugs (NSAIDs), such as *indomethacin* (Indocin) 25 to 50 mg PO three times daily.

Cellulitis. Cellulitis is most often caused by *Staphylococcus* or *Streptococcus*. Because it can be difficult to determine which is responsible, treatment to cover both organisms is usual. Small, localized areas of cellulitis with intact skin may be treated with cloxacillin, cephalexin, or erythromycin, all at doses of 250 to 500 mg PO four times daily. If the patient is febrile, if the area of cellulitis is extensive, or if the patient is diabetic, IV antibiotics should be considered. A good choice is *cephalothin* 1 to 2 g IV every 6 hours.

Cellulitis associated with skin ulcers in the diabetic patient should be swabbed for Gram's stain, culture, and sensitivity. In the diabetic patient, such infections are commonly caused by multiple organisms and often respond to *cefoxitin* 1 to 2 g IV every 8 hours.

Benign Nocturnal Leg Cramps. The cause of this condition is unknown. They frequently respond to *quinine sulfate* 300 mg PO at bedtime PRN.

References

1. Hull RD, Raskob GE, Pinco GF, et al: Subcutaneous low-molecular-weight heparin compared with continuous intravenous heparin in the treatment of proximal-vein thrombosis. N Engl J Med 1992;326:975–982.
2. The Columbus Investigators: Low-molecular-weight heparin in the treatment of venous thromboembolism. N Engl J Med 1997;337:657–662.
3. Weinmann E, Salzman EW: Deep-vein thrombosis. N Engl J Med 1994;331:1630–1641.
4. Hay SM, Allen MJ, Barnes MR: Acute compartment syndromes resulting from anticoagulant treatment. BMJ 1992;305:1474–1475.

20

LINES, TUBES, AND DRAINS

Almost every patient admitted to the hospital will have some form of intravenous (IV) line, tube, or drain inserted during his or her stay. These devices are useful in the care of patients but on occasion clog, leak, or otherwise malfunction, requiring your expertise and common sense to remedy the problem.

Because the corrective measures that you may have to take when problems arise with lines, tubes, and drains carry the risk of contact with blood and body fluids, make sure you are familiar with and follow your institution's infection control guidelines.

This chapter describes some of the problems that can occur with commonly used lines, tubes, and drains.

Central Lines

Chest Tubes

Urethral Catheters

T-Tubes, J-Tubes, and Penrose Drains

Nasogastric and Enteral Feeding Tubes

CENTRAL LINES

Blocked Central Lines

■ PHONE CALL

Questions

1. How long has the line been blocked?
2. What are the vital signs?
3. What was the reason for admission?

Orders

Ask the RN for a dressing set, two pairs of sterile gloves in your size, chlorhexidine (Hibitane) skin disinfectant, a 5-ml syringe, and a size 20- or 21-gauge needle to be at the bedside. You will probably have to remove the dressing that is securing the central line, and you must keep the site sterile. A second pair of sterile gloves is useful. It is easy to contaminate your gloves when on call at night.

Inform RN

"Will arrive at the bedside in . . . minutes."

A blocked central line requires you to see the patient immediately.

■ ELEVATOR THOUGHTS (What causes a central line to block?) (Fig. 20–1)

1. Kinked tubing
2. Thrombus at the catheter tip

■ MAJOR THREAT TO LIFE

- Failure of delivery of medications
  Interruption of delivery of essential medications may temporarily deprive the patient of required treatment.

■ BEDSIDE

Quick Look Test

Does the patient look well (comfortable), sick (uncomfortable or distressed), or critical (about to die)?

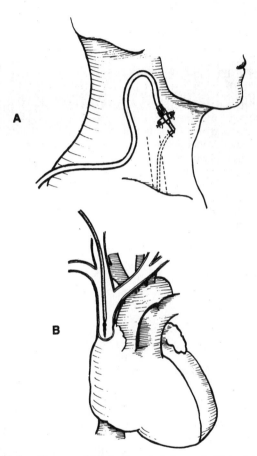

Figure 20–1 □ Causes of blocked central lines. *A,* Kinked tubing. *B,* Thrombosis at the catheter tip.

A blocked central line, by itself, should not cause the patient to look sick or critical. If the patient looks unwell, search for another cause.

Airway and Vital Signs

A blocked central line should not compromise the airway or other vital signs.

Selective Physical Examination and Management

Inspect the central line. **Is the line kinked?**

If so, remove the dressing securing the line, straighten the line, and see whether there now is flow of IV fluid. If the problem is a kinked line, clean the area using sterile technique and secure the line with a plastic occlusive dressing without rekinking it.

If there is no flow of IV fluid with the line wide open, proceed as follows.

1. Turn off the IV line.
2. Place the patient in the Trendelenburg position (head down). Take the 5-ml syringe and size 20- or 21-gauge capped needle and get ready to disconnect the central line from the IV tubing.
3. During the expiration phase of respiration, disconnect the central line from the IV tubing. Quickly attach the syringe to the central line and the capped needle to the IV tubing. The latter keeps the tubing sterile. The disconnection must be performed quickly to avoid an air embolus, which may result from air being sucked into the line due to negative intrathoracic pressure generated during inspiration. The risk of an air embolus is diminished by clamping the IV tubing, placing the patient in Trendelenburg position, and disconnecting the line only during expiration.
4. Draw back gently on the syringe because too much force will collapse the central line tubing. If the line is blocked with a small thrombus, this maneuver often is sufficient to dislodge the clot.
5. Draw back 3 ml of blood if possible. During the expiratory phase of respiration, remove the capped needle from the end of the IV tubing, remove the syringe from the central line, and reattach the IV tubing to the central line. Turn the IV on again. Blocked central lines should never be flushed. Flushing may dislodge a clot attached to the catheter tip, with subsequent pulmonary embolism.

If the previous maneuvers have been unsuccessful in unblocking the central line, determine whether the central line is still necessary. Is the patient receiving medications that can be delivered only via a central line (e.g., amphotericin, dopamine, total parenteral nutrition [TPN])? Was the central line started because of lack of peripheral vein access? If so, reexamine the patient to see whether there now are any peripheral veins suitable for IV access.

If central venous access is essential, the next step is to insert a new central line at a different site. A new central line should not be inserted over a guidewire placed through the blocked central line because the insertion of the guidewire may also dislodge a clot.

In situations where central venous access is essential and no alternative sites are available, streptokinase or urokinase has been used to dissolve the obstructing clot. Significant risks are involved with the use of these agents, and routine use is not recommended.

Bleeding at the Central Line Entry Site

■ PHONE CALL

Questions

1. **What are the vital signs?**
2. **What was the reason for admission?**

Orders

Ask for a dressing set, two pairs of sterile gloves in your size, and chlorhexidine (Hibitane) skin disinfectant to be at the bedside. You will probably have to remove the plastic occlusive dressing that is securing the central line, and you must keep the site sterile.

Inform RN

"Will arrive at the bedside in . . . minutes."

Bleeding at the central line site requires you to see the patient immediately.

■ ELEVATOR THOUGHTS (What causes bleeding at the line insertion site?)

1. Oozing of subcutaneous and cutaneous blood vessels (capillaries)
2. Coagulation disorders

a. Drugs (warfarin, heparin, aspirin, nonsteroidal anti-inflammatory drugs [NSAIDs], streptokinase, tissue plasminogen activator [tPA])
b. Thrombocytopenia, platelet dysfunction
c. Clotting factor deficiency

■ MAJOR THREAT TO LIFE

- Upper airway obstruction
  Bleeding into the soft tissues of the neck may cause tracheal compression, resulting in life-threatening upper airway obstruction. The patient may look sick or critical if excessive blood loss has occurred.

■ BEDSIDE

Quick Look Test

Does the patient look well (comfortable), sick (uncomfortable or distressed), or critical (about to die)?
   These patients look well unless there is an upper airway obstruction or excessive blood loss has occurred.

Airway and Vital Signs

Check the airway. **What is the respiratory rate (RR)?**
If there is any evidence of an upper airway obstruction (inspiratory stridor or significant soft tissue swelling of the neck), call your resident for help immediately.

Selective Physical Examination and Management

1. Remove the dressing and try to identify a specific area of bleeding.
2. If you are unable to identify a specific site of bleeding, clean the site using sterile technique and reinspect the area. Usually, generalized oozing of blood is seen at the entry site, with no one specific skin vessel identified as the culprit.
3. Apply continuous pressure to the entry site for the next 20 minutes. This is performed by applying, with a gloved hand, a folded, sterile 2 cm × 2 cm gauze dressing to the site with firm, continuous pressure. Do not release this pressure during the 20 minutes because the platelet plug you are allowing to form may be broken (Fig. 20–2).

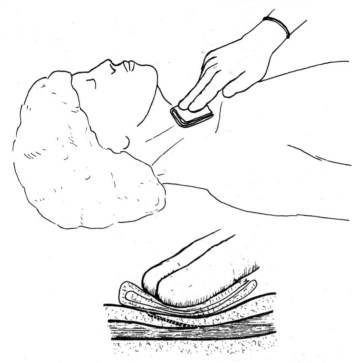

Figure 20–2 □ Continuous firm local pressure is required for 20 minutes to stop the oozing of blood from the central line entry site. Make sure the pressure is applied over the puncture site in the vein and not at the skin entry site.

4. Reinspect the entry site. If the bleeding has stopped, clean the area using sterile technique and secure the line with plastic occlusive dressing. If there is still bleeding at the site, repeat the previous maneuver for an additional 20 minutes. Provided that continuous pressure has been applied, any bleeding should have stopped. In the unusual circumstance where bleeding has not stopped, a coagulation disorder should be suspected. (Refer to Chapter 31 for management of coagulation problems.) Alternatively, a single suture may be placed at the site of bleeding in an attempt to provide hemostasis.
5. Removal of the central line should be considered if bleeding at the insertion site is excessive and resistant to the previous measures.

Shortness of Breath After Central Line Insertion

■ PHONE CALL

Questions

1. How long has the patient had SOB?
2. What are the vital signs?
3. What was the reason for admission?

Orders

1. Ask the RN for a dressing set, two pairs of sterile gloves in your size, chlorhexidine (Hibitane) skin disinfectant, and a size 16 IV catheter to be at the bedside. If the patient has a tension pneumothorax, you will need to insert a size 16 IV catheter into the second intercostal space on the hyperresonant side, with your resident's guidance.
2. If you suspect a pneumothorax, order a stat portable chest x-ray (CXR) in the upright position in expiration. Hypotension, tachypnea, and pleuritic chest pain after central line insertion are suggestive of a pneumothorax.
3. Order an O_2 mask at 10 L/min.

Inform RN

"Will arrive at bedside in . . . minutes."

SOB after central line insertion requires you to see the patient immediately.

■ ELEVATOR THOUGHTS (What causes shortness of breath after central line insertion?) (Fig. 20–3)

1. Pneumothorax or tension pneumothorax
2. Massive soft tissue hematoma from inadvertent carotid artery puncture, resulting in upper airway obstruction
3. Cardiac tamponade
4. Air embolus
5. Pleural effusion

■ MAJOR THREAT TO LIFE

- Upper airway obstruction
- Tension pneumothorax
- Cardiac tamponade

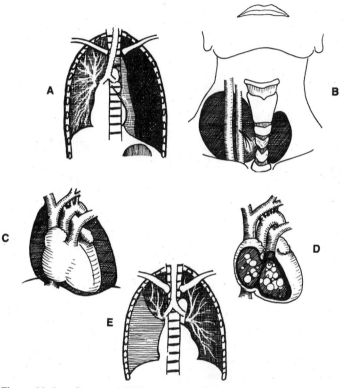

Figure 20–3 □ Causes of SOB after central line insertion. *A,* Pneumothorax. *B,* Massive soft tissue hematoma from inadvertent carotid artery puncture, resulting in upper airway obstruction. *C,* Cardiac tamponade. *D,* Air embolus. *E,* Pleural effusion.

- Air embolus

Upper airway obstruction may result from a massive soft tissue hematoma (e.g., from inadvertent carotid artery puncture). A *tension pneumothorax* may develop minutes to days after the insertion of a central line if pleural perforation occurred during insertion. Rarely, *cardiac tamponade* results from perforation by the catheter of the right atrium or right ventricle. Air may be inadvertently introduced if the line is disconnected incorrectly, resulting in an *air embolus*.

■ BEDSIDE

Quick Look Test

Does the patient look well (comfortable), sick (uncomfortable or distressed), or critical (about to die)?

A patient with a tension pneumothorax, upper airway obstruction, cardiac tamponade, or air embolus looks sick or critical.

Airway and Vital Signs

Check the airway. If there is any evidence of an upper airway obstruction (i.e., inspiratory stridor or significant soft tissue swelling of the neck), call the intensive care unit/cardiac care unit (ICU/CCU) team immediately for possible intubation.

What are the blood pressure (BP) and RR?

Hypotension and tachypnea in a patient with a recently inserted central line may indicate a tension pneumothorax or cardiac tamponade, inadvertently caused at the time of line insertion. See page 181 for the assessment and page 207 for the management of tension pneumothorax and cardiac tamponade.

Selective Physical Examination

Resp	Tracheal deviation (tension pneumothorax or massive pleural effusion)
	Unilateral hyperresonance to percussion with decreased breath sounds (pneumothorax)
	Stony dullness to percussion, decreased breath sounds, decreased tactile fremitus (pleural effusion)
CVS	Pulsus paradoxus (cardiac tamponade or tension pneumothorax)
	Pulsus paradoxus is present when the decrease

in systolic BP with inspiration is > 10 mm Hg (the normal variation in systolic BP with quiet respiration is 0 to 10 mm Hg). A pulsus paradoxus is definitely present if the radial pulse disappears during inspiration is.

Elevated JVP (cardiac tamponade or tension pneumothorax)

Distant heart sounds (pericardial effusion or cardiac tamponade)

Mill wheel murmur, hypotension, elevated JVP (major air embolism)

Central line — Check all IV connections to ensure that they are not loose (air embolus).

Management

Tension pneumothorax is a medical emergency requiring urgent treatment. You will need supervision by your resident or attending physician.

1. Identify the second intercostal space in the midclavicular line on the affected (hyperresonant) side.
2. Mark this point with the pressure from a capped needle or ballpoint pen.
3. Open the dressing set and pour the chlorhexidine (Hibitane) into the appropriate space.
4. Put on the sterile gloves and clean the identified area.
5. Insert the size 16 IV catheter into the designated site. Remove the inner needle, leaving the plastic cannula in the chest. If a tension pneumothorax is present, there will be a loud sound of air rushing out through the catheter. You will not need to connect the catheter to suction because the lung will decompress itself.
6. Order a chest tube sent to the room immediately. The definitive treatment is the insertion of a chest tube.

Small pneumothoraces usually undergo spontaneous reabsorption over a few days.

Large or symptomatic pneumothoraces require chest tube drainage.

Cardiac tamponade is a medical emergency.

1. Clamp the IV tubing and turn off the IV line.
2. Call the ICU/CCU team immediately for possible urgent pericardiocentesis. An emergency echocardiogram, if available, will confirm the diagnosis before pericardiocentesis.
3. Volume expansion with normal saline (NS) through a large-bore IV may be a useful temporizing measure to help maintain adequate CO.

Air embolism may be helped by placing the patient on the right side in Trendelenburg position (head down) to trap the air bubbles in the right ventricle and prevent them from entering the pulmonary artery. The patient should be kept in this position until the air bubbles have been reabsorbed. (Aspiration of air bubbles from the right ventricle is advocated by some experts.) Reinspect all the IV connections and make certain they are secure. If necessary, a new central line may have to be inserted.

Massive unilateral pleural effusion should be managed as follows.
1. Clamp the IV tubing and stop the IV fluid.
2. Thoracentesis will be required if the patient has marked SOB.

CHEST TUBES

Chest tubes are inserted to drain air (pneumothoraces), blood (hemothoraces), fluid (pleural effusions), or pus (empyemas) (Fig. 20–4). They should always be connected to an underwater seal. They may be left to straight drainage (no suction) or, more commonly, to suction. Figure 20–5 illustrates the various chest tube

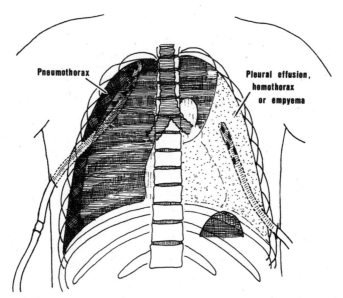

Figure 20–4 □ Chest tubes are inserted to drain air (pneumothoraces), blood (hemothoraces), fluid (pleural effusions), and pus (empyemas).

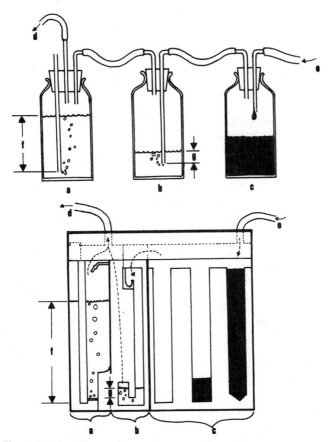

Figure 20–5 □ Chest tube apparatus. a, Suction control chamber. b, Underwater seal. c, Collection chamber. d, To suction. e, From patient. f, Height equals amount of suction in cm H_2O. g, Height equals underwater seal in cm H_2O.

drainage apparatuses. Common chest tube problems are illustrated in Figure 20–6.

Persistent Bubbling in the Drainage Container (Air Leak)

■ PHONE CALL

Questions

1. Why was the chest tube inserted?
2. What are the vital signs?
3. Does the patient have SOB?
4. What was the reason for admission?

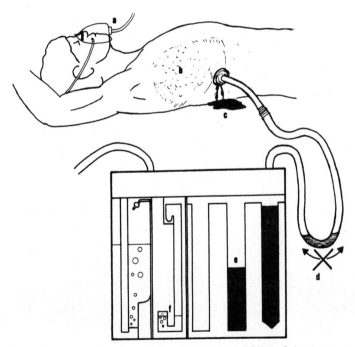

Figure 20–6 □ Common chest tube problems. a, SOB. b, Subcutaneous emphysema. c, Bleeding at the entry site. d, Loss of fluctuation. e, Excessive drainage. f, Persistent bubbling.

Orders

None.

Inform RN

"Will arrive at the bedside in . . . minutes."
Persistent bubbling in the drainage container is a potential emergency, requiring you to see the patient as soon as possible. Any malfunctioning of the chest tube, if associated with SOB, requires you to see the patient immediately.

■ ELEVATOR THOUGHTS (What causes persistent bubbling in the drainage compartment?)

1. Loose tubing connection
2. Air leaking into the chest around the chest tube at the insertion site
3. Traumatic tracheobronchial injury. A large, persistent air leak in traumatic pneumothorax suggests a concomitant tracheobronchial injury.
4. Persistent bronchopleural air leak
   a. Postlobectomy
   b. Ruptured bleb or bulla (e.g., asthma, emphysema)
   c. After intrathoracic procedures (e.g., needle biopsy, thoracentesis)

■ MAJOR THREAT TO LIFE

A persistent air leak suggests either a pneumothorax from intrathoracic injury or a loose connection of the drainage apparatus. Hence, the major threat to life is the underlying intrathoracic disease process responsible for the persistent air leak. As long as air continues to bubble through the collection chamber, one can be reasonably certain that excessive intrapleural air will not accumulate.

■ BEDSIDE

Quick Look Test

Does the patient look well (comfortable), sick (uncomfortable or distressed), or critical (about to die)?
If a small air leak is the problem, the patient may look well.

A patient who looks sick may be developing a larger pneumothorax or may look sick for unrelated reasons.

Airway and Vital Signs

Provided that all tubing connections are snug and the chest tube dressing is airtight, a persistent air leak means that the patient has a pneumothorax. As long as air continues to bubble through the collection chamber, the pneumothorax should drain and thus not result in alteration of vital signs.

Selective History and Chart Review

Why was the chest tube inserted?
   If the chest tube was inserted to drain a pneumothorax, the tube should be bubbling unless the lung is fully expanded and the leak has sealed.
   If the chest tube was inserted to drain a hemothorax, a pleural effusion, or an empyema with straight drainage (no suction), new onset of bubbling in the collection chamber represents either loose tubing connections, air leaking into the chest from around the chest tube insertion site, or the development of a pneumothorax.

Selective Physical Examination and Management

Provided that a pneumothorax is not present, a persistent air leak is indicated by air bubbles in the underwater seal section of the Pleur-Evac while the suction is turned off. If the air leak is small, it may be seen only with measures that increase intrapleural pressure (e.g., coughing) (Fig. 20–7).

Clamping of chest tubes before obtaining an x-ray may be dangerous, especially if there is a persistent pneumothorax. *Never leave a patient with a clamped chest tube unattended.* A tension pneumothorax may develop rapidly if a ball-valve mechanism is present.

The following procedure is recommended when there is persistent bubbling in the drainage compartment.

1. Inspect the tubing connections to ensure that all seals are airtight.
2. Remove the dressing at the entry site of the chest tube, listen for sucking sounds, and observe the incision area. If the incision is too large and inadequately closed, insert one or two sterile 2-0 sutures to seal the opening. If the incision is adequately closed with sutures, reapply a pressure dressing,

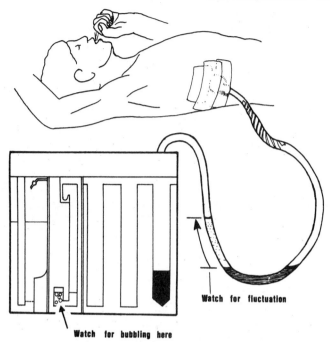

Watch for fluctuation

Watch for bubbling here

Figure 20–7 □ Loss of fluctuation of the underwater seal. Ask the patient to cough, and observe for any fluctuation or bubbling.

ensuring that the petrolatum (Vaseline) gauze occlusive dressing seals the incision.

3. Disconnect the suction from the Pleur-Evac. Persistent air leak (spontaneous or with coughing) usually means an air leak from the lung (persistent pneumothorax).

4. Obtain a CXR to ensure correct tube placement. The chest tube holes should be inside the thorax, and the tip of the tube should be away from mediastinal and subclavicular structures.

5. If on CXR the lung is not reexpanded, call surgery for consideration of placing a second chest tube and for management of the persistent air leak from the lung.

Bleeding Around the Chest Tube Entry Site

■ PHONE CALL

Questions

1. **Why was the chest tube inserted?**
2. **What are the vital signs?**

3. Does the patient have SOB?
4. What was the reason for admission?

Orders

Ask the RN for a dressing set, two pairs of sterile gloves in your size, and chlorhexidine (Hibitane) skin cleanser to be at the bedside. You will have to remove the dressing around the chest tube, and you must keep the site sterile.

Inform RN

"Will arrive at the bedside in . . . minutes."

Bleeding around the chest tube entry site is a potential emergency, requiring you to see the patient as soon as possible. Any malfunctioning chest tube in association with SOB requires you to see the patient immediately.

■ ELEVATOR THOUGHTS (What causes bleeding around the chest tube entry site?)

1. Inadequate pressure bandage
2. Inadequate closure of the incision with suture
3. Coagulation disorders
4. Trauma to intercostal vessels or lung during insertion of the chest tube
5. Blockage of chest tube or inadequately sized chest tube with drainage of the hemothorax around the entry site

■ MAJOR THREAT TO LIFE

- Hemorrhagic shock

  Continuous oozing, if allowed to progress, may eventually lead to intravascular volume depletion and, in the extreme case, hemorrhagic shock.

■ BEDSIDE

Quick Look Test

Does the patient look well (comfortable), sick (uncomfortable or distressed), or critical (about to die)?

If there is only a small amount of bleeding from the chest tube entry site, the patient will probably look well. A patient who has lost more blood may look sick or critical.

Airway and Vital Signs

What are the BP and RR?

Hypotension and tachycardia may indicate major loss of blood. Tachypnea may indicate a large hemothorax.

Selective History and Chart Review

1. Why was the chest tube inserted?
2. Check the following recent laboratory results: hemoglobin (Hb), prothrombin time (PT), activated partial thromboplastin time (aPTT), and platelet count.

Selective Physical Examination and Management

Remove the dressing at the chest tube entry site and inspect the incision. If the incision is too large and inadequately closed, insert one or two sutures to seal the opening. If the incision is adequately closed with sutures, reapply a pressure dressing over the site, taking care to ensure that the pressure is maintained. Such maneuvers, when performed adequately, will stop the bleeding in the majority of situations.

Is the chest tube obstructed, resulting in blood draining around the entry site? Try milking the chest tube. Reinspect to see if this maneuver reestablished fluctuation in the underwater seal. The connecting tube is made of rubber and may be carefully stripped using the chest tube strippers. These two maneuvers help dislodge blood clots and debris that may be blocking the tube.

Is the chest tube too small, thus unable to drain a large hemothorax adequately? A larger size chest tube may be required.

Drainage of an Excessive Volume of Blood

■ PHONE CALL

Questions

1. Why was the chest tube inserted?
2. What are the vital signs?
3. Does the patient have SOB?
4. What was the reason for admission?

Orders

None.

Inform RN

"Will arrive at the bedside in . . . minutes."

Drainage of an excessive volume of blood via the chest tube

is a potential emergency and requires you to see the patient immediately. Any malfunctioning chest tube, if associated with SOB, requires you to see the patient immediately.

■ ELEVATOR THOUGHTS (What causes excessive blood to drain via the chest tube?)

- Intrathoracic bleeding

■ MAJOR THREAT TO LIFE

- Hemorrhagic shock
  Hemorrhagic shock may result from excessive intrathoracic blood loss.

■ BEDSIDE

Quick Look Test

Does the patient look well (comfortable), sick (uncomfortable or distressed), or critical (about to die)?
  A patient with hemorrhagic shock will look pale, sweaty, and restless.

Airway and Vital Signs

What are the BP and HR?
  Hypotension and tachycardia may indicate hemorrhagic shock.

What is the RR?
  Tachypnea and hypotension may indicate a tension pneumothorax.

Management I

1. Give supplemental oxygen, e.g., 4 L/min by nasal prongs.
2. If the patient is hypotensive, draw 20 ml of blood and start a large-bore IV (size 16 if possible). Give 500 ml of NS or Ringer's lactate IV as fast as possible.
3. Send blood for an immediate crossmatch for 4 to 6 units of packed red blood cells (RBCs) on hold, Hb, PT, aPTT, and platelet count.
4. Order a stat CXR.

Selective Chart Review and Management II

Is the patient receiving anticoagulant medication (heparin, warfarin)?

If so, review the initial indication for anticoagulation. Can the anticoagulant be safely discontinued or reversed? Consult the hematology department for assistance in the management of this difficult and potentially life-threatening situation.

Estimate how much blood the patient has lost over the past 48 hours by reviewing the intake/output chart.

If the patient has lost > 500 ml over 8 hours, consultation with a thoracic surgeon is recommended. The patient may need immediate transfer to the operating room for an emergency thoracotomy to localize the site of hemorrhage and achieve hemostasis.

If the patient has lost < 500 ml over 8 hours, order hourly monitoring of the blood lost via the chest tube, noting that a physician needs to be informed if the blood loss is > 50 ml/hr.

Loss of Fluctuation of the Underwater Seal

■ PHONE CALL

Questions

1. Why was the chest tube inserted?
2. What are the vital signs?
3. Does the patient have SOB?
4. What was the reason for admission?

Orders

None.

Inform RN

"Will arrive at the bedside in . . . minutes."

Loss of fluctuation of the underwater seal is a potential emergency and requires you to see the patient as soon as possible. Any malfunctioning chest tube, if associated with SOB, requires you to see the patient immediately.

■ ELEVATOR THOUGHTS (What causes loss of fluctuation of the underwater seal?)

1. Kinked chest tube
2. Plugged chest tube
3. Improper chest tube positioning

The underwater seal is essentially a one-way, low-resistance valve. During expiration, the intrapleural pressure increases, becoming higher than atmospheric pressure, forcing air or fluid that is in the pleural space through the chest tube and underwater seal (see Fig. 20–7).

■ MAJOR THREAT TO LIFE

- Tension pneumothorax
  Inadequate drainage of a pneumothorax because of a blocked chest tube may lead to a tension pneumothorax (Figs. 20–8 and 20–9).

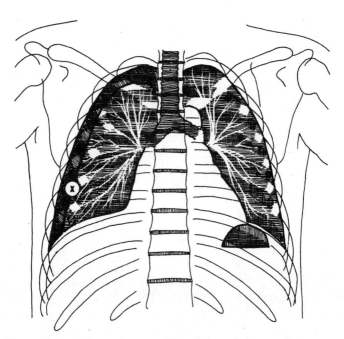

Figure 20–8 □ Pneumothorax. *x*, Edge of visceral pleura or lung.

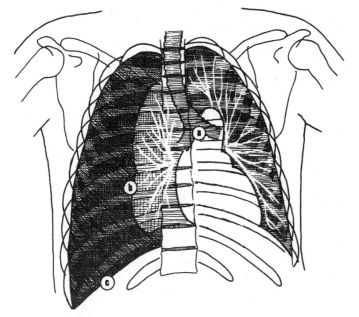

Figure 20–9 □ Tension pneumothorax. a, Shifted mediastinum. b, Edge of collapsed lung. c, Low flattened diaphragm.

■ BEDSIDE

Quick Look Test

Does the patient look well (comfortable), sick (uncomfortable or distressed), or critical (about to die)?
   A patient who looks sick may be developing a tension pneumothorax or may look sick for unrelated reasons.

Airway and Vital Signs

What are the BP and RR?
   Hypotension and tachypnea may indicate a tension pneumothorax.

Selective History and Chart Review

1. Why was the chest tube inserted?
2. How long ago did the chest tube stop fluctuating?
3. What has been draining from the chest tube? What volume has drained over the past 24 hours?

Selective Physicial Examination and Management

1. Inspect the underwater seal. Is there any fluctuation? Ask the patient to cough, and observe the tube for any fluctuation. A chest tube with its distal aperture located within the pleural space fluctuates with respiration.
2. Inspect the chest tube for kinking. You may need to remove the dressing at the chest tube site. If the chest tube is kinked, reposition and reinspect it for fluctuation of the underwater seal.
3. Try milking the chest tube. Reinspect to see if this maneuver reestablishes fluctuation in the underwater seal. The connecting tubing is rubber and may be carefully stripped using chest tube strippers. These two maneuvers help dislodge blood clots and debris that may be blocking the tube.
4. Order a portable CXR. Improper positioning of the chest tube may result in loss of fluctuation of the underwater seal.
5. If the tube is not fluctuating after all the aforementioned maneuvers are attempted, a new chest tube may have to be inserted.

Subcutaneous Emphysema

■ PHONE CALL

Questions

1. **Why was the chest tube inserted?**
2. **What are the vital signs?**
3. **Does the patient have SOB?**
4. **What was the reason for admission?**

Orders

Ask the RN for a dressing set, two pairs of sterile gloves in your size, and chlorhexidine (Hibitane) skin cleanser to be at the bedside. You will have to remove the dressing around the chest tube, and you must keep the site sterile.

Inform RN

"Will arrive at the bedside in . . . minutes."

Subcutaneous emphysema is a potential emergency requiring you to see the patient immediately. Any malfunctioning chest tube, if associated with SOB, requires you to see the patient immediately.

■ ELEVATOR THOUGHTS (What causes subcutaneous emphysema?)

1. Chest tube may be too small for the size of the leak
2. Inadequate suction
3. One of the chest tube apertures may be in the chest wall
4. Chest tube may be in the chest wall or abdominal cavity
5. Insignificant localized subcutaneous emphysema around the entry site is not uncommon after chest tube insertion

■ MAJOR THREAT TO LIFE

- Upper airway obstruction
  Subcutaneous emphysema extending up into the neck rarely results in tracheal compression.

■ BEDSIDE

Quick Look Test

Does the patient look well (comfortable), sick (uncomfortable or distressed), or critical (about to die)?
  The patient with upper airway obstruction will look sick or critical, and there may be audible inspiratory stridor.

Airway and Vital Signs

1. Inspect and palpate the neck for subcutaneous emphysema.
2. What is the RR? The patient with upper airway obstruction will be tachypneic.
3. What are the BP and HR? Subcutaneous emphysema may be accompanied by a tension pneumothorax. If so, the patient will be tachycardic.

Selective History and Chart Review

Why was the chest tube inserted?

Selective Physical Examination and Management

1. If there is significant upper airway obstruction (palpable subcutaneous emphysema over the trachea, inspiratory stridor, tachypnea), call the ICU/CCU team immediately for probable intubation and transfer to the ICU/CCU. Cardio-

thoracic surgery may be required if mediastinal decompression is indicated.

2. **What size chest tube has been inserted? Is the chest tube too small in diameter?** Multifenestrated vinyl chest tubes are available in two sizes: 20F and 36F. The 20F may not be large enough, and air may escape from the pleural cavity into the chest wall, resulting in subcutaneous emphysema. If the chest tube is too small, a larger one will need to be inserted. Sometimes, two large chest tubes may be required for adequate drainage.

3. **Is the chest tube connected to suction?** A large pneumothorax may not be drained adequately if it is connected only to an underwater seal, as opposed to suction.

4. Remove the dressing at the chest tube site and inspect the chest tube. **Are any of the drainage holes in the distal end of the chest tube visible?** None of the drainage lines should be visible. They should all be inside the pleural cavity. Subcutaneous emphysema may be caused by misplacement of the chest tube, with one of the drainage holes inadvertently in the soft tissues of the chest wall. A new chest tube should be inserted. Do not reintroduce the partially extruded chest tube, since you may introduce infection into the pleural space.

Shortness of Breath

■ PHONE CALL

Questions

1. Why was the chest tube inserted?
2. What are the vital signs?
3. What was the reason for admission?

Orders

Ask the RN for a dressing set, two pairs of sterile gloves in your size, chlorhexidine (Hibitane) skin cleanser, and a size 16 IV catheter. A tension pneumothorax, if present, is most effectively treated with insertion of a size 16 IV catheter into the pleural space on the affected side.

Inform RN

"Will arrive at the bedside in . . . minutes."

SOB in a patient with a chest tube in place is a potential emergency and requires you to see the patient immediately.

■ ELEVATOR THOUGHTS (What causes shortness of breath in a patient with a chest tube?)

Causes Related to the Chest Tube

1. Tension pneumothorax; this may occur because of
   a. Inadequate suction
   b. Misplaced tube (i.e., chest tube not in the pleural cavity)
   c. Blocked or kinked tube
   d. Bronchopulmonary fistula
2. Increasing pneumothorax; this may result from the same causes as tension pneumothorax
3. Subcutaneous emphysema
4. Increasing pleural effusion or hemothorax
5. Reexpansion pulmonary edema (sometimes this occurs after rapid expansion of a pneumothorax, drainage of pleural fluid, or both)

Causes Unrelated to the Chest Tube

See Chapter 24, page 266.

■ MAJOR THREAT TO LIFE

- Tension pneumothorax
- Upper airway obstruction

Inadequate drainage of a pneumothorax produced through a ball-valve mechanism may result in a life-threatening *tension pneumothorax*. Tracheal compression from interstitial emphysema rarely causes *upper airway obstruction*.

■ BEDSIDE

Quick Look Test

Does the patient look well (comfortable), sick (uncomfortable or distressed), or critical (about to die)?
  A sick or critical looking patient may have a tension pneumothorax or may have an unrelated reason for SOB (Chapter 24).

Airway and Vital Signs

1. Inspect and palpate the neck for subcutaneous emphysema.
2. What is the RR? Rates > 20/min suggest hypoxia, pain, or

anxiety. Look for thoracoabdominal dissociation, which may indicate impending respiratory failure. Remember that the rib cage and abdominal wall normally move in the same direction during inspiration and expiration.

3. What are the BP and HR? Hypotension and tachycardia may indicate a tension pneumothorax or another unrelated cause of SOB (Chapter 24).

Selective Physical Examination

Does the patient have a tension pneumothorax?

Vitals	Tachypnea
	Hypotension
HEENT	Tracheal deviation away from the hyperresonant side
Resp	Unilateral hyperresonance
	Decreased air entry on hyperresonant side
CVS	Elevated JVP
Chest tube	Is there bubbling in the collection chamber? Absence of bubbling suggests malposition or malfunction of the chest tube.

Selective Chart Review

Why was the chest tube inserted?

Management

1. If there is *significant upper airway obstruction* (palpable subcutaneous emphysema over the trachea, inspiratory stridor, tachypnea), call the ICU/CCU team immediately for probable intubation and transfer to the ICU/CCU.
2. *Tension pneumothorax* is a medical emergency requiring urgent treatment. You will need supervision by your resident or attending physician.
   a. Identify the second intercostal space in the midclavicular line on the affected (hyperresonant) side.
   b. Mark this point using pressure from the cap of a needle or ballpoint pen.
   c. Open the dressing set and pour the chlorhexidine (Hibitane) into the appropriate container.
   d. Put on sterile gloves.
   e. Clean the area previously identified.
   f. Insert the size 16 IV catheter into the designated area. If a tension pneumothorax is present, there will be a loud sound of air rushing out through the catheter. You will

not need to connect the catheter to suction, since the pleural space will decompress itself.

g. Order a chest tube sent to the room immediately. The definitive treatment is insertion of a chest tube.

3. If there is an increasing pneumothorax but no evidence of a tension pneumothorax, order a stat upright CXR in expiration. Meanwhile, look for any correctable causes, e.g., kinked or blocked tubing, inadequate suction, and dislodged chest tube.

4. For the management of other causes of SOB (i.e., causes unrelated to chest tubes), see Chapter 24.

URETHRAL CATHETERS

There are five types of urethral catheters (Fig. 20–10). The *Foley* (balloon retention) *catheter* is the most commonly used of these. It consists of a double-lumen tube. The larger lumen drains urine, and the smaller lumen admits 5 to 30 ml of water to inflate the balloon tip. *Straight (Robinson) catheters* are used to obtain in-and-out collections of urine, to obtain sterile specimens in patients who are unable to void voluntarily, and to obtain postvoiding residual urine volume measurements. A *Coudé catheter* has a curved tip that facilitates insertion when a urethral obstruction (e.g., benign prostatic hypertrophy) makes passage of a Foley catheter difficult. *Three-way irrigation catheters* have, in addition to lumens for urine drainage and balloon inflation, a third lumen for bladder irrigation. These catheters are used commonly after transurethral prostate resection to facilitate bladder irrigation and drainage of blood clots. A *Silastic catheter* is similar to a Foley catheter but is constructed of softer, less-reactive plastic. It is used when a urethral catheter is required on a long-term basis.

Blocked Urethral Catheter

■ PHONE CALL

Questions

1. **How long has the catheter been blocked?**
2. **What are the vital signs?**
3. **Does the patient have suprapubic pain?**
   Urinary retention secondary to a blocked catheter can result in suprapubic pain due to bladder distention.
4. **What was the reason for admission?**

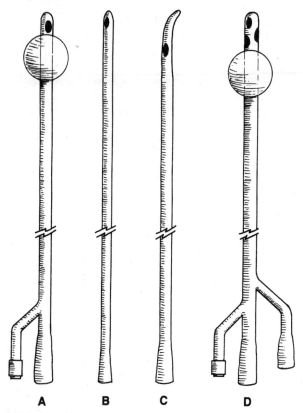

Figure 20–10 □ Urethral catheters. *A*, Foley catheter. *B*, Straight (Robinson) catheter. *C*, Coudé catheter. *D*, Three-way irrigation catheter.

Orders

Ask the RN to try flushing the catheter with 30 to 40 ml of sterile NS if this has not been done.

Inform RN

"Will arrive at the bedside in . . . minutes."

Provided that the patient does not have suprapubic pain (bladder distention), assessment of a blocked urinary catheter can wait an hour or two if other problems of higher priority exist.

■ ELEVATOR THOUGHTS (What causes blocked urethral catheters?)

1. Urinary sediment
2. Blood clots
3. Kinked catheter (look under the bedsheets!)
4. Improperly placed or dislodged catheter

■ MAJOR THREAT TO LIFE

- Bladder rupture
- Progressive renal insufficiency

Bladder rupture may occur if bladder distention progresses without decompression. Because bladder distention is painful, bladder rupture from this cause usually is seen only in the unconscious or paraplegic patient. Persistent lower urinary tract obstruction may lead to hydronephrosis and renal failure.

■ BEDSIDE

Quick Look Test

Does the patient look well (comfortable), sick (uncomfortable or distressed), or critical (about to die)?

Most patients with blocked urethral catheters look well. However, patients with acute bladder distention may look distressed because of abdominal pain.

Airway and Vital Signs

A blocked urethral catheter is not usually responsible for alterations in vital signs unless pain due to bladder distention causes tachypnea or tachycardia.

Selective Physical Examination and Management

1. Percuss and palpate the abdomen to determine whether the bladder is distended. Suprapubic dullness and tenderness suggest a distended bladder.
2. Examine the tubing for kinking of the catheter, blood clots, or sediment.
3. Order a sterile dressing tray, a 50-ml bulb syringe (or a 50-ml syringe and an adapter), and two pairs of sterile gloves in your size. Aspirate and irrigate the catheter with 30 to 40 ml of sterile NS as follows.

a. Ask an assistant to hold the distal part of the catheter close to the connection between the tubing and urinary drainage bag.
b. Wear sterile gloves and clean the distal catheter and the proximal connecting tubing with chlorhexidine.
c. Disconnect the drainage tubing from the catheter. Ask an assistant to hold the connecting tubing in the air to maintain a sterile tip.
d. Using a 50-ml syringe, aspirate the catheter vigorously to dislodge and extract any blood clots or sediment that may have blocked the catheter. If the maneuver is unsuccessful, flush the catheter with 30 to 40 ml of sterile NS. Several attempts at aspiration should be made before abandoning this technique.
e. Reconnect the catheter to the connecting tubing, using sterile technique. The majority of blocked Foley catheters will become unplugged with this maneuver.

4. If flushing of the catheter fails to relieve obstruction, a new catheter should be inserted if one is still required.

Gross Hematuria

■ PHONE CALL

Questions

1. Why was the urethral catheter inserted?
2. What are the vital signs?
3. Is the patient receiving anticoagulant drugs or cyclophosphamide?
4. What was the reason for admission?

Orders

None.

Inform RN

"Will arrive at the bedside in . . . minutes."

Gross hematuria in the anticoagulated patient requires you to see the patient immediately.

■ ELEVATOR THOUGHTS (What causes gross hematuria in the catheterized patient?)

1. Urethral trauma

a. Inadvertent or partial removal of the catheter with the balloon still inflated

b. Trauma during catheter insertion (false passage)

2. Drugs
   a. Anticoagulants (heparin, warfarin)
   b. Thrombolytic agents (streptokinase, tPA, urokinase)
   c. Cyclophosphamide

3. Coagulation abnormalities
   a. Disseminated intravascular coagulation (DIC)
   b. Specific factor deficiencies
   c. Thrombocytopenia

4. Unrelated problems
   a. Renal stones
   b. Carcinoma of the kidney, bladder, or prostate
   c. Glomerulonephritis
   d. Prostatitis
   e. Rupture of a bladder vein

■ MAJOR THREAT TO LIFE

- Hemorrhagic shock

  Although gross hematuria is dramatic and most distressing to the patient, it is rare for bleeding to be sufficiently significant to result in hemorrhagic shock. It only requires 1 ml of blood in 1 L of urine to change the color from yellow to red.

■ BEDSIDE

Quick Look Test

Does the patient look well (comfortable), sick (uncomfortable or distressed), or critical (about to die)?

It is unusual for these patients to look other than well. If they look sick or critical, search for a separate unrecognized problem.

Airway and Vital Signs

What is the BP?

Hypotension in the patient with gross hematuria may be a sign of hemorrhagic shock.

What is the HR?

A resting tachycardia, though a nonspecific finding, may indicate hypovolemia if significant blood loss has occurred.

Selective History and Chart Review

Is the patient receiving any of the following medications?
Heparin, warfarin
Streptokinase, tPA, urokinase
Cyclophosphamide

Is there any abnormality in the coagulation profile?
PT, aPTT, platelet count

Is there a history of urethral trauma?
Recent inadvertent removal of Foley catheter with the balloon still inflated (especially in the elderly, confused patient)
Recent genitourinary (GU) surgery
Recent difficulty with insertion of a urethral catheter

Has there been a recent decrease in the Hb value? How much blood has the patient lost?
Bleeding via the urinary tract is unlikely to cause significant hemodynamic changes unless there has been recent GU surgery.

Management

1. If the patient is anticoagulated, review the initial indication for the anticoagulation. Decide, in consultation with your resident and a hematologist, whether the risk of anticoagulation is still warranted.
2. If a coagulation abnormality is identified, refer to Chapter 31 for discussion of investigation and management.
3. If there is a history of recent urethral trauma, continued significant blood loss is unlikely. Have the vital signs taken every 4 to 6 hours for the next 24 hours. Significant bleeding may be manifested by tachycardia and orthostatic hypotension.

Inability to Insert a Urethral Catheter

■ PHONE CALL

Questions

1. Why was the urethral catheter ordered?
2. What are the vital signs?
3. Does the patient have suprapubic pain?
4. How many attempts have been made to catheterize the patient?
5. What was the reason for admission?

Orders

Ask the RN for a catheter insertion set, two pairs of sterile gloves in your size, and chlorhexidine (Hibitane) skin disinfectant to be at the bedside.

Inform RN

"Will arrive at the bedside in . . . minutes."

Provided that the patient does not have suprapubic pain (bladder distention), insertion of a urethral catheter can wait an hour or two if other problems of higher priority exist.

■ ELEVATOR THOUGHTS (What causes difficulty in urethral catheterization?)

1. Urethral edema
   a. Multiple insertion attempts
   b. Inadvertent removal of a Foley catheter with the balloon still inflated
2. Urethral obstruction
   a. Benign prostatic hypertrophy
   b. Carcinoma of the prostate
   c. Urethral stricture
   d. Anatomic anomaly (diverticulum, false passage)

■ MAJOR THREAT TO LIFE

- Bladder rupture
- Progressive renal insufficiency

Bladder rupture may occur if bladder distention is not relieved by placement of a urinary catheter. A suprapubic catheter may be required if urethral catheterization is impossible. Persistent bladder obstruction may lead to hydronephrosis and *renal failure*.

■ BEDSIDE

Quick Look Test

Does the patient look well (comfortable), sick (uncomfortable or distressed), or critical (about to die)?

Patients with acute bladder distention may look distressed because of abdominal pain.

Airway and Vital Signs

Inability to insert a urethral catheter should not compromise the vital signs.

Selective History and Chart Review

1. Is there a history of recent, multiple attempts at catheterization or removal of a catheter with the balloon still inflated (urethral edema)?
2. Is there a history of benign prostatic hypertrophy, carcinoma of the prostate, urethral stricture, or an anatomic abnormality of the urethra?
3. What was the original indication for urethral catheter placement? Does the indication still exist?

Selective Physical Examination and Management

1. Percuss and palpate the abdomen to determine whether the bladder is distended. Suprapubic tenderness and dullness are suggestive of a distended bladder.
2. If urethral edema is suspected, try inserting a smaller catheter.
3. If there is a history of urethral obstruction, try inserting a Coudé catheter.
4. If you are unable to catheterize the patient, consult the urology department for assistance.

T-TUBES, J-TUBES, AND PENROSE DRAINS

T-tubes are usually used for postoperative drainage of the common bile duct after common bile duct exploration or choledochotomy (Fig. 20–11). A T-tube cholangiogram is commonly performed on the 7th to 10th postoperative day. If the cholangiogram is normal, the T-tube is removed. If a blockage (strictures, tumors, retained common duct stones) exists, the T-tube is left in place.

J-tubes are jejunostomy tubes, surgically inserted to provide enteral nutrition on a long-term basis. They are particularly useful when gastroesophageal reflux and aspiration are a problem.

Gastrostomy tubes may be inserted percutaneously under direct vision (e.g., gastroscopy or fluoroscopy) and are used for long-term feeding when there is no gastroesophageal reflux.

Penrose drains are flat rubber drains inserted into wounds or operative sites with potential dead spaces to prevent the accumulation of pus, intestinal contents, blood, bile, or pancreatic juice.

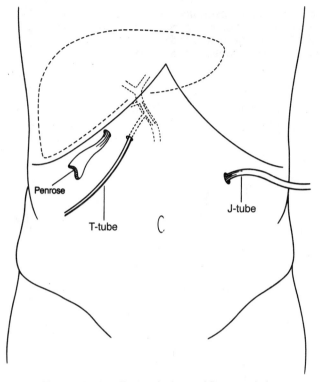

Figure 20–11 ▫ T-tube, J-tube, and Penrose drain.

Closed suction (Davon or Jackson-Pratt) *drains* are used with operative, large potential dead spaces where bacterial ingress may contaminate sterile cavities.

Sump drains have filters incorporated into them to prevent airborne bacteria from entering. They are usually used to drain peripancreatic fluid collections. Interventional radiologists sometimes insert various percutaneous drains into the biliary tree and intra-abdominal abscesses. Problems with these drains should be referred to the radiologist or surgeon.

Blocked T-Tubes and J-Tubes

■ PHONE CALL

Questions

1. How long has the tube been blocked?
2. What type of tube is in place?

3. **Has the tube been dislodged?**
4. **What operation was performed, and how many days ago?**
5. **What are the vital signs?**
6. **What was the reason for admission?**

Orders

Ask the RN for a dressing set, two pairs of gloves in your size, and chlorhexidine (Hibitane) skin disinfectant to be at the bedside. You will have to remove the dressing around the drainage tube, and you must keep the site sterile.

Inform RN

"Will arrive at the bedside in . . . minutes."

Provided that you are certain the tube has not been dislodged, assessment of blocked T-tubes and J-tubes can wait an hour or two if other problems of higher priority exist.

■ ELEVATOR THOUGHTS (What causes blocked T-tubes or J-tubes?)

1. Blood clots within the tube
2. Debris within the tube
3. Failure to irrigate the tube regularly

■ MAJOR THREAT TO LIFE

- Sepsis with blocked T-tubes

  Blocked T-tubes may lead to postoperative infection with resultant abscess formation or systemic sepsis. Provided that they are not dislodged, blocked J-tubes present no immediate threat to life. The risk of further surgery exists if replacement of the tube is required.

■ BEDSIDE

Quick Look Test

Does the patient look well (comfortable), sick (uncomfortable or distressed), or critical (about to die)?

The patient with a blocked T-tube or J-tube will look well unless the underlying problem causes the patient to look sick or critical.

Airway and Vital Signs

A blocked T-tube or J-tube should not compromise the airway or vital signs.

Selective Physical Examination and Management

Aspirate and irrigate the tube as follows.

1. Ask an assistant to hold the distal part of the T-tube or J-tube close to the connection between the tube and the drainage bag.
2. Wear sterile gloves and clean the distal end of the T-tube or J-tube and the proximal connecting tubing with chlorhexidine (Hibitane).
3. Disconnect the tube from the connecting tubing and give the connecting tubing to the assistant to maintain a sterile field.
4. Using a 5-ml syringe, aspirate very gently (i.e., withdraw the syringe plunger) to dislodge and extract the obstruction.
5. If this maneuver is unsuccessful, fill a second 5-ml syringe with 3 ml of sterile NS and very gently flush the T-tube or J-tube by applying slow, careful pressure to the syringe plunger. Only gentle pressure should be used. After flushing with saline, attempt to aspirate gently. If this maneuver fails, do not try again.
6. Reconnect the T-tube or J-tube and the drainage bag, maintaining sterile technique.

If the aspiration and irrigation are unsuccessful, the surgeon should be informed immediately. The decision between a T-tube cholangiogram to visualize the problem and a closed exploration of the obstructed tube with a Fogarty catheter will have to be made. Closed exploration should be performed only by someone experienced in the procedure. It can be done only when a large, intact T-tube has been used or when the back wall of the T-limb has been cut away. An adequately functioning T-tube usually drains 100 to 250 ml/8 hr.

Dislodged T-Tubes, J-Tubes, and Penrose Drains

■ PHONE CALL

Questions

1. How long ago was the tube or drain dislodged?
2. What type of tube is in place?
3. What operation was performed, and how many days ago?
4. What are the vital signs?
5. What was the reason for admission?

Orders

Ask the RN for a dressing set, two pairs of gloves in your size, and chlorhexidine (Hibitane) skin cleanser to be at the bedside. You will have to remove the dressing around the drainage tube, and you must keep the site sterile.

Inform RN

"Will arrive at the bedside in . . . minutes."

Assessment of dislodged T-tubes and J-tubes requires you to see the patient immediately because urgent replacement of the tube is mandatory if it was inserted recently. A delay in this replacement may result in the patient's requiring emergency surgery to replace the tube.

■ ELEVATOR THOUGHTS (What causes dislodgment of tubes and drains?)

1. Failure to secure the tube or drain adequately
2. Confused, uncooperative patient

■ MAJOR THREAT TO LIFE

- Sepsis

  Dislodged T-tubes and Penrose drains may lead to postoperative sepsis with resultant abscess formation or systemic sepsis. Dislodged J-tubes and T-tubes that cannot be replaced early may require surgical replacement, thus increasing the risk of morbidity and mortality from a second anesthetic.

■ BEDSIDE

Quick Look Test

Does the patient look well (comfortable), sick (uncomfortable or distressed), or critical (about to die)?

  The patient with a recently dislodged T-tube, J-tube, or Penrose drain will look well unless the underlying problem causes the patient to look sick or critical.

Airway and Vital Signs

A dislodged T-tube, J-tube, or Penrose drain should not compromise the vital signs acutely.

Selective Physical Examination and Management

A dislodged *T-tube* draining the common bile duct is a potentially life-threatening situation because septic shock can follow rapidly. If dislodgment is suspected, order an immediate T-tube cholangiogram and inform the surgeon. The patient will need surgery to reestablish drainage if dislodgment is confirmed by the cholangiogram.

A dislodged *J-tube* (enterostomy tube) must be reinserted immediately as follows.

1. Wear sterile gloves and clean and drape the tube exit site.
2. If the tube is only partially dislodged, carefully clean the exposed tubing and gently advance the tube to the appropriate (previous) depth.
3. If the tube has been completely dislodged, select a similar sterile tube and introduce it gently through the track left by the previous tube. Do not force the tube.
4. If this maneuver is successful, secure the tube well by suturing it in place with a 3-0 suture.
5. Order a water-soluble radiocontrast x-ray to confirm the correct positioning of the replaced or repositioned tube.

If replacement of the J-tube (enterostomy tube) is unsuccessful, notify the surgeon, who will decide whether an urgent reoperation is indicated.

Dislodged *Penrose drains* should not be reinserted into the wound because bacteria will be introduced into the site. Secure the Penrose drain in the position you find it and examine the area for abscess formation (heat, tenderness, swelling) daily for the next few days. Inform the surgeon that the Penrose drain has become dislodged.

NASOGASTRIC AND ENTERAL FEEDING TUBES

Blocked Nasogastric and Enteral Tubes

■ PHONE CALL

Questions

1. How long has the tube been blocked?
2. What type of tube is in place?
3. Has the tube been dislodged?
4. What are the vital signs?
5. What was the reason for admission?

Orders

Ask the RN for a 50-ml syringe, sterile NS, and a bowl to be at the bedside.

Inform RN

"Will arrive at the bedside in . . . minutes."

A blocked NG or enteral tube is not an emergency. Assessment can wait an hour or two if other problems of higher priority exist.

■ ELEVATOR THOUGHTS (What causes blocked nasogastric or enteral feeding tubes?)

1. Debris within the tube
2. Blood clots within the tube
3. Failure to irrigate the tube regularly

■ MAJOR THREAT TO LIFE

- Aspiration pneumonia
  If the NG tube is blocked and thus fails to drain the stomach, gastric contents can be aspirated into the lungs.

■ BEDSIDE

Quick Look Test

Does the patient look well (comfortable), sick (uncomfortable or distressed), or critical (about to die)?

Failure to drain the gastric contents by a blocked NG tube may result in the patient's developing nausea and vomiting, thus looking sick.

Airways and Vital Signs

What is the RR?

A blocked NG tube should not compromise the airway unless gastric contents accumulate and are aspirated into the lungs.

Selective Physical Examination and Management

1. Irrigate the tube with 25 to 50 ml of NS. As the tube is being irrigated, listen over the stomach region for the gurgling of fluid that indicates that the tube is in the stomach.

2. If the previous maneuver is unsuccessful, remove the tube and replace it with a new tube if there is ongoing gastric stasis with the potential for aspiration.
3. Ensure that the usual nursing protocols are being followed for regular irrigation of the tube.

Dislodged Nasogastric and Enteral Feeding Tubes

■ PHONE CALL

Questions

1. How long has the tube been dislodged?
2. What type of tube is in place?
3. What are the vital signs?
4. What was the reason for admission?

Orders

None.

Inform RN

"Will arrive at the bedside in . . . minutes."
Assessment of a dislodged NG or enteral feeding tube may wait an hour or two if other problems of higher priority exist. Be careful, however, not to leave the diabetic patient who has received insulin without caloric intake for too long.

■ ELEVATOR THOUGHTS (What causes a nasogastric or enteral feeding tube to become dislodged?)

1. Failure to secure the tube adequately
2. Confused, uncooperative patient

■ MAJOR THREAT TO LIFE

- Aspiration pneumonia
  If the NG tube is dislodged and thus fails to drain the stomach, gastric contents may accumulate and can be aspirated into the lung. The danger of a dislodged or misplaced enteral feeding tube is the risk of infusing the enteral feeding solution into the lung.

■ BEDSIDE

Quick Look Test

Does the patient look well (comfortable), sick (uncomfortable or distressed), or critical (about to die)?

Patients who have aspirated because ot a dislodged NG tube or a malpositioned feeding tube may appear tachypneic and unwell.

Airway and Vital Signs

A dislodged NG or enteral feeding tube should not compromise the vital signs unless aspiration of gastric contents or enteral feeding solutions has occurred.

Selective Physical Examination and Management

1. Inspect the tube. **Are there any markings on the tube that indicate how far the tube is situated?** If you are not familiar with these markings, ask the RN to bring a similar tube so you will be able to estimate how far in the tube is.
2. Aspirate the tube to see if gastric contents can be obtained. Instill 25 to 50 ml of air using the 50-ml syringe while listening over the stomach region with your stethoscope. If the tube is properly positioned, you should be able to hear a gurgling swoosh as air is introduced into the stomach.
3. A small-bore enteral feeding tube should not be pushed farther down if it has been dislodged. Do *not* insert the guidewire down the tube blindly, as laceration or perforation of the esophagus, stomach, or duodenum may occur if the tip of the guidewire exits from one of the distal apertures in the tube. Dislodged enteral feeding tubes must be removed and replaced. The same tube may be reused, with the guidewire being inserted into the tube under direct vision ex vivo. The tube, stiffened by the guidewire, may then be reinserted.
4. Ensure that the usual nursing protocols are being followed for regular irrigation of the tube.

21

POLYURIA, FREQUENCY, AND INCONTINENCE

You will receive many calls at night regarding patients' urinary volumes; the patients are voiding either too much or too little. It is often difficult for a patient to differentiate between problems of *polyuria* and *frequency*, and for many elderly patients, either of these problems may present as *incontinence*. Once you clarify which one of the three problems is present, you will find the remainder easy.

■ PHONE CALL

Questions

1. Clarify the symptom.
   Polyuria refers to a urine output > 3 L/day. This usually comes to the attention of the nurse when reviewing the fluid balance record or when the urinary drainage bag requires frequent emptying. *Frequency* of urination refers to the frequent passage of urine, whether of large or small volume, and may occur in concert with polyuria or urinary incontinence. *Urinary incontinence* refers to the involuntary loss of urine.

2. What are the vital signs?

3. What was the admitting diagnosis?

Orders

Polyuria, frequency, and incontinence are seldom urgent problems. Urinary incontinence is a common problem in hospitalized elderly patients and is a frequent source of frustration for nurses. Avoid ordering a Foley catheter as the first line of treatment.

Inform RN

"Will arrive at the bedside in . . . minutes."

If the patient's vital signs are stable and other sick patients require assessment, a patient with polyuria, frequency, or incontinence need not be seen immediately.

■ ELEVATOR THOUGHTS

What causes polyuria?
- Diabetes mellitus
- Diabetes insipidus (central, nephrogenic)
- Psychogenic polydipsia
- Large volumes of oral or intravenous (IV) fluids
- Diuretics
- Diuretic phase of acute tubular necrosis
- Postobstructive diuresis
- Salt-losing nephritis
- Hypercalcemia

What causes frequency?
- Urinary tract infection (UTI)
- Partial bladder outlet obstruction (e.g., prostatism)
- Bladder irritation (tumors, stones, infections)

What causes incontinence?
- Urge incontinence (UTI, diabetes mellitus, urolithiasis, dementia, stroke, normal pressure hydrocephalus, benign prostatic hypertrophy [BPH], pelvic tumor, depression, anxiety)
- Stress incontinence (in multiparous women, lax pelvic bladder support; in men, after prostatic surgery)
- Overflow incontinence (bladder outlet obstruction as in BPH, urethral stricture; spinal cord disease, autonomic neuropathy, fecal impaction)
- Environmental factors (inaccessibility to call bell, obstacles to the bathroom)
- Iatrogenic factors (diuretics, sedatives, anticholinergics, alpha blockers, calcium channel blockers, angiotensin-converting enzyme [ACE] inhibitors)

■ MAJOR THREAT TO LIFE

- *Polyuria*: intravascular volume depletion. If polyuria is not due to fluid excess and continues without adequate fluid replacement, the intravascular volume will drop and the patient may become hypotensive.
- *Frequency* or *incontinence*: sepsis. Frequency or incontinence does not pose a major threat to life unless an underlying UTI goes unchecked and progresses to pyelonephritis or sepsis.

■ BEDSIDE
Quick Look Test

Does the patient look well (comfortable), sick (uncomfortable or distressed), or critical (about to die)?

Most often, patients with polyuria, frequency, or incontinence look well. If the patient looks sick or critical, search for a previously unrecognized problem. For example, if *polyuria* is due to previously undetected diabetes mellitus, the patient may be ketoacidotic and appear sick. Similarly, *frequency* or *incontinence* may prove to be the presenting manifestation of UTI in a patient who appears sick.

Airway and Vital Signs

Check for postural changes. A rise in heart rate (HR) > 15 beats/min or a fall in systolic blood pressure (BP) > 5 mm Hg or any fall in diastolic BP indicates significant hypovolemia. *Caution:* A resting tachycardia alone may indicate decreased intravascular volume.

Fever suggests possible UTI.

Selective Physical Examination I

Is the patient volume depleted?
CVS   Pulse volume, JVP
           Skin temperature and color
Neuro   Level of consciousness

Management

What immediate measure must be taken to correct or prevent intravascular volume depletion?
Replace intravascular volume. If the patient is volume depleted, give IV normal saline (NS) or Ringer's lactate, aiming for a JVP of 2 to 3 cm H_2O above the sternal angle and normalization of the vital signs. Remember that aggressive fluid repletion in a patient with a history of congestive heart failure (CHF) may compromise cardiac function. Do not overshoot the mark!

Selective History and Chart Review

Identify the specific problem.

Polyuria. Polyuria may be suspected by history but can be accurately confirmed only through scrutiny of meticulously kept fluid balance sheets. If these are not available, order strict intake/output monitoring. It is worthwhile to document polyuria (> 3 L/day) before embarking on an exhaustive workup of a possibly nonexistent problem.
1. Ask about associated symptoms. "Polyuria + polydipsia" suggests diabetes mellitus, diabetes insipidus, or compulsive

water drinking (psychogenic polydipsia). Of these, diabetes mellitus is the most common.

2. Check the chart for recent laboratory results.
   a. Blood glucose (diabetes mellitus)
   b. Potassium
   c. Calcium

   Hypokalemia and hypercalcemia are important reversible causes of nephrogenic diabetes insipidus. (Refer to Chapter 33 for management of hypokalemia and Chapter 30 for management of hypercalcemia.)

3. Make sure the patient is not on any drugs that may cause either nephrogenic diabetes insipidus (lithium carbonate, demeclocycline) or diuresis (diuretics, mannitol).

Frequency. Frequency can be assessed by questioning the patient. Estimate from the nursing notes or fluid balance sheets whether the patient is a reliable historian. Ask about associated symptoms. Fever, dysuria, hematuria, and foul-smelling urine suggest UTI. Poor stream, hesitancy, dribbling, or nocturia suggests prostatism.

Incontinence. Incontinence is obvious when it occurs and is often embarrassing to the patient. You need an honest history from the patient to make a proper diagnosis. Address the subject nonjudgmentally. Review the patient's medications to ensure that he or she is not receiving medications that may cause incontinence.

Selective Physical Examination II

Look for specific causes and complications of polyuria, frequency, or incontinence.

Vitals	Fever (UTI)
HEENT	Visual fields (pituitary neoplasm)
Resp	Kussmaul's respiration (diabetic ketoacidosis); Kussmaul's respirations are characterized by deep, pauseless breathing at a rate of 25 to 30/min
ABD	Enlarged bladder (neurogenic bladder, bladder outlet obstruction with overflow incontinence)
	Suprapubic tenderness (cystitis)
Neuro	Level of consciousness
	Localizing findings
	An alert, conscious person with polyuria and with free access to fluids and salt will not become volume depleted. If volume depletion is present, suspect metabolic or structural neurologic abnormalities impairing the normal response to thirst. Perform a complete neurologic examination,

looking for evidence of stroke, subdural hemorrhage, or metabolic abnormalities.

Skin   Perineal skin breakdown (a complication of repeated incontinence and a source of infection)

Rectal   Enlarged prostate (bladder outlet obstruction)

Perineal sensation, resting tone of anal sphincter, anal wink

An anal wink is elicited by gently stroking the perineal mucosa with a tongue depressor. A normal response is manifested by contraction of the external sphincter.

If abnormalities in perineal sensation, anal sphincter tone, or anal wink are discovered, the bulbocavernosus reflex should also be tested. To elicit this reflex, the index finger of the examining hand is introduced into the rectum, and the patient is asked to relax the sphincter as much as possible. The glans penis is then squeezed with the opposite hand, which normally results in involuntary contraction of the anal sphincter. Innervation of the anus is similar to that of the lower urinary tract; therefore, abnormalities in perineal sensation or in the sacral reflexes may provide a clue that a spinal cord lesion is responsible for the incontinence.

Management

What more needs to be done tonight?

Polyuria

1. Once intravascular volume is restored, ensure adequate continuing replacement (usually IV) fluid as estimated by urinary, insensible (400 to 800 ml/day), and other (nasogastric suction, vomiting, diarrhea) losses. Recheck the volume status periodically to ensure that your mathematic estimates for replacement correlate with an appropriate clinical response.

2. Order strict intake/output records to be kept.

3. Order serum glucose, Chemstrip, or glucose meter testing. This will identify diabetes mellitus before it progresses to ketoacidosis (type 1 diabetes) or hyperosmolar coma (type 2 diabetes). The presence of glycosuria on urinalysis will provide more rapid evidence of hyperglycemia as a possible cause of polyuria. Random blood glucose levels of < 10 mmol/L are seldom accompanied by osmotic diuresis. If hyperglycemia of > 10 mmol/L exists, refer to Chapter 32, pages 347 to 349, for further management.

4. Serum calcium level often is not available as a stat test at

night. If there is strong suspicion of hypercalcemia (polyuria or lethargy in a patient with malignancy, hyperparathyroidism, or sarcoidosis), contact the laboratory for permission to measure the serum calcium level on an urgent basis.

5. Maximal urine concentrating ability measured by the water deprivation test can help differentiate among central diabetes insipidus, nephrogenic diabetes insipidus, and psychogenic polydipsia. This test can be arranged on an elective basis in the morning.

Frequency

1. If other symptoms (urgency, dysuria, low-grade fever, suprapubic tenderness) of UTI (cystitis) are present, empirical treatment with antibiotics may be warranted, pending urine culture and sensitivity results, which will usually take 48 hours to complete. Scrutiny of the patient's chart may reveal a previous urine culture or previous antibacterial therapy that may affect the selection of empirical treatment.

   Any of the following may be effective therapy in an uncomplicated case (i.e., no evidence of upper UTI, no evidence of prostatitis, no renal disease, and no recent urinary tract instrumentation). These antibiotics are generally used for 3 days in women and for 7 days in men. However, women with diabetes, a structural urinary tract abnormality, or a recently treated UTI should receive a 7-day course.

   a. *Trimethoprim-sulfamethoxazole* (160 mg/800 mg) 1 tab PO twice daily
   b. *Trimethoprim* 100 mg PO twice daily
   c. *Nitrofurantoin* 100 mg PO twice daily
   d. *Norfloxacin* 400 mg PO twice daily
   e. *Phenazopyridine* 200 mg PO three times daily after meals may help alleviate dysuria in cases of urethritis during the first day or two of treatment. Warn the patient that this drug may turn the urine orange. Also, encourage high fluid intake to promote washout of the urinary tract.

2. If history and physical examination suggest partial bladder outlet obstruction, examine the abdomen carefully for an enlarged bladder. If the patient has urinary retention, a Foley catheter should be placed. (Refer to Chapter 9, pages 76 to 77, for further investigation and management of urinary retention.)

   Always check for heart murmurs before catheterizing a patient. Patients with cardiac valvular abnormalities are at risk for the development of infective endocarditis after genitourinary (GU) procedures, including catheterization with a Foley catheter. High-risk patients (prosthetic heart valves, previous endocarditis, cyanotic congenital heart disease) should receive *ampicillin* 2 g IV or IM plus *gentamicin* 1.5 mg/kg IV/IM. Both antibiotics should be given 30 minutes before catheterization. Then, 6 hours later, give *ampicillin* 1 g IV/IM or *amoxicillin* 1 g PO. Moderate-risk patients (mitral valve prolapse [MVP] with regurgitation, hypertrophic cardiomyopathy, acquired valvular dysfunction, most noncyanotic congenital cardiac malformations) should receive *amoxicillin* 2 g PO 1 hour before catheterization or ampicillin 2 g IV/IM 30 minutes before catheterization. High-risk patients allergic to ampicillin/amoxicillin may be given *vancomycin* 1 g IV over 1 to 2 hours plus *gentamicin* 1.5 mg/kg IV/IM. In moderate-risk patients allergic to ampicillin/amoxicillin, vancomycin should be given, but the gentamicin can be omitted.[1]

A brief in-and-out catheterization, in the presence of sterile urine, may not require antibiotic prophylaxis. If, however, the patient has a prosthetic cardiac valve, you may want to err on the safe side and administer prophylactic antibiotics. Ask your resident or the patient's cardiologist for advice in this situation.

3. Other causes of frequency, such as bladder irritation by stones or tumors, can be addressed by urologic consultation in the morning. You may be able to expedite the diagnosis of bladder tumor by ordering a collection of urine for cytologic study.

Incontinence

1. Even if incontinence is the only symptom, order a urinalysis and urine culture to ensure that a UTI is not contributing to the patient's symptoms.
2. Check for hyperglycemia, hypokalemia, and hypercalcemia if there is a question of polyuria. These conditions may present as incontinence in the elderly or bedridden patient, and specific treatment may alleviate the incontinence.
3. If neurologic examination (e.g., abnormal sacral reflexes, diminished perineal sensation, lower limb weakness or spasticity) suggests the presence of a *spinal cord lesion*, consultation should be arranged with a neurologist.
4. In the case of *overflow incontinence*, one must differentiate between overflow due to bladder outlet obstruction (e.g., BPH, uterine prolapse) and impaired ability of detrusor contraction (e.g., lower motor neuron bladder). This is best done in the morning by assessment of urinary bladder dynamics under the direction of a urologist. If the bladder is palpably enlarged and the patient is distressed, bladder catheterization may be attempted. Forceful attempts at catheterization should be avoided, and a urologist should be called for assistance if the catheter does not pass easily (see Chapter 20, page 230). If no correctable obstruction is found, long-term treatment may involve intermittent straight catheteriza-

tion, which is less likely to cause infection than a chronic indwelling Foley catheter. Aim for a urine volume < 400 ml every 4 to 6 hours. Greater volumes result in ureterovesical reflux, which promotes ascending UTI. A young motivated patient with a neurogenic bladder can be taught to self-catheterize. In these cases, a silicone elastomer (Silastic) Foley catheter should be used. This type has the advantage of less predisposition to calcification and encrustation and may be kept in place up to 6 weeks at a time.

5. *Urge incontinence* (detrusor instability) is a condition in which the bladder escapes central inhibition, resulting in reflex contractions. It is the most common cause of incontinence in the elderly population and is often manifested by involuntary micturition preceded by a warning of a few seconds or minutes. Ensure that there are no physical barriers preventing the patient from reaching the bathroom or commode in time. Is there easy access to the call bell? Are the nurses responding promptly? Are the bedrails kept up or down? Does the patient have a medical condition (e.g., Parkinson's disease, stroke, arthritis) that prevents easy mobilization when the urge to void occurs? If there is no evidence of perineal skin breakdown, *urinary incontinence pads* with frequent checks and changes by the nursing staff are adequate. (Babies exist for years in such a state!) If perineal skin breakdown or ulceration is present, a Foley or condom catheter is justified to allow skin healing. Long-term treatment involves regular toileting every 2 to 3 hours while awake and limiting the evening fluid intake.

6. Urinary spillage with coughing or straining suggests *stress incontinence*. Again, if there is no evidence of perineal skin breakdown, urinary incontinence pads are adequate until urologic consultation can assess the need for medical versus surgical management.

■ REMEMBER

Urinary incontinence is an understandable source of frustration for nurses caring for these patients. Listen to the concerns of the nurses looking after your patients and discuss with them the reasons for your actions.

Reference

1. Prevention of bacterial endocarditis. JAMA 1997;277:1794–1801.

22

PRONOUNCING DEATH

One of the required duties of medical students and residents on call at night is the pronouncement of death in patients who have recently died. This is a situation that is seldom addressed in medical school, and you will certainly wonder what needs to be done to pronounce a patient dead. Unfortunately, there has long been uncertainty surrounding what constitutes the medical and legal definitions of death.

Traditionally, the determination of death has been solely a medical decision. In the United States, legislative action on the criteria of death falls within state jurisdiction. Many states have opted to follow the recommendations set forth by the Harvard Medical School Ad Hoc Committee,[1] Capron and Kass,[2] or the Kansas legislation of 1971.[3] It is best to be familiar with the medical and legal criteria accepted for the determination of death in the state in which you work.

The recommended criteria of death to be used for all purposes within the jurisdiction of the Parliament of Canada, issued by the Law Reform Commission of Canada[4] in 1981, were as follows:

1. A person is dead when an irreversible cessation of all that person's brain function has occurred.
2. The irreversible cessation of brain function can be determined by the prolonged absence of spontaneous circulatory and respiratory functions.
3. When the determination of the prolonged absence of spontaneous circulatory and respiratory functions is made impossible by the use of artificial means of support, the irreversible cessation of the brain function can be determined by any means recognized by the ordinary standards of current medical practice.

Although criterion 1 alone may imply that a complete neurologic examination is required for pronouncement of death, we know that this is neither practical nor necessary. Criterion 2 accounts for this by assuming that when "prolonged absence of spontaneous circulatory and respiratory functions" exists, irreversible cessation of the patient's brain function has occurred. Hence, there will be no question in the majority of cases that most of the patients you will be asked to pronounce dead will indeed be medically and legally dead because they will fulfill the criterion set out in 2 alone. Thus, legally, in most cases, all that is required of you to pronounce a patient dead is to verify that there has been a prolonged absence of spontaneous circulatory and respiratory functions. A slightly more detailed assessment is recommended, however, and will take only a few minutes to complete.

The RN will page you and inform you of the death of the patient, requesting that you come to the unit and pronounce the patient dead.

1. Identify the patient by the hospital identification tag worn on the wrist.
2. Ascertain that the patient does not rouse to verbal or tactile stimuli.
3. Listen for heart sounds and feel for the carotid pulse. The deceased patient is pulseless and without heart sounds.
4. Look and listen to the patient's chest for evidence of spontaneous respirations. The deceased patient shows no evidence of breathing movements or of air entry on examination.
5. Record the position of the pupils and their reactions to light. The deceased patient shows no evidence of pupillary reaction to light. Though the pupils are usually dilated, this position is not invariable.
6. Record the time at which your assessment was completed. Although other emergencies take precedence over pronouncing a patient dead, one should try not to postpone this task too long, since the time of death is legally the time at which you pronounce the patient dead.
7. Document your findings on the chart. A typical chart entry may read as follows: Called to pronounce Mr. Doe dead. Patient unresponsive to verbal or tactile stimuli. No heart sounds heard, no pulse felt. Not breathing, no air entry heard. Pupils fixed and dilated. Patient pronounced dead at 2030 hours, December 7, 2000.
8. Notify the family physician, attending physician, or both if the nurses have not already done so. Decide together with the attending physician whether an autopsy would be useful and appropriate in this patient's case.
9. Notify relatives. Next of kin should be notified as soon as possible after you have pronounced the patient dead and notified the family physician, attending physician, or both. Normally, it is the responsibility of the family physician to notify the relatives once he or she has been told of the patient's death. Occasionally, you may experience the situation where the family physician has signed over his or her nighttime call to a partner or another physician who does not know the patient or family. In this situation, it is best to inform the physician on call, and if he or she is uncomfortable with speaking to the family, a member of the house staff who knows the patient or family best should then notify the next of kin. The family will appreciate hearing the news from a familiar voice.

If neither the family physician on call nor the housestaff knows the patient, spend a few minutes familiarizing yourself with the patient's medical history and mode of death. If you are appointed to deliver the news to the family, the following guidelines may be helpful.

- Identify yourself, e.g., "This is Dr. Jones calling from St. Paul's Hospital."
- Ask for the next of kin, e.g., "May I speak with Mrs. Doe, please?"
- Deliver the message, e.g., "Mrs. Doe, I am sorry to inform you that your husband died at 8:30 this evening."
- You may be surprised to find that in many instances this news is not unexpected. It is, however, always comforting to a family to know that a relative has died peacefully—e.g., "As you know, your husband was suffering from a terminal illness. Although I was not with your husband at the time of his death, the nurses looking after him assure me that he was very comfortable at the time of his death and that he passed away peacefully."
- If an autopsy is desired by one of the medical staff, this question should be broached now—e.g., "Your husband had an unusual illness, and if you are agreeable, it would be very useful to us to perform an autopsy. Although it obviously will not change the course of events in terms of your husband's illness, it may provide some valuable information for other patients suffering from similar problems to your husband's." If there is any hesitation on the part of the next of kin, emphasize that he or she is under no obligation to grant permission for an autopsy to be performed if it is against the perceived wishes of the patient or family. If the next of kin refuses, do not argue, no matter how interested you may be in the outcome of the case. Accept the family's decision graciously—e.g., "We understand completely, and, of course, we will respect your wishes."
- Ask the next of kin if he or she would like to come to the hospital to see the patient one last time. Inform the nurses of this decision. Questions pertaining to funeral homes and the patient's personal belongings are best referred to the nurse in charge.

■ SPECIAL SITUATIONS

Medical technology has introduced two other scenarios in the pronouncement of a patient's death.

The Mechanically Ventilated Patient Without Circulatory Function

There is general understanding that those patients whose hearts have stopped beating despite being mechanically ventilated will all meet the criteria for legal death through a lack of spontaneous ventilation once the ventilator is turned off. Thus, it is reasonable practice to

1. Ensure that connections are intact and properly attached if the patient is on the ECG monitor. (This ensures that the absence of cardiac electrical activity is not an artifact due to faulty electrical connections.)
2. Follow the usual procedure for pronouncing death.
3. Discuss your findings with the attending physician *before* disconnecting the ventilator.
4. After agreement with the attending physician, disconnect the ventilator. Observe the patient for 3 minutes for evidence of spontaneous respiration.
5. Document your findings in the chart—e.g., "Called to pronounce Mr. Doe dead. Patient unresponsive to verbal or tactile stimuli. No heart sounds heard, no pulse felt. Pupils fixed and dilated. Patient being mechanically ventilated. Ventilator disconnected at 2030 hours after discussion with attending physician, Dr. Smith. No spontaneous respirations noted for 3 minutes. Patient pronounced dead at 2033 hours, December 7, 2000."

The Mechanically Ventilated Patient with Circulatory Function Intact

This type of patient is usually being cared for in the intensive care unit. A variety of controversial criteria exists for the determination of brain death,[5-8] and criteria may differ between geographic locations. The task of pronouncing a mechanically ventilated patient dead and the discussion of organ procurement are best left to the intensive care unit staff and associated subspecialists in consultation with the patient's family.

References

1. Report of the Ad Hoc Committee of the Harvard Medical School to Examine the Definition of Brain Death. JAMA 1968;205:337.
2. Capron and Kass: A Statutory Definition of the Standards for Determining Human Death, 121 U. Pa. L. Rev. 87 (1972a).
3. Kan. Stat. Ann. 77–202 (Supp. 1974).
4. Report on the Criteria for the Determination of Death. Law Reform Commission of Canada, 1981.

5. Conference of Royal College and Faculties of the United Kingdom: Diagnosis of brain death. Lancet 1976;2:1069–1070.
6. Guidelines for the diagnosis of brain death. Can Med Assoc J 1987;136:200A–200B.
7. Halevy A, Brody B: Brain death: Reconciling definitions, criteria, and tests. Ann Intern Med 1993;119:519–525.
8. Spoor MT, Sutherland FR: The evolution of the concept of brain death. Ann RCPSC 1995;28:30–32.

23

SEIZURES

A seizure is one of the more dramatic events you may witness while on call. Usually, everyone around you will be in a panic. The key to controlling the situation is to remain calm.

■ PHONE CALL

Questions

1. **Is the patient still seizing?**
2. **What type of seizure was witnessed?**
   Was the seizure generalized tonic-clonic, or was it focal?
3. **What is the patient's level of consciousness?**
4. **Has there been any obvious injury?**
5. **What was the reason for admission?**
6. **Does the patient have diabetes mellitus?**

Orders

1. Ask the RN to make sure the patient is positioned on his or her side. During both the seizure and the postictal state, the patient should be kept in the lateral decubitus position to prevent aspiration of gastric contents.
2. Ask the RN to have the following available at the bedside:
   a. Oral airway
   b. Intravenous (IV) setup with normal saline (NS) (flushed through and ready for immediate use)
   c. Two blood tubes (one for chemistry and one for hematology)
   d. *Diazepam* (Valium) 20 mg
   e. *Thiamine* 100 mg
   f. 50% dextrose in water (D50W) 50 ml (1 ampule)
   g. Chart
3. If the patient is postictal, ask the RN to remove any dentures, suction the oropharynx, and insert an oral airway.
4. Order a stat blood glucose, Chemstrip, or glucose meter reading if the patient is in the postictal state (unconscious).

Inform RN

"Will arrive at bedside in . . . minutes."
A seizure requires you to see the patient immediately.

■ ELEVATOR THOUGHTS
(What causes seizures?)

1. Drugs
   a. Drug withdrawal
      (1) Antiepileptic medication inadvertently discontinued or nontherapeutic level
      (2) Alcohol withdrawal. Caution: *Does the patient have delirium tremens in addition to the seizures?*
      (3) Benzodiazepine or barbiturate withdrawal
   b. Drug toxicity (does not necessarily imply "overdose")
      (1) Meperidine (Demerol) overdose (an easily missed diagnosis in the elderly postoperative patient)
      (2) Penicillin at high doses
      (3) Theophylline toxicity
      (4) Lidocaine HCl infusion
      (5) Isoniazid
      (6) Lithium carbonate
      (7) Neuroleptics (e.g., chlorpromazine)
      (8) Cocaine, amphetamines
2. Central nervous system
   a. Tumor
   b. Previous stroke
   c. Previous head injury
   d. Meningitis/encephalitis
   e. Idiopathic epilepsy
3. Endocrine: The Four Hypos
   a. Hypoglycemia
   b. Hyponatremia
   c. Hypocalcemia
   d. Hypomagnesemia
4. Miscellaneous
   a. Uremia
   b. Central nervous system (CNS) vasculitis
   c. Hypertensive encephalopathy
   d. Hypoxia/hypercapnia
   e. Pseudoseizure
5. Common causes of seizures in patients with acquired immunodeficiency syndrome (AIDS)
   a. Mass lesions (toxoplasmosis, CNS lymphoma)
   b. Human immunodeficiency virus (HIV) encephalopathy
   c. Meningitis (cryptococcal, herpes zoster, toxoplasmosis, aseptic)
   d. Any of the usual causes of seizures seen in immunocompetent hosts

■ MAJOR THREAT TO LIFE

- Aspiration
- Hypoxia

The patient should be lying in the lateral decubitus position to prevent the tongue from falling posteriorly and blocking the airway and to minimize the risk of aspiration of gastric contents while in the postictal state. Patients usually keep breathing throughout seizure activity. Most patients can be in status epilepticus for 30 minutes with no subsequent neurologic damage.

IF THE SEIZURE HAS STOPPED

The majority of seizures will have stopped by the time you arrive at the bedside. The procedures and protocols to follow if the seizure has stopped are discussed subsequently. The procedures and protocols to follow if the seizure persists begin on page 261.

■ BEDSIDE

Quick Look Test

Does the patient look well (comfortable), sick (uncomfortable or distressed), or critical (about to die)?

Most patients after a generalized tonic-clonic seizure are unconscious (the postictal state).

Airway, Vital Signs, and Blood Glucose Results

In what position is the patient lying?

The patient should be positioned in the lateral decubitus position to prevent aspiration of gastric contents (Fig. 23–1).

Remove any dentures and suction the airway. Insert an oral airway if one is not already in place (Fig. 23–2). The patient is not out of danger yet! The patient might begin to experience another seizure, so make sure the airway is protected.

Give oxygen by face mask or nasal prongs.

What is the Chemstrip result?

Hypoglycemia needs to be treated immediately to prevent further seizures.

Management I

Draw blood (20 ml) and establish IV access. Send the blood for the following tests.

- *Chemistry tube:* electrolytes, urea, creatinine, random blood

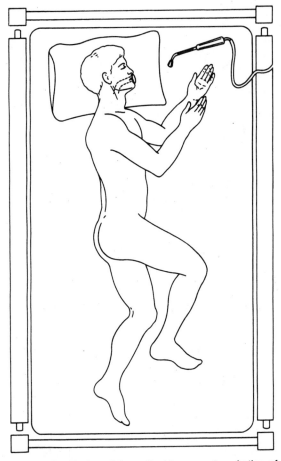

Figure 23–1 □ Positioning of the patient to prevent aspiration of gastric contents.

glucose, Ca, Mg, albumin, and antiepileptic drug levels (if the patient is receiving these medications). If the patient is undergoing a 3-day fast for investigation of possible hypoglycemia, order an insulin level as well.

- *Hematology tube:* complete blood cell count (CBC) and manual differential.

Once the IV is established, keep the line open with NS. NS is the IV fluid of choice, as phenytoin is not compatible with dextrose-containing solutions.

If the *Chemstrip* result or *glucose meter* reading reveals hypogly-

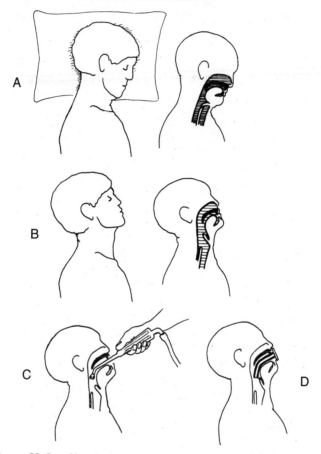

Figure 23–2 □ Airway management. Correct positioning of the head, correct suctioning, and correct inserting of an oral airway. *A*, Neck flexion closes the airway. *B*, Neck extension to sniffing position opens the airway. *C*, Suctioning. *D*, Placement of the airway.

cemia, give *thiamine* 100 mg IV by slow, direct injection over 3 to 5 minutes, followed by D50W 50 ml IV by slow, direct injection. Thiamine is given before administration of glucose to protect against an exacerbation of Wernicke's encephalopathy.

Draw arterial blood gases (ABGs) if the patient appears cyanotic.

Selective Physical Examination I

Assess level of consciousness. **Does the patient respond to verbal or painful stimuli? Is the patient in a postictal state (i.e., de-**

creased level of consciousness [LOC])? *Remember:* If the patient does not regain consciousness between seizures, after 30 minutes the diagnosis becomes *status epilepticus*.

Selective History and Chart Review

1. *Ask any witnesses the following details about the seizure.*
   a. Length of time?
   b. Generalized tonic-clonic or focal?
   c. Onset generalized or focal? A focal onset of a generalized tonic-clonic seizure suggests structural brain disease, which may be old or new.
   d. Any injury observed during the seizure?
2. *Is there a history of epilepsy, alcohol or sedative withdrawal, head injury (e.g., recent fall while in hospital), stroke, CNS tumor (primary or secondary), or diabetes mellitus?*
3. *Is the patient receiving any of the following medications, which may induce seizures?*
   a. Penicillin
   b. Meperidine (Demerol)
   c. Insulin
   d. Oral hypoglycemics
   e. Antidepressants, lithium carbonate
   f. Isoniazid
   g. Lidocaine
   h. Neuroleptics (e.g., chlorpromazine)
   i. Theophylline
4. *Is the patient positive for HIV or otherwise immunosuppressed?* Seizures are a common manifestation of CNS disease in the HIV-positive patient.
5. *What are the most recent laboratory results?*
   a. Glucose
   b. Na
   c. Ca
   d. Albumin
   e. Mg
   f. Antiepileptic drug levels
   g. Urea
   h. Creatinine

The chart is reviewed before the physical examination because an immediate, treatable cause (e.g., insulin or meperidine overdose, hyponatremia) is more likely to be found in the chart.

Selective Physical Examination II

Vitals	Repeat now
HEENT	Tongue or cheek lacerations, nuchal rigidity
Resp	Signs of aspiration

Neuro	Complete CNS examination within the limits of level of consciousness
	Can the patient speak, follow commands?
	Is there any asymmetry of pupils, visual fields, reflexes, or plantar responses? Asymmetry suggests structural brain disease.
MSS	Palpate skull and face, spine and ribs
	Passive ROM of all four limbs
	Are there any lacerations, hematomas, or fractures?

Management II

Establish the *provisional* and *differential diagnoses* of the seizure—this must be a causally defined diagnosis (e.g., "generalized tonic-clonic seizure secondary to hypoglycemia").

Are there any *complications* of the seizure giving rise to a second diagnosis? For example, if a head injury has been sustained, the provisional diagnosis might be "forehead hematoma," and the differential diagnosis would include subdural hematoma and frontal bone fracture.

Treat the underlying cause! Seizure is a sign, not a diagnosis.

Maintain IV access for 24 hours with NS. If there is a concern regarding volume overloading, use a heparin lock instead of maintaining the IV line open with NS.

In most patients with a single seizure, it is not necessary to administer antiepileptic medications, particularly if a rapidly correctable metabolic cause is found. Exceptions include the patient already on antiepileptic medication but with inadequate serum concentrations, the patient with suspected structural CNS abnormality, and the HIV-positive patient (in whom seizures tend to be recurrent). If further seizures are anticipated, a long-acting antiepileptic drug (e.g., phenytoin rather than diazepam) is recommended (see page 263 for dosage). Although diazepam is useful as an anticonvulsant to halt seizures, it is not useful as a prophylactic. The antiepileptic medication of choice is *phenytoin*.

The *elderly* and other patients suspected of having *structural CNS disease* as a cause of their seizure should have a computed tomography (CT) head scan performed.

The *HIV-positive patient* should have a CT head scan (because of the high incidence of CNS mass lesions), and if there is no risk of herniation, a lumbar puncture (LP) also should be performed. Occasionally, cryptococcal meningitis may coexist in an HIV-positive patient who also has a mass lesion on CT head scan.

Seizure precautions should be instituted for the next 48 hours and then reviewed (Table 23–1).

Table 23–1 □ SEIZURE PRECAUTIONS

1. Place bed in lowest position
2. Provide oral airway at head of bed
3. Keep side rails up when patient is in bed. In case of generalized tonic-clonic seizure, pad side rails
4. Provide patient with firm pillow
5. Provide suction at bedside
6. Provide oxygen at bedside
7. Allow bathroom use with supervision only
8. Allow baths or showers only with a nurse in attendance
9. Take axillary temperature only
10. Provide direct supervision when patient uses sharp objects, such as straight razor, nail scissors

IF THE PATIENT IS STILL SEIZING

Don't panic (almost everybody else will)! Most seizures will resolve without treatment within 2 minutes.

■ BEDSIDE

Quick Look Test

Does the patient look well (comfortable), sick (uncomfortable or distressed), or critical (about to die)?

A patient having a generalized tonic-clonic seizure often engenders anxiety in the observer. Remember, if the patient is seizing, you can be assured that he or she has both a blood pressure (BP) and a pulse.

Ask the RN to notify your resident of the situation—a seizure is a medical emergency.

Airway, Vital Signs, and Blood Glucose Result

In what position is the patient lying?

The patient should be positioned and maintained in the lateral decubitus position to prevent aspiration of gastric contents. One or two assistants may be required to hold the patient in this position if the seizure is violent.

Suction the airway. Do not insert an oral airway or attempt to remove dentures if force is required; you might break the patient's teeth.

Give oxygen by face mask or nasal prongs.

What is the patient's BP?

It is virtually impossible to take a BP during a generalized tonic-clonic seizure, so palpate the femoral pulse. (You may need an assistant to hold the patient's knee against the bed.) A palpable femoral pulse usually indicates a systolic BP > 60 mm Hg.

What is the Chemstrip result?

Hypoglycemia, if present, needs to be treated immediately.

Management I

How long has the patient been seizing?
- If the seizure has stopped, refer to page 256.
- If the seizure has lasted < 3 minutes
  - Do not give diazepam yet.
  - Recheck the airway.
  - Observe the seizure activity.
  - Do *not* attempt to start an IV line yet; it will be much easier in 1 or 2 minutes, after the seizure has stopped.
  - Ensure that IV tubing is flushed through with NS and that thiamine, D50W, diazepam, and two blood tubes are all available at the bedside.
- If the seizure has lasted > 3 minutes
  - Draw blood (20 ml) and establish IV access.

Tips on Starting the IV Line. When the patient is seizing, it is very difficult to start an IV line. This is an emergency and not the time for a novice to try his or her hand at starting the IV. Appoint the most experienced person present to obtain IV access. The patient's arm should be held firmly by one or two assistants (Fig. 23–3) while maintaining the patient on the side. Sit down—it is much easier to start an IV line when sitting rather than standing. Try for the largest vein available but not the antecubital vein unless forced because the elbow will then have to be splinted to avoid losing the IV access.

Medications. Order the following medications to be given immediately.
- *Thiamine* 100 mg IV by slow, direct injection over 3 to 5 minutes.
- *D50W* 50 ml IV by slow, direct injection. If hypoglycemic, the patient will become conscious abruptly while receiving the first 30 ml of D50W. Do not proceed with any further medication; change the IV fluid to D5W. Thiamine is given before the administration of glucose to protect against an exacerbation of Wernicke's encephalopathy.
- *Diazepam* (Valium) at a rate of 2 mg/min IV until the seizure stops or to a maximum dose of 20 mg. It will take 10 minutes to deliver 20 mg of diazepam at this rate. (An Ambu bag should be available at the bedside whenever diazepam is

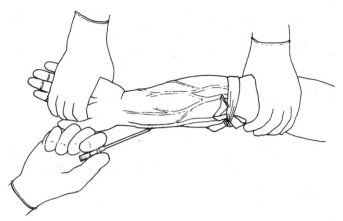

Figure 23–3 □ Positioning required when starting an IV line during a generalized tonic-clonic seizure.

being given IV because diazepam may cause respiratory depression.) If diazepam is not available, a good alternative is *lorazepam* (Ativan) 2 to 4 mg IV over 3 to 5 minutes.
- Phenytoin. Ask an assistant to obtain the following.
  - A second IV setup with NS (Fig. 23–4). Diazepam and phenytoin are not compatible, so they cannot be given via the same IV line.
  - *Phenytoin,* loading dose 18 mg/kg (1250 mg for a 70-kg patient), to be available at the bedside. The phenytoin loading dose may be injected directly via NS IV at a rate no faster than 25 to 50 mg/min or as an infusion (add the loading dose to 100 ml of NS) given at a rate not greater than 25 to 50 mg/min. After phenytoin administration, the IV line should be flushed through with NS to avoid local venous irritation due to the alkalinity of the drug. Phenytoin may cause hypotension and cardiac dysrhythmias. Monitor the femoral pulse for decrease of volume (hypoten-

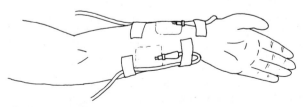

Figure 23–4 □ Two IV lines are needed if both diazepam (Valium) and phenytoin (Dilantin) are to be administered.

sion) and for irregularities of rhythm (Fig. 23–5). If either of these problems occurs, slow the phenytoin infusion rate.

If seizing continues despite administering half the maximum dose of diazepam (10 mg), begin administering the loading dose of phenytoin (Dilantin) (no faster than 25 to 50 mg/min) but continue with the diazepam until the maximum dose has been given.

If the patient has *already received phenytoin* or has an inadequate level, give *half* the phenytoin loading dose IV. The most frequent side effects of overshooting with an extra loading dose are dizzi-

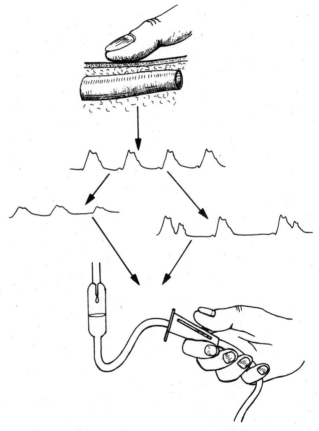

Figure 23–5 □ Phenytoin (Dilantin) may cause hypotension or cardiac dysrhythmias, detectable by palpating the femoral pulse. If either one is present, the phenytoin infusion rate should be slowed.

ness, nausea, and blurred vision for a few days. These are not major risks.

If the seizure now stops, stop giving the diazepam but give the full loading dose of phenytoin. It now becomes practical to arrange for continuous electrocardiographic monitoring and repeated measurements of BP, which is important while the remainder of the phenytoin is being infused. See page 256 for further instructions. Most seizures can be controlled with diazepam and phenytoin. If not, CNS infection or structural brain disease should be considered.

If the seizure has persisted for 30 minutes, the patient is now in *status epilepticus.* This is an emergency! A neurologist, intensivist, or anesthesiologist should be consulted immediately. The patient should be transferred to the intensive care unit/ cardiac care unit (ICU/CCU) for management of the airway and probable intubation.

Status epilepticus is rare. It is defined as a single seizure lasting 30 minutes or repetitive seizures without intervening periods of normal consciousness, lasting more than 30 minutes.

Additional treatment in the ICU/CCU may include an IV phenobarbital infusion or, rarely, general anesthesia with halothane and neuromuscular blockade.

24

SHORTNESS OF BREATH

Calls at night to assess a patient's breathing are common. Do not become overwhelmed by the myriad causes of shortness of breath (SOB) that you learned in medical school. In hospitalized patients, as you will see, there are only four common causes of SOB.

■ PHONE CALL

Questions

1. **How long has the patient had SOB?**
2. **Did the SOB begin gradually or suddenly?**
   The sudden onset of SOB suggests pulmonary embolus or pneumothorax.
3. **Is the patient cyanotic?**
4. **What are the vital signs?**
5. **What was the reason for admission?**
6. **Does the patient have chronic obstructive pulmonary disease (COPD)?**
   What you need to know is whether the patient is a CO_2 retainer. In most cases, this will apply to patients with COPD or with a history of heavy smoking.
7. **Does the patient have O_2 ordered?**

Orders

1. *Oxygen.* If you are certain that the patient is not a CO_2 retainer, you may safely order any concentration of O_2 in the short-term situation. If you are not certain, order O_2 28% by Venturi mask and reassess on arrival at the bedside.
2. If the admitting diagnosis is asthma and the patient has not received an inhaled bronchodilator within the last 2 hours, order nebulized *salbutamol* 2.5 to 5 mg in 5 ml of normal saline (NS) or 180 μg (2 puffs) by metered dose inhaler, immediately.
3. *Arterial blood gas* (ABG) set at bedside. Not all patients with SOB will require ABG determination, but it is best to have the equipment ready on arrival if needed. Alternatively, ask for an urgent measurement of pulse oximetry, if available.

Inform RN

"Will arrive at bedside in . . . minutes."
SOB requires you to see the patient immediately.

■ ELEVATOR THOUGHTS
(What causes SOB?)

1. Cardiovascular causes
   a. Congestive heart failure (CHF)
   b. Pulmonary embolism
2. Pulmonary causes
   a. Pneumonia
   b. Bronchospasm (asthma and COPD)
3. Miscellaneous causes
   a. Anxiety, upper airway obstruction, pneumothorax, massive pleural effusions, massive ascites, postoperative atelectasis, cardiac tamponade, and aspiration of gastric contents

■ MAJOR THREAT TO LIFE

- Hypoxia
  Inadequate tissue oxygenation is the most worrisome end result of any process causing SOB. Hence, you must direct your initial assessment toward determining whether hypoxia is present.

■ BEDSIDE

Quick Look Test

Does the patient look well (comfortable), sick (uncomfortable or distressed), or critical (about to die)?
This simple observation will help determine the necessity of immediate intervention. If the patient looks sick, order ABGs, O_2, and an IV of D5W TKVO. Ask the RN to bring the cardiac arrest cart to the bedside, attach the patient to the ECG monitor, and prepare for possible intubation. Consult the ICU immediately.

Airway and Vital Signs

Check that the upper airway is clear.

What is the respiratory rate (RR)?
Rates < 12/min suggest a central depression of ventilation, which is usually due to a stroke, narcotic overdose, or some other drug overdose. Rates > 20/min suggest hy-

poxia, pain, or anxiety. Look also for thoracoabdominal dissociation that may indicate impending respiratory failure. Remember that the chest cage and abdominal wall normally move in the same direction.

What is the heart rate (HR)?

Sinus tachycardia is an expected accompaniment of hypoxia. This is because vascular beds supplying hypoxic tissue dilate, and a compensatory sinus tachycardia occurs in an effort to increase cardiac output and thereby improve oxygen delivery.

What is the temperature?

An elevated temperature suggests infection (pneumonia, pyothorax, or bronchitis) but is consistent with pulmonary embolism.

What is the blood pressure (BP)?

Hypotension may indicate CHF, septic shock, massive pulmonary embolism, or tension pneumothorax (see Chapter 18). Suspicion of any of these conditions should prompt you to call your resident for help. Also, measure the amount of pulsus paradoxus, which, in asthmatics, roughly correlates with the degree of airflow obstruction. Pulsus paradoxus also may be a clue to the presence of cardiac tamponade.

Pulsus paradoxus is an inspiratory fall in systolic BP > 10 mm Hg. To determine whether a pulsus paradoxus is present, inflate the BP cuff 20 to 30 mm Hg above the palpable systolic BP. Deflate the cuff slowly. Initially, Korotkoff's sounds will be heard only in expiration. At some point during cuff deflation, Korotkoff's sounds will appear in inspiration as well. The number of millimeters of mercury (mm Hg) between the initial appearance of Korotkoff's sounds and their appearance throughout the respiratory cycle represents the degree of pulsus paradoxus (Fig. 24–1).

Selective Physical Examination

Is the patient hypoxic?

Vitals	Repeat now. Again, ensure airway patency.
HEENT	Check for central cyanosis (blue tongue and mucous membranes).
	Check that the trachea is midline.
Resp	Are breath sounds present and of normal intensity? Check for crackles, wheezing, consolidation, or pleural effusion.
Neuro	Check level of sensorium. Is the patient alert, confused, drowsy, or unresponsive?

Cyanosis often does not occur until there is severe hemoglobin

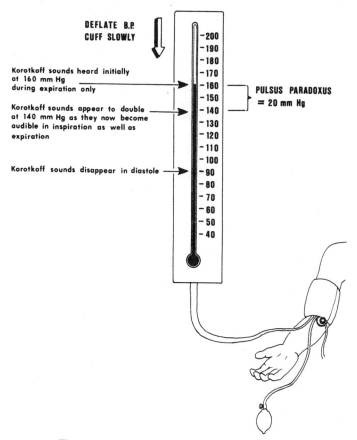

DEFLATE B.P. CUFF SLOWLY

Korotkoff sounds heard initially at 160 mm Hg during expiration only

Korotkoff sounds appear to double at 140 mm Hg as they now become audible in inspiration as well as expiration

Korotkoff sounds disappear in diastole

PULSUS PARADOXUS = 20 mm Hg

Figure 24–1 □ Determination of pulsus paradoxus.

desaturation and may not occur at all in the anemic patient. If hypoxia is suspected, confirm by ABG measurement. *Remember*: Cyanosis is helpful only if it is present—its absence does not mean that the P_{O_2} is adequate.

Management

What immediate measure needs to be taken to correct hypoxia?
Supply adequate O_2. The initial concentration of O_2 ordered depends on your judgment of how sick the patient is. An accurate assessment can be made by drawing ABG samples, beginning empirical O_2 treatment, and adjusting F_{IO_2},

depending on the results of subsequent ABGs or pulse oximetry. If pulse oximetry is available, gradually increase the FIO_2 until the O_2 saturation is $> 94\%$; then, recheck with ABGs. Remember that pulse oximetry tells you nothing about PCO_2, pH, or $(A-a)O_2$ gradient. In most cases, a $PO_2 > 60$ mm Hg or an O_2 saturation of 94% is adequate.

What harm can your treatment cause?

Some patients with COPD are CO_2 retainers and are dependent on mild hypoxia to stimulate the respiratory center. An $FIO_2 > 0.28$ may remove this hypoxic drive to breathe. Unless there is or has been hypercarbia (check the patient's old chart), it is difficult to predict which patients with COPD will be CO_2 retainers, and it is therefore prudent to assume that all patients with COPD and heavy smoking histories are CO_2 retainers until proven otherwise.

Administration of 100% O_2 can cause atelectasis or O_2 toxicity if given over a period of days. This is of more concern in the mechanically ventilated patient because these FIO_2 levels are impossible to attain unless the patient is intubated.

Why is the patient SOB or hypoxic?

There are four common causes of SOB in hospitalized patients, as follows:

- Cardiovascular causes
  1. CHF
  2. Pulmonary embolism
- Pulmonary causes
  3. Pneumonia
  4. Bronchospasm (asthma and COPD)

In most cases, you will find it easy to distinguish among these four conditions. Look for specific associated signs and symptoms, as outlined in Table 24–1, that will help you identify which one of the four major causes of SOB your patient is most likely to have and treat him or her accordingly. Once you have established which pattern of SOB your patient most likely has, take a more thorough selective history and physical examination.

CARDIOVASCULAR CAUSES

Congestive Heart Failure

Selective History

- Is there a history of CHF or cardiac disorder?
- Is there orthopnea?

Table 24-1 □ DISCRIMINATING FEATURES IN THE HISTORY AND PHYSICAL EXAMINATION OF A PATIENT WITH SOB

	CHF	Pulmonary Embolism and Infarction	Pneumonia	Asthma/COPD
History				
Onset	Gradual	Sudden	Gradual	Gradual
Other	Orthopnea PND	Risk factors (see p 275)	Cough Fever Sputum production	Previous history
Physical Examination				
Temperature	Normal	Normal or slightly elevated	High	Normal
Pulsus paradoxus	No	No	No	Yes
JVP	Elevated	Elevated or normal	Normal	Normal
S_3	Present	Occasional RVS_3 present	Absent	Absent
Respiratory				
Crackles	Bibasal	Unilateral	Unilateral	No
Wheezes	±	±	±	Present
Friction rub	No	±	±	No
Other	Pleural effusions		Consolidation Bronchial breath sounds Whispering pectoriloquy	

- Is there paroxysmal nocturnal dyspnea (PND)?
- Are there trends in daily weight or fluid balance records that may heighten your suspicion of fluid retention and hence CHF?

Selective Physical Examination

Assess the *volume status*. **Is the patient volume overloaded?**

Vitals	Tachycardia, tachypnea
HEENT	Elevated JVP
Resp	Inspiratory crackles ± pleural effusions (more often on the right side)
CVS	Cardiac apex displaced laterally
	S₃
	Systolic murmurs (aortic stenosis, mitral regurgitation, VSD, tricuspid regurgitation)
ABD	Hepatomegaly with positive HJR
Ext	Presacral or ankle edema

Crackles and S_3 are the most reliable indication of left-sided heart failure, whereas elevated jugular venous pressure (JVP), enlarged liver, positive hepatojugular reflex (HJR), and peripheral edema indicate right-sided heart failure.

Chest X-ray (CXR) (Fig. 24–2)
- Cardiomegaly
- Perihilar congestion

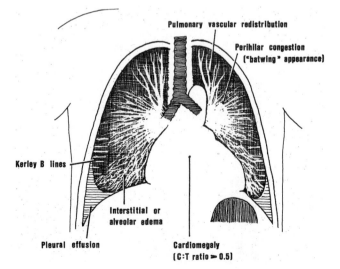

Figure 24–2 □ Chest x-ray features of congestive heart failure.

- Bilateral interstitial (early) or alveolar (more advanced) infiltrates
- Redistribution of pulmonary vascular markings
- Kerley's B lines
- Pleural effusions

Treatment

General Measures

- IV D5W TKVO. IV access is required to deliver medications. Switch to heparin lock when the acute episode has resolved.
- O_2
- Restricted sodium diet
- Bedrest
- SC heparin (5000 U SC every 12 hours). Patients with CHF are predisposed to venous thrombosis and pulmonary emboli and should receive prophylactic SC heparin while at bedrest.
- Fluid balance charting
- Daily weight

Specific Measures. Cardiac function can be improved by altering preload, afterload, or contractility. In the acute situation, intervention initially involves decreasing the preload.

- Sit the patient up; this position pools blood in the legs.
- Give *morphine sulfate* 2 to 4 mg IV every 5 to 10 minutes up to 10 to 12 mg pools blood in the splanchnic circulation. Morphine sulfate may cause hypotension or respiratory depression. Take the BP and RR before and after each dose is given. If necessary, *naloxone hydrochloride* 0.2 to 2.0 mg IV, IM, or SC may be used to reverse the hypotension or respiratory depression of morphine, up to a total of 10 mg. Nausea or vomiting also may occur and usually can be controlled with *dimenhydrinate* 25 mg IV/IM or 50 mg PO every 4 hours as needed (PRN).
- Give *nitroglycerin ointment* 2.5 to 5.0 cm (1 to 2 inches) topically every 6 hours. If nitroglycerin ointment is not readily available, you may instead give *nitroglycerin tablets* 0.3 to 0.6 mg SL or *nitroglycerin spray* 1 puff SL every 5 minutes until the patient feels less SOB, as long as the systolic BP remains > 90 mm Hg. All nitroglycerin preparations pool blood in the peripheral circulation. Nitroglycerin preparations commonly cause headaches, which can be treated with *acetaminophen* 325 to 650 mg PO every 4 hours PRN.

These three measures are temporary, shifting the excessive intravascular volume from the central veins. Only the diuretics, furosemide and metolazone, actually reduce extracellular volume.

- Give *furosemide* 40 mg IV given over 2 to 5 minutes. If there is no response (e.g., a lessening of the symptoms and signs of CHF, a diuresis), double the dose every 1 hour (i.e., 40, 80, and then 160 mg) to a total dose of about 400 mg. Larger initial doses (e.g., 80 to 120 mg) may be required if the patient has renal insufficiency, is in severe CHF, or is already on maintenance furosemide. Doses of furosemide > 100 mg should be infused at a rate not exceeding 4 mg/min to avoid ototoxicity. Smaller initial doses (e.g., 10 mg) may suffice for frail, elderly (80- to 90-year-old) patients.

- If furosemide is not effective, diuresis may be achieved with *metolazone* 2.5 to 10 mg PO. Metolazone has been shown to result in a dramatic diuresis when combined with furosemide.

The diuretics mentioned may cause hypokalemia, which is of particular concern in the patient receiving digitalis. Monitor the serum potassium level once or twice daily in the acute situation. High doses of these diuretics also may lead to serious sensorineural hearing loss, especially if the patient is also receiving other ototoxic agents, such as aminoglycoside antibiotics.

If diuretics are ineffective, it is unlikely that the patient is going to produce urine. Other methods of removing intravascular volume, such as *phlebotomy* (200 to 300 ml) and *rotating tourniquets*, are seldom required in the hospital setting. If there is a persistent component of bronchospasm (cardiac asthma), an inhaled beta agonist may improve oxygenation.

Digoxin is not of benefit acutely unless the CHF was precipitated by a bout of supraventricular tachycardia (e.g., atrial fibrillation or flutter with rapid ventricular response rates), which can be slowed by digoxin. (Refer to Chapter 15 for the management of tachydysrhythmias.)

Causes of CHF. *CHF is a symptom* and a very serious one! After you have treated the symptom, sit down and determine *why* the patient developed CHF. This requires you to identify the *etiologic factor*, of which there are six possibilities.

1. Coronary artery disease
2. Hypertension
3. Valvular heart disease
4. Cardiomyopathy (dilated, restrictive, hypertrophic)
5. Pericardial disease
6. Congenital heart disease

If the patient has a *history* of CHF, the *etiologic factor* may already be identified for you in the patient's chart. However, the job does not end there, for now you must also identify a *precipitating factor*, of which the following 10 are most common:

1. Myocardial infarction (MI) or ischemia
2. Fever, infection
3. Dysrhythmia
4. Pulmonary embolism

5. Increased sodium load (dietary, medicinal, parenteral)
6. Cardiac depressant drugs (e.g., beta blockers, disopyramide, calcium entry blockers)
7. Sodium-retaining agents (e.g., nonsteroidal anti-inflammatory drugs [NSAIDs])
8. Noncompliance with diet or medication
9. Renal disease
10. Anemia

Remember that any *new etiologic factor* may also act as a *precipitating factor* in a patient with a history of CHF. Document the suspected *etiologic* and *precipitating* factors in the chart.

Pulmonary Embolism

The classic triad of SOB, hemoptysis, and chest pain actually occurs in only a minority of cases. The best way to avoid missing this diagnosis is to consider it in each patient with SOB whom you see.

Selective History

Look for predisposing causes.

Stasis
- Prolonged bedrest
- Immobilized limb
- Obesity
- CHF
- Pregnancy

Vein Injury
- Trauma (especially hip fractures)
- Surgery (especially abdominal, pelvic, and orthopedic procedures)

Hypercoagulability
- Malignancy
- Inflammatory bowel disease
- Nephrotic syndrome
- Use of birth control pills
- Deficiencies of antithrombin III, protein C or S; antiphospholipid antibodies; Factor V Leiden mutation

Selective Physical Examination

Features suggestive of pulmonary embolism include the following:
- Pleural friction rub
- Pulmonary consolidation

- Unilateral or bilateral pleural effusion
- Sudden-onset cor pulmonale
- New-onset tachydysrhythmia
- Simultaneous deep venous thrombosis (DVT)

CXR (Fig. 24–3). If clinically stable, the patient should have an upright posteroanterior (PA) and lateral CXR rather than a portable CXR to ensure optimal imaging and prevent masking of pleural fluid, which can occur when images are taken with the patient in the supine position. CXR may reveal the following:

- Atelectasis (loss of volume)
- Unilateral wedge-shaped pulmonary infiltrate
- Unilateral pleural effusion
- Raised hemidiaphragm
- Areas of oligemia
- Entirely normal

ECG. Only a massive pulmonary embolism will give you the classic right ventricular strain pattern of S_1, Q_3, right-axis deviation, and right bundle-branch block (RBBB). The most common ECG finding is a *sinus tachycardia*, but other supraventricular tachycardias also may occur.

ABGs. The most common finding on ABG determination is

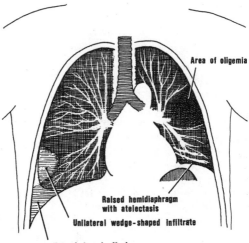

Area of oligemia

Raised hemidiaphragm with atelectasis

Unilateral wedge-shaped infiltrate

Unilateral pleural effusion

Figure 24–3 □ Variable chest x-ray features of pulmonary embolism. Positive findings on radiography depend on the presence of pulmonary infarction. An entirely normal chest x-ray, in the setting of severe SOB, however, is very suggestive of a pulmonary embolism.

acute respiratory alkalosis. Of patients with pulmonary embolism, 85% have $Po_2 < 80$ mm Hg on room air. If the Po_2 is > 80 mm Hg and pulmonary embolism is still suspected, look for an elevated $P(A-a)O_2$. (See Appendix E, pages 410 to 411, for calculation.)

Management

If your suspicion of pulmonary embolism is high and the patient is hypotensive, then thrombolytic therapy should be considered.[1] In this case, call your resident now. The aim of thrombolytic therapy is to dissolve the pulmonary embolism; either *streptokinase* 250,000 IU given IV over 30 minutes followed by 100,000 IU/hr for 24 hours or *tissue plasminogen activator (tPA)* 100 mg IV over 2 hours may be given, but streptokinase is less expensive. Pulmonary arteriotomy with embolectomy may also be life-saving in centers where this procedure is immediately available.[2]

If your suspicion for pulmonary embolism is high and the patient is hemodynamically stable, you are obligated to begin anticoagulation therapy without further confirmation of the diagnosis at this point. The aim of anticoagulation is not to dissolve the pulmonary embolism but rather to prevent further embolization from the site of venous thrombosis, which may prove fatal.

However, before ordering a thrombolytic or an anticoagulant, ensure that the patient has no history of bleeding disorders, peptic ulcers, and intracranial disease, such as recent stroke, subarachnoid hemorrhage (SAH), tumor, and recent surgery. All are contraindications to anticoagulation. These patients will require confirmation of pulmonary embolism with ventilation-perfusion ($\dot{V}/\dot{Q}$) scan or pulmonary angiography and, if embolism is documented, consultation for consideration of interruption of the inferior vena cava by the insertion of a transvenous intracaval device.

Draw a blood sample for complete blood count (CBC), activated partial thromboplastin time (aPTT), PT, and platelet count immediately. If there are *no contraindications,* begin *heparin* 100 U/kg IV bolus (usual dose, 5000 to 10,000 U IV) and follow with a maintenance infusion of 1000 to 1600 U/hr, with the lower range selected for patients with a higher risk of bleeding.

Heparin should be delivered by infusion pump, with maintenance dosing ordered as in the following example: heparin 25,000 U/500 ml D5W to run at 20 ml/hr = 1000 U/hr. It is dangerous to put large doses of heparin in small-volume IV bags because runaway IV bags filled with heparin can result in serious overdose.

Heparin and warfarin are dangerous drugs because of their potential for causing bleeding disorders. Write and double-check your heparin orders carefully. Also, measure platelet counts once or twice a week to detect reversible heparin-induced thrombocytopenia, which may occur at any time while a patient is on heparin.

Low-molecular-weight heparin (LMWH) is a safe and effective alternative to IV unfractionated heparin in the treatment of selected patients with pulmonary embolism.[3] Several formulations of LMWH exist, with different distributions of molecular weight resulting in differences in their inhibitory activities against factor Xa and thrombin, the extent of plasma protein binding, and their plasma half-lives. You should familiarize yourself with the LMWH formulation used in your hospital. Also, be careful to note that the dose of LMWH used in the *treatment* of pulmonary embolism is considerably higher than that used for *prophylaxis* of DVT. One formulation used for the *treatment* of pulmonary embolism is *tinzaparin* 175 U/kg SC daily.

After starting heparin, obtain a $\dot{V}/\dot{Q}$ scan as soon as possible to confirm the diagnosis of pulmonary embolism. A *high-probability* $\dot{V}/\dot{Q}$ scan indicates an approximately 90% probability for pulmonary embolism[4] and is sufficient evidence to continue anticoagulation. A *normal* $\dot{V}/\dot{Q}$ scan rules out clinically important pulmonary embolism. A *low-* or *intermediate-probability* $\dot{V}/\dot{Q}$ scan in the presence of high clinical suspicion should be confirmed by pulmonary angiography before committing the patient to long-term anticoagulation. Alternatively, the demonstration of simultaneous DVT by nuclear or contrast venography, impedance plethysmography, or duplex ultrasonography is sufficient evidence to continue anticoagulation.

In patients receiving IV unfractionated heparin, monitor the aPTT every 4 to 6 hours and adjust the heparin maintenance dose until the aPTT is in the therapeutic range (1.5 to 2.5 times normal). After this, daily aPTT measurements are sufficient. Initial measurements of aPTT are made only to ensure adequate anticoagulation. Because of the more predictable anticoagulant response of LMWHs, patients receiving this medication do not require monitoring of the aPTT.

Continue IV heparin for 5 days. Add oral warfarin on the first day, beginning at 10 mg PO and titrating the dose to achieve a prothrombin time (PT) with an international normalized ratio (INR) of 2.0 to 3.0. (This corresponds to a PT of 1.3 to 1.5 times control, using rabbit brain thromboplastin. If you are unsure of the method used by your laboratory, call them and ask.) Measure aPTT *and* PT daily during this initial adjustment phase. The attainment of a therapeutic PT will usually take 5 days, at which time the heparin can be discontinued.

Numerous drugs interfere with warfarin metabolism to increase or decrease the PT. Before prescribing any drug to a patient on warfarin, look up its effect on warfarin metabolism and monitor PTs carefully if an interaction is anticipated.

Except in unusual circumstances, a patient receiving heparin should receive no aspirin-containing drugs, sulfinpyrazone, dipyridamole, or thrombolytic agents and no IM injections.

Ask your patient daily about signs of bleeding or bruising. Instruct your patient that prolonged pressure after venipuncture will be required to prevent local bruising while on anticoagulation.

PULMONARY CAUSES

Pneumonia

Selective History and Physical Examination

- Cough: A cough productive of purulent sputum is typical. However, the cough may be dry in the early stages of pneumonia.
- Fever, chills
- Pleuritic chest pain
- Is the patient immunocompromised?
- Pulmonary consolidation ± pleural effusion

Laboratory Data

CBC. A white blood cell (WBC) count > 15,000/mm³ suggests a bacterial infection. Lower counts, however, do not exclude a bacterial cause of pneumonia. Lymphopenia (absolute lymphocyte count < 1000/mm³) or a low CD4 cell count (< 200/mm³) suggests that you are dealing with pneumonia in a human immunodeficiency virus (HIV)–infected patient.[5]

CXR. There are variable findings, from patchy diffuse infiltrates to consolidation (pleural effusion). Remember that a volume-depleted patient may not manifest the typical CXR findings of pneumonia until the intravascular volume is restored to normal. Trust your clinical examination.

Identify the Organism

- Sputum Gram's stain and culture. If the patient is not able to spontaneously cough up sputum, you may induce it with ultrasonic nebulization or chest physical therapy. Take a sputum sample to the laboratory yourself and examine the Gram's stain. (See Appendix E, page 417, for interpretation of the Gram's stain.) Sputum should also be sent for staining and culture for acid-fast bacilli and *Legionella* culture or direct fluorescent antibody test.

- Blood culture ($\times$ 2)
- Blood for measurement of *Mycoplasma* IgM
- Thoracentesis. Moderate to large pleural effusions should be tapped to exclude empyema. Pleural biopsy also will be necessary if tuberculosis (TB) is a consideration. Send pleural fluid to the laboratory for
  - Gram's stain and aerobic and anaerobic cultures
  - Ziehl-Neelsen (ZN) stain and TB cultures
  - Cell count and differential
  - Lactate dehydrogenase (LDH)
  - Protein
  - Glucose
- If appropriate, send for
  - Fungal cultures
  - pH
  - Cytology
  - Amylase
  - Triglycerides

A simultaneous serum glucose, protein, and LDH should be drawn immediately after the pleural tap has been completed. These serum determinations are necessary to compare with pleural fluid values in assessing whether the fluid is a transudate or exudate.

Always consider TB in your differential diagnosis. Order ZN stains and sputum for culture if TB is suspected.

Pneumocystis carinii is the most common cause of pneumonia in the patient who is positive for HIV. This organism occasionally may be demonstrated by immunofluorescent staining of a sputum sample obtained by inducing sputum production, although bronchoalveolar lavage is still the best method of confirming the diagnosis.

Management

General Measures
- O_2
- Chest physical therapy

Specific Measures
- Antimicrobial agents

Your choice will depend on the results of Gram's stain or other available stains. However, in the absence of a definitive smear, your choice of antimicrobial agent should be made by considering rapidity of progression, the severity of the pneumonia, and the presence of comorbid conditions.

For **community-acquired pneumonia** in immunocompetent individuals of a severity to require hospitalization, the probable organisms include

Streptococcus pneumoniae

"Atypical" agents *(Mycoplasma pneumoniae, Chlamydia pneumoniae, Legionella)*

Hemophilus influenzae

A useful antibiotic choice is *erythromycin* 500 mg PO or IV every 6 hours. Erythromycin IV is painful. This can be reduced by diluting each 500-mg dose in 500 ml of fluid and giving slowly over 6 hours. If *S. pneumoniae* (pneumococci) is diagnosed, the antibiotic of choice, in sensitive strains, remains *penicillin G* 1 to 2 million units IV every 4 to 6 hours.

For **rapidly progressing pneumonia, aspiration pneumonia** (oral anaerobes), pneumonia complicating **COPD,** and pneumonia acquired in **hospital or nursing homes,** the following *additional* organisms are possible:

Oral anaerobes

Gram-negative bacilli

Staphylococcus aureus

A useful antibiotic choice in these situations is one of the following:

Cefuroxime 500 mg PO or IV every 12 hours, or

Cefixime 400 mg PO every 24 hours, or

Trimethoprim-sulfamethoxazole 160 mg/800 mg PO every 8 to 12 hours, or

Amoxicillin/clavulanate 500 mg PO every 8 hours

For **severe pneumonia** (defined by the presence of cavitation, involvement of more than one lobe, respiratory failure, or sepsis), the additional organism that may be the cause is

Pseudomonas aeruginosa

A useful antibiotic choice is

Ceftazidime 1 to 2 g IV every 8 hours, or

Imipenem/cilastatin 500 mg every 6 to 8 hours

Either of these choices may be combined with an aminoglycoside such as *gentamicin* 2 to 3 mg/kg as a loading dose followed by maintenance doses determined by the creatinine clearance.

Aspiration pneumonias should be considered in any situation in which a decreased level of consciousness or an interference with the cough reflex has occurred (e.g., alcoholism, stroke, seizure, postsurgery). Episodes of aspiration do not require antibiotic treatment unless there are clinical signs of bacterial infection (e.g., fever, sputum production, leukocytosis).

Alcoholics, in addition to patients with aspiration pneumonias, have a high frequency of *Klebsiella pneumoniae.* This should be treated with two drugs—usually a cephalosporin and an aminoglycoside, such as *cefazolin* 1 to 2 g IV every 8 hours and *gentamicin* 1.5 to 2 mg/kg IV loading dose, followed by 1 to 1.5 mg/kg IV every 8 hours of gentamicin if renal function is normal. Aminoglycosides can cause nephrotoxicity and ototoxicity. Avoid these side effects by following serum aminoglycoside levels, usually after the third or fourth maintenance dose, and serum creatinine levels. If the patient already has renal insufficiency, *give the same loading dose* but adjust the maintenance dose interval according to the creatinine clearance (see Appendix E, page 410).

The most common infecting pulmonary pathogen in **HIV-positive** patients is *P. carinii*. Urgent diagnostic bronchoscopy is advisable when this organism is suspected, although induced sputum samples may sometimes demonstrate the organism. If the patient looks sick and bronchoscopy is not immediately available, the attending physician may want to give one dose of *trimethoprim-sulfamethoxazole* or *pentamidine isethionate* and arrange for bronchoscopy as soon as possible. Steroids also may be helpful in patients who are particularly ill with *P. carinii* pneumonia.[6]

Pentamidine has numerous side effects, including hypotension, tachycardia, nausea, vomiting, unpleasant taste, and flushing. Some of these side effects can be minimized by administering the dose in 500 ml D5W over 2 to 4 hours. In addition, biochemical abnormalities may include hyperkalemia, hypocalcemia, megaloblastic anemia, leukopenia, thrombocytopenia, hyperglycemia or hypoglycemia, elevated liver enzyme levels, and dose-related, reversible nephrotoxicity.

Patients with HIV infection are also predisposed to bacterial infections, particularly by encapsulated organisms such as *S. pneumoniae* and *H. influenzae*.[7] Pulmonary infection with *Mycobacterium avium* and fungi (cryptococci, *Histoplasma*, coccidioides) is frequently part of disseminated disease involving these organisms. *Mycobacterium tuberculosis* may occur as localized or disseminated disease.

Bronchospasm (Asthma and Chronic Obstructive Pulmonary Disease)

Asthma is a condition characterized by airflow obstruction that varies significantly over time.

COPD may take the form of *chronic bronchitis*, which is a clinical diagnosis (production of mucoid sputum on most days for 3 months of the year in 2 consecutive years), or *emphysema*, which is a pathological diagnosis (enlargement of airways distal to the terminal bronchioles). Most patients with COPD have features of both.

Selective History

- Does the patient smoke cigarettes?
- Is the patient on theophylline or steroids?
- Has the patient ever required intubation?

- Can precipitating factors (e.g., specific allergies, nonspecific irritants, upper respiratory tract infection [URTI], pneumonia, beta blocker administration) be identified?
- Is the patient having an anaphylactic reaction? Look for evidence of systemic autocoid (e.g., histamine) release (i.e., wheezing), itch (urticaria), and hypotension. Anaphylactic reactions in hospitalized patients are most commonly seen after the administration of IV dye, penicillin, or aspirin. If there is suspicion of anaphylaxis, refer immediately to Chapter 18, page 180, for appropriate management. This is an emergency!

Selective Physical Examination

Is there evidence of obstructive airways disease?

Vitals	Pulsus paradoxus
HEENT	Cyanosis
	Elevated JVP (cor pulmonale): Cor pulmonale is defined as right-sided heart failure secondary to pulmonary disease.
	Position of trachea: A pneumothorax may be a complication of asthma/COPD and results in a shift of the trachea away from the affected side.
Resp	Intercostal indrawing
	Use of accessory muscles of respiration
	Increased anteroposterior (AP) diameter
	Hyperinflated lungs with depressed hemidiaphragms
Wheez-ing	Diffuse wheezing is most often a manifestation of asthma or COPD but may also be seen in CHF (cardiac asthma), pulmonary embolism, pneumonia, or anaphylactic reactions. Ensure that the patient has not undergone IV dye studies within the past 12 hours.
	Prolonged expiratory phase
CVS	Loud P_2
	Right ventricular (RV) heave, RV S_3 (pulmonary hypertension, cor pulmonale)

CXR
- Hyperinflation of lung fields
- Flattened diaphragms
- Increased AP diameter
- Look also for infiltrates (suggesting concomitant pneumonia), atelectasis (suggesting mucous plugging), pneumothorax, or pneumomediastinum.

Spirometry. Spirometry provides an objective measurement of the severity of airflow limitation and is helpful in evaluating the efficacy of your therapy in patients with mild to moderate asthma. Some patients with severe asthma will be too unwell to perform spirometry. The common parameters followed are the forced expiratory volume in 1 second (FEV_1) and the peak expiratory flow rate (PEFR). The results from the best of three attempts should be recorded.

Management

General Measures
- O_2
- Hydration
- Pulse oximetry monitoring

Specific Measures

STEP 1: Inhaled beta agonists, such as *salbutamol* 2.5 to 5.0 mg in 5 ml of NS by nebulizer or 180 μg (2 puffs) by metered-dose inhaler every 4 hours. When delivered properly (Table 24–2) under supervision, therapy given by a metered-dose inhaler is as effective as, and less expensive than, nebulizer treatments.[8] If a patient is too dyspneic and distressed to coordinate the efforts required to allow effective delivery of a beta-2 agonist by metered-dose inhaler, nebulization of the drug may be preferable. An anticholinergic agent, such as *ipratropium bromide* 250 to 500 μg (1.0 to 2.0 ml) in 3 ml of NS by nebulizer, may also improve oxygenation but should always be preceded or followed by an inhaled beta agonist because it occasionally can worsen bronchoconstriction.

Although standard dosing intervals for beta agonists are every 4 to 6 hours, they may be given almost continuously in severe bronchospasm, as long as you watch closely for potential side effects (supraventricular tachycardias, premature ventricular contractions [PVCs], muscle tremors).

Table 24–2 □ TECHNIQUE FOR INHALATION OF BETA₂-ADRENERGIC AGONISTS FROM METERED-DOSE INHALERS

Shake the cannister thoroughly.
Hold the mouthpiece of the inhaler 4 cm in front of the open mouth, or use a spacer between the inhaler and the mouth.
Breathe out slowly and completely.
Discharge the inhaler while taking a slow, deep breath (5 to 6 seconds).
Hold the breath at full inspiration for 10 seconds.

Reprinted with permission from Nelson, HS: β-Adrenergic bronchodilators. N Engl J Med 1995;333:501. Copyright 1995 Massachusetts Medical Society. All rights reserved.

STEP 2: *Steroids* (most useful in patients with pure asthma). In hospitalized patients, IV steroids have no advantage over oral steroids in hastening the resolution of bronchospasm.[9] The optimal steroid preparation and dosage are controversial. However, because pure asthma is predominantly a response to airway inflammation, steroids should be used early in the management of exacerbations. In addition, steroids may take 6 hours to work, so they must be given now if persistent wheezing is anticipated in the next 6 to 24 hours. *Prednisone* 40 to 60 mg PO daily is recommended. If the patient is unable to swallow or absorb oral medications, then *methylprednisolone* 40 to 60 mg IV every 6 hours or *hydrocortisone* 250 to 500 mg IV bolus, followed by a maintenance dose of 100 mg IV every 6 hours, may be given. Beclomethasone dipropionate (Beclovent) is not useful in acute bronchospasm.

Steroids have few side effects in the short-term situation. Sodium retention is of concern in the patient with CHF or hypertension; hyperglycemia may occur in diabetics.

There has been a great deal of concern about tapering steroids too rapidly. A person on steroids for less than 2 weeks can have the steroids discontinued abruptly without fear of steroid withdrawal. Of more concern is exacerbation of wheezing as steroids are tapered. This may limit the rate at which steroids can be withdrawn.

When a patient develops an exacerbation of bronchospasm, a general rule is to administer medications *beyond* what is usually required as an outpatient. For example, an asthmatic patient normally controlled on a salbutamol inhaler at home will probably require both more frequent inhaled beta agonist ± ipratropium, and steroids during an exacerbation. If a patient with COPD is wheezing despite outpatient treatment with a beta agonist and a theophylline preparation or if the patient is already on a small dose of prednisone, he or she should be given higher doses of prednisone during the acute attack.

Theophylline preparations do not provide more bronchodilation than that achieved by beta-2 agonists in patients with acute severe asthma and are no longer recommended.[10, 11]

Look for evidence of bronchitis or pneumonia as the precipitant of bronchospasm. In patients so affected, bronchospasm may persist until appropriate *antibiotics* are given.

Five Warnings in Asthma

1. Sudden acute deterioration in an asthmatic patient may represent a *pneumothorax*.
2. *Rising* P_{CO_2}. Patients with an acute attack of asthma hyperventilate. A normal P_{CO_2} of 40 mm Hg in the acute situation may signify impending respiratory failure.
3. *Disappearance of wheezing* in the acute situation is an ominous

sign, indicating that the patient is not moving sufficient air in and out to generate a wheeze.

4. *Sedatives are contraindicated in asthma and COPD.* The RN may not be aware of this and may unknowingly request a sleeping pill from your colleague while you are off duty. To avoid this pitfall, write clearly in your orders "No sedatives or sleeping pills."

5. Some asthmatic patients have a triad of asthma, nasal polyps, and aspirin sensitivity. When prescribing analgesics in asthmatics, it is best to *avoid NSAIDs,* including aspirin, because fatal anaphylactoid reactions have occurred in some patients given these medications.

RESPIRATORY FAILURE

Any of the four conditions causing SOB and a variety of others may lead to respiratory failure. Suspect that this is occurring if the RR $< 12/$min or if there is thoracoabdominal dissociation. Confirm the diagnosis of acute respiratory failure by ABG determination. A $P_{O_2} < 60$ mm Hg or $P_{CO_2} > 50$ mm Hg with a pH < 7.30 while breathing room air indicates *acute respiratory failure.*

1. Ensure that the patient has not received narcotic analgesics in the past 24 hours, which may depress the RR. Pupillary constriction may give you a hint that a narcotic is the culprit. If a narcotic has been given or if you are uncertain, order *naloxone hydrochloride* 0.2 to 2.0 mg IV immediately.

2. If no response to naloxone occurs, arrange for transfer of the patient to the ICU/CCU. Acute respiratory acidosis with pH < 7.30 may respond to aggressive treatment of the underlying respiratory or neuromuscular disorder. Noninvasive pressure support ventilation delivered by face mask may be useful for acute exacerbations of COPD (if the RR is $> 30/$min and the pH < 7.35) and may prevent the need for intubation.[12] However, if there is no rapid improvement, make arrangements for possible endotracheal intubation. Acute respiratory acidosis with pH < 7.20 usually requires mechanical ventilation until the precipitating cause of respiratory deterioration can be reversed.

■ REMEMBER

1. Abdominal problems can masquerade as SOB. [One of us (S.M.) was once called to see a patient whose SOB resolved as soon as urinary retention was relieved by placement of a Foley catheter and 1300 ml of urine was drained.] Massive ascites and obesity may also compromise respiratory function.

2. Do not be worried about your inexperience with endotracheal intubation. A patient in respiratory failure can be bagged and masked effectively for hours until someone with intubation experience is available to assist you.

3. Notice that *epinephrine* does not appear in the protocol for treatment for asthma. There is no need to use epinephrine in the adult with an attack of asthma or COPD unless bronchospasm as a component of an anaphylactic reaction is present. Epinephrine given inadvertently in cases of cardiac asthma has resulted in fatal MI.

4. An occasional patient has SOB as a manifestation of anxiety. In this instance, SOB is often qualitatively unique, in that the patient describes "shortness of the *deep* breath," with the sensation that he or she cannot get a satisfactory deep breath. Sighing and yawning are common accompaniments.

References

1. Wolfe M, Skibo CK, Goldenhaber SZ: Pulmonary embolic disease: Diagnosis, pathophysiologic aspects, and treatment with thrombolytic therapy. Curr Probl Cardiol 1993 Oct; 18(10):625–627, 630.

2. Gulba DC, Schmid C, Borst HG, et al: Medical compared with surgical treatment for massive pulmonary embolism. Lancet 1994;343:576–577.

3. Simonneau G, Sors H, Charbonnrer B, et al: A comparison of low-molecular-weight heparin with unfractionated heparin for acute pulmonary embolism. N Engl J Med 1997;337:663–669.

4. The PIOPED Investigators: Value of the ventilation/perfusion scan in acute pulmonary embolism. JAMA 1990;263:2753–2759.

5. Bartlett JG, Mundy LM: Community acquired pneumonia. N Engl J Med 1995;333:1618–1624.

6. The National Institutes of Health–University of California Expert Panel for Corticosteroids as Adjunctive Therapy for Pneumocystis Pneumonia: Consensus statement on the use of corticosteroids as adjunctive therapy for pneumocystis pneumonia in the acquired immunodeficiency syndrome. N Engl J Med 1990;323:1500–1504.

7. Shelhamer JH, Toews GB, Masur H, et al: NIH conference. Respiratory disease in the immunosuppressed patient. Ann Intern Med 1992; 117:415–431.

8. Bowton DL, Goldsmith WM, Haponik EF: Substitution of metered dose inhalers for hand-held nebulizers: Success and cost savings in a large, acute care hospital. Chest 1992;101:305–308.

9. Beveridge RC, et al: Guidelines for the emergency management of asthma in adults. Can Med Assoc J 1996;155:25–36.

10. Kelly HW, Murphy S: Beta-adrenergic agonists for acute, severe asthma. Ann Pharmacother 1992;26:81–91.

11. Siegel D, Sheppard D, Gelb A, Weinberg PF: Aminophylline increases the toxicity but not the efficacy of inhaled beta-adrenergic agonist in the treatment of acute exacerbations of asthma. Am Rev Respir Dis 1985;132:283–286.

12. Brochard L, Mancebo J, Wysocki M, et al: Nonivasive ventilation for acute exacerbations of chronic obstructive pulmonary disease. N Engl J Med 1995;333:817–822.

25

SKIN RASHES AND URTICARIA

This chapter will not transform you into a dermatologist, able to diagnose any rash with one quick glance. It will, however, help you to accurately describe rashes about which you are called at night. This ability will facilitate confirmation of the diagnosis in the morning by more experienced physicians. You may be called because a rash has appeared abruptly (e.g., drug reaction), or the patient has been admitted with a rash and the nursing staff is concerned that the rash may be infectious (e.g., scabies or lice). Urticarial rashes are rare in hospitalized patients; however, they are important to recognize because they may be the prodrome of anaphylactic shock.

■ PHONE CALL

Questions

1. **How long has the patient had the rash?**
   If the rash has appeared abruptly, a drug reaction is most likely.
2. **Is there any urticaria (hives)?**
   Urticaria is often the first sign of an impending anaphylactic reaction. Urticaria of the central part of the face is a common manifestation of angioedema.
3. **Is there any facial swelling, audible wheezing, or shortness of breath (SOB)?**
   These features suggest impending airway obstruction.
4. **What are the vital signs?**
5. **What drugs has the patient received within the past 12 hours? Has the patient received blood products or intravenous (IV) contrast material within the past 12 hours?**
   Remember that patients undergoing computed tomography (CT) scans are often given IV contrast material.
6. **Does the patient have any known allergies?**
7. **What was the reason for admission?**

Orders

If the patient has evidence of anaphylaxis or angioedema (urticaria, wheezing, SOB, or hypotension), order the following to be available at the bedside immediately.

1. IV line to be started immediately with normal saline (NS).
2. *Epinephrine* 5 ml (0.5 mg) of 1:10,000 for IV administration (this is available in a predrawn syringe from the emergency cart) or epinephrine 0.5 ml (0.5 mg) of 1:1000 for SC administration. Epinephrine may be required *either* IV *or* SC depending on the severity of the reaction. Do not confuse these doses and routes of administration.
3. *Diphenhydramine* (Benadryl) 50 mg IV
4. *Hydrocortisone* (Solu-Cortef) 250 mg IV

Inform RN

"Will arrive at bedside in . . . minutes."

Evidence of facial urticaria (which may be the first manifestation of angioedema) or of anaphylaxis (urticaria, wheezing, SOB, or hypotension) requires you to see the patient immediately. Also, if the rash is acute and the patient has or is receiving systemic medication, blood, or IV contrast material, you should go directly to the bedside. Assessment of a rash with no associated symptoms of anaphylaxis can wait an hour or two if other problems of higher priority exist.

■ ELEVATOR THOUGHTS
(What causes skin rashes?)

The majority of calls at night regarding acute-onset skin rashes pertain to drug reactions. The lesions may be urticarial and occasionally are associated with life-threatening anaphylaxis. Other drug reactions can have widely varied morphology but are usually symmetric and often start on the buttocks. Early drug reactions are often localized.

1. Urticaria (rare but life threatening)
   a. Drugs
      (1) IV contrast material
      (2) Opiates (codeine, morphine, meperidine)
      (3) Antibiotics (penicillins, cephalosporins, sulfonamides, tetracycline, quinine, polymyxin, isoniazid)
      (4) Anesthetic agents (curare)
      (5) Angiotensin-converting enzyme (ACE) inhibitors (captopril, enalapril, lisinopril, monopril)
      (6) Aspirin and other nonsteroidal anti-inflammatory drugs (NSAIDs)
   b. Blood transfusion reaction
   c. Food allergies—especially nuts, fruits, tomatoes, lobster, shrimp
   d. Physical urticarias—e.g., cold, heat, pressure, vibration
2. Erythematous, maculopapular (morbilliform) rashes

    a. Antibiotics (penicillin, ampicillin, sulfonamides, chloramphenicol). Erythematous maculopapular rashes are common in patients with acquired immunodeficiency syndrome (AIDS) receiving sulfonamides and characteristically occur around day 10 of treatment for *Pneumocystis* pneumonia. Ampicillin commonly causes a generalized maculopapular eruption 2 to 4 weeks after administration of the first dose; thus, it is important to check not only the current drugs the patient is receiving but also all recently discontinued drugs, because the eruption may appear several weeks after the drug has been stopped.

    b. Antihistamines

    c. Antidepressants (amitriptyline)

    d. Diuretics (thiazides)

    e. Oral hypoglycemics

    f. Anti-inflammatory drugs (gold, phenylbutazone)

    g. Sedatives (barbiturates)

    h. Scabies and lice. These organisms commonly produce excoriated papules. The lesions of scabies are usually present in finger webs, wrists, waist, axillae, areolae, genitals, and feet. Lesions from lice may occur anywhere on the body but are common in the scalp, pubic hair, neck, flanks, waistline, and axillae. Both organisms are associated with intense itching.

3. Vesicobullous rashes

    a. Antibiotics (sulfonamides, dapsone)

    b. Anti-inflammatory drugs (penicillamine)

    c. Sedatives (barbiturates)

    d. Halogens (iodides, bromides)

    e. Herpes zoster

    f. Toxic epidermal necrolysis (sulfonamides, allopurinol)

4. Purpura. Drug-induced thrombocytopenia causes nonpalpable purpura, whereas vasculitis causes palpable purpura.

    a. Antibiotics (sulfonamides, chloramphenicol)

    b. Diuretics (thiazides)

    c. Anti-inflammatory drugs (phenylbutazone, indomethacin, salicylates)

5. Exfoliative rashes. If a drug eruption is not recognized early and the drug is not discontinued, the patient may develop mucosal erosions and profound skin injury with blistering and extensive loss of epidermis (Stevens-Johnson syndrome or toxic epidermal necrolysis).

    a. Antibiotics (sulfa derivatives, cotrimoxazole, penicillins, streptomycin)

    b. Anti-inflammatory drugs (phenylbutazone, piroxicam)

    c. Antiseizure medication (carbamazepine, phenytoin)

    d. Sedatives/anxiolytics (barbiturates, chlormezanone)

    e. Miscellaneous (allopurinol)

6. Fixed drug eruption. Certain drugs may produce a skin lesion in a specific area. Repeat administration of the drug reproduces the skin lesion in the same location. The lesion is usually composed of dusky red patches distributed over the trunk or proximal limbs.

 a. Antibiotics (sulfonamides, metronidazole)
 b. Anti-inflammatory drugs (phenylbutazone)
 c. Analgesics (phenacetin)
 d. Sedatives (barbiturates, chlordiazepoxide)
 e. Laxatives (phenolphthalein)

■ MAJOR THREAT TO LIFE

- Upper airway obstruction due to angioedema
- Anaphylactic shock

 Urticarial skin rash may be a prodrome of angioedema or anaphylaxis, whereas other types of skin rashes are not. Drugs and IV contrast material are the usual causes of anaphylactic shock in hospitalized patients—unless the allergic patient was unlucky enough to have been stung by a wasp or to have eaten shrimp.

- Toxic epidermal necrolysis

 The patient will look scalded, with peeling of the outer surface of the skin. Frequently, fever will be difficult to control. If you suspect toxic epidermal necrolysis, you should call for a dermatology consultation immediately, and the patient should be transferred to a burn unit or intensive care unit (ICU)—do not procrastinate and do not give systemic steroids. Common drugs involved include allopurinol, sulfonamides, and anticonvulsants. With *toxic shock syndrome* (see page 182) and *necrotizing fasciitis* (see page 191), the patient is more ill or complains more of local pain than you would expect from objective signs. Obtain a dermatology or infectious disease consult immediately.

■ BEDSIDE

Quick Look Test

Does the patient look well (comfortable), sick (uncomfortable or distressed), or critical (about to die)?

 The patient with upper airway obstruction due to angioedema and the patient with an anaphylactic reaction look apprehensive and usually have SOB and are sitting upright in bed.

Airway and Vital Signs

What is the respiratory rate (RR)?

Tachypnea, particularly if associated with audible stridor or wheezing, is an ominous sign. Inspiratory stridor suggests impending upper airway obstruction—notify your resident and an anesthetist immediately.

What is the blood pressure (BP)?

Hypotension suggests impending or established anaphylactic shock, and the patient requires immediate treatment. If anaphylaxis is suspected, insert a large-bore IV (size 16 when possible), if not already done, and run in normal saline (NS) as fast as possible.

What is the temperature?

Skin rashes are often more prominent when the patient is febrile.

Selective Physical Examination

Is there evidence of an impending anaphylactic reaction?

HEENT	Tongue, pharyngeal, or facial edema (angioedema)
Resp	Wheezing (anaphylaxis)
	If evidence of an impending anaphylactic reaction exists, refer to page 180 for immediate treatment.
Skin	When an urticarial rash appearing as a manifestation of angioedema or anaphylaxis has been ruled out, the remaining task is to describe the rash accurately to help you diagnose the lesion and perhaps to help someone else diagnose it if it disappears or changes by the morning.

Describe the location of the rash.

Is it *generalized, acral* (hands, feet), or *localized*? Remember always to examine the buttocks, a common site for the onset of drug eruptions.

Describe the color of the rash.

- Red, pink, brown, white

Describe the primary lesion (Fig. 25–1).

- *Macule*—flat (noticeable from the surrounding skin because of the color difference)
- *Patch*—a large macule
- *Papule*—solid, elevated, size < 1 cm
- *Plaque*—solid, elevated, size > 1 cm
- *Vesicle*—elevated, well-circumscribed, size < 1 cm

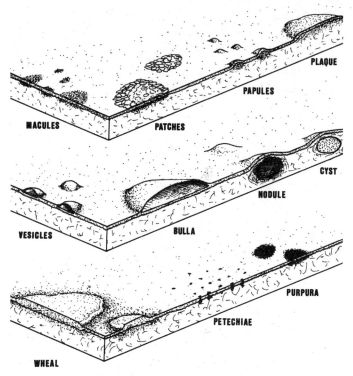

Figure 25–1 □ Primary skin lesions.

- *Bulla*—elevated, well-circumscribed, size > 1 cm
- *Nodule*—deep-seated mass, indistinct borders, size < 0.5 cm in both width and depth
- *Cyst*—nodule filled with expressible fluid or semisolid material
- *Wheal (hives)*—well-circumscribed, flat-topped, firm elevation (papule, plaque, or dermal edema) ± central pallor, and irregular borders
- *Petechia*—red or purple, nonblanchable macule, size < 3 mm
- *Purpura*—red or purple, nonblanchable macule or papule, size > 3 mm

Describe the secondary lesion *(Fig. 25–2).*
- *Scale*—dry, thin plate of thickened keratin layers (white color differentiates it from crust)

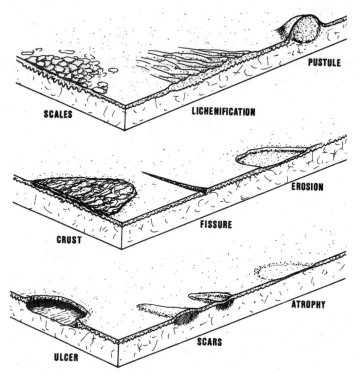

Figure 25–2 □ Secondary skin lesions.

- *Lichenification*—dry, leathery thickening, shiny surface, accentuated skin markings
- *Pustule*—vesicle containing purulent exudate
- *Crust*—dried, yellow exudate of plasma (result of broken vesicle, bulla, or pustule)
- *Fissure*—linear, epidermal tear
- *Erosion*—wide, epidermal fissure, moist and well-circumscribed
- *Ulcer*—erosion into the dermis
- *Scar*—flat, raised, or depressed area of fibrosis
- *Atrophy*—depression secondary to thinning of the skin

Describe the configuration of the rash.
- *Annular*—circular
- *Linear*—in lines
- *Grouped*—clusters, e.g., vesicular lesions of herpes zoster or herpes simplex

Selective History and Chart Review

- How long has the rash been present?
- Does it itch?
- How has it been treated?
- Is this a new or a recurrent problem?
- Which drugs was the patient receiving before the rash started?

Management

1. If the rash is associated with urticaria and thought to be secondary to a drug reaction, the drug should be withheld until confirmation of the diagnosis in the morning.
2. Seemingly minor nonurticarial maculopapular rashes may occasionally be the initial presentation of a more serious reaction such as toxic epidermal necrolysis. Ideally, if the rash is thought to be a drug reaction, the offending drug should be stopped. If the offending medication is essential to the patient's management overnight, a suitable alternative may be chosen. Sometimes no suitable alternative exists, and the decision to stop or continue the offending medication must be made with the help of your resident or attending physician.
3. When the skin rash is not a drug eruption and the diagnosis is clear, the standard recommended treatment can be instituted. (Refer to a dermatology text for specific treatment.)
4. Often, housestaff have difficulty in diagnosing skin rashes with confidence. If uncertain, it is often sufficient to describe the lesion accurately and refer the patient to a dermatologist in the morning. Several important exceptions exist:
   a. A *petechial rash* suggests a disorder of platelet number or function. A *purpuric rash* may indicate a coagulation disorder; activated partial thromboplastin time (aPTT), prothrombin time (PT), and platelet studies should be ordered where appropriate.
   b. *Herpes zoster* appearing in the immunocompromised patient (e.g., the patient with AIDS) may require urgent treatment because of the risk of systemic dissemination, especially to the central nervous system. If you suspect herpes zoster (initially erythematous macules and papules in a dermatomal distribution progressing to grouped vesicles and hemorrhagic crusts) in an immunocompromised patient, consult your resident or attending physician for consideration of beginning treatment with IV acyclovir.

c. Patients with hereditary *deficiency of protein C* may develop skin necrosis, typically 3 to 5 days after beginning warfarin therapy. The skin lesions usually begin as painful red plaques overlying areas of fat. In these cases, warfarin needs to be stopped immediately, its effect reversed with vitamin K, and heparin substituted as an anticoagulant.

26

SYNCOPE

Syncope is a brief loss of consciousness due to sudden reduction in cerebral blood flow. An additional term, "presyncope," has been coined to refer to the situation in which there is reduction in cerebral blood flow sufficient to result in a sensation of impending loss of consciousness, although the patient does not actually pass out. Presyncope and syncope represent degrees of the same disorder and should be addressed as manifestations of the same underlying problem. Your task is to discover the cause of the syncopal attack.

■ PHONE CALL

1. **Did the patient actually lose consciousness?**
2. **Is the patient still unconscious?**
3. **What are the vital signs?**
4. **Is the patient diabetic?**
5. **Was the patient recumbent, sitting, or standing when the episode occurred?**

   Syncope while the patient is in the recumbent position is almost always cardiac in origin.
6. **Was any seizure-like activity witnessed?**
7. **What is the admitting diagnosis?**

   An admitting diagnosis of seizure disorder, transient ischemic attack, or cardiac disease may help direct you to the cause of the syncopal attack.
8. **Has the patient sustained any evidence of injury?**

Orders

If the patient is still *unconscious,* order the following.
1. IV D5W TKVO immediately, if IV line not already in place.
2. Turn the patient on the left side. This maneuver prevents the tongue from falling back into the throat and thus obstructing the upper airway, and minimizes the risk of aspiration should vomiting occur.
3. Stat 12-lead electrocardiogram (ECG) and rhythm strip. Although almost all patients with syncope will regain consciousness within a few minutes, you are more likely to be able to

297

document a cardiac dysrhythmia early while the patient is still symptomatic.
4. If the patient is diabetic, order a stat glucose meter reading, then give 50 ml of D50W IV.
5. If the patient has *regained consciousness*, if there is no evidence of head or neck injury, and if the vital signs are stable, do the following:
   a. To return the patient to bed, ask the RN to slowly raise the patient to a sitting position, then a standing position.
   b. The patient should be placed back in bed, with instructions to remain there until you are able to assess the problem.
   c. Order an ECG and a rhythm strip.
   d. Have the vital signs taken every 15 minutes until you arrive at the bedside. Ask the RN to call you back immediately should the vital signs become unstable before you are able to assess the patient.

Inform RN

"Will arrive at bedside in . . . minutes."

Syncope requires you to see the patient immediately if the patient is still unconscious or if there are abnormalities in the heart rate (HR) or blood pressure (BP). If the patient is alert and conscious with normal vital signs (and if there are other more urgent problems to be assessed), the RN may observe the patient and call you if a problem arises before you are able to assess the patient.

■ ELEVATOR THOUGHTS
(What causes syncope?)

1. Cardiac causes
   a. Dysrhythmias
      (1) Tachycardias
         (a) Ventricular tachycardia
         (b) Ventricular fibrillation
      (2) Bradycardias
         (a) Sinus bradycardia
         (b) Second- and third-degree atrioventricular (AV) block
         (c) Sick sinus syndrome (SSS)
   b. Pacemaker syncope
      (1) Pacemaker failure to capture
      (2) Pacemaker syndrome (i.e., uncoordinated AV contractile sequence)
   c. Syncope with exertion
      (1) Aortic stenosis

       (2) Pulmonic stenosis
       (3) Hypertrophic obstructive cardiomyopathy
       (4) Subclavian steal syndrome
2. Neurologic causes
   a. Brainstem transient ischemic attack (TIA) or stroke (drop attacks)
   b. Seizure
   c. Subarachnoid hemorrhage (SAH)
   d. Cervical spondylosis
3. Neurally mediated (reflex) syncope
   a. The common faint (vasodepressor reaction)
   b. Situational syncope (e.g., cough, micturition, defecation, sneezing, postprandial)
   c. Carotid sinus syncope
4. Orthostatic hypotension
   a. Drug induced
   b. Volume depletion
   c. Autonomic failure
5. Miscellaneous
   a. Pulmonary embolism
   b. Hyperventilation
   c. Anxiety attacks

■ MAJOR THREAT TO LIFE

- Aspiration

  If the patient is still unconscious, aspiration is a major threat to life.

- Dysrhythmia

  If the patient is conscious, recurrence of potentially fatal cardiac dysrhythmia is a major threat.

- Aspiration pneumonia or adult respiratory distress syndrome (ARDS)

  Because most patients recover from syncopal attacks within a few minutes, the actual loss of consciousness experienced by the patient is not the major problem. Of greater importance is that while the patient is unconscious, the patient's tongue may block the oropharynx or the patient may aspirate oral or gastric contents into the lungs, an occurrence that may result in the development of aspiration pneumonia or ARDS. Therefore, in the unconscious patient, your primary goal is to protect the airway until the patient regains consciousness and the cough reflexes are again effective.

- Recurrence of an unrecognized potentially fatal cardiac dysrhythmia.

  Once the patient has regained consciousness, the major threat to life is the recurrence of an unrecognized potentially fatal cardiac dysrhythmia. This can be best identified and managed by transferring the patient to an intensive care unit/cardiac care unit (ICU/CCU) or other setting with ECG monitors if there is suspicion that a dysrhythmia was responsible for the syncopal episode.

■ BEDSIDE

Quick Look Test

Does the patient look well (comfortable), sick (uncomfortable or distressed), or critical (about to die)?

This simple observation helps determine the necessity of immediate intervention. Most patients who have had episodes of syncope and have regained consciousness look perfectly well.

Airway and Vital Signs

Airway

If the patient is still unconscious, ensure that the RN has placed him or her on the left side and that the patient's tongue has not fallen into the back of the throat. Most causes of syncope are very short lived, and by the time you arrive at the bedside, the patient will have regained consciousness. Look for abnormalities in the vital signs, which may help make your diagnosis of the specific cause of syncope much easier.

What is the heart rate?

Supraventricular or ventricular tachycardia should be documented on ECG tracings, and the patient should be treated immediately. (Refer to Chapter 15, page 144, for treatment of supraventricular tachycardia and Chapter 15, page 147, for treatment of ventricular tachycardia.)

Any patient with a transient or persistent supraventricular or ventricular tachycardia or its history when no other cause of syncope can be found should be transferred to the ICU/CCU or other setting with ECG monitoring for appropriate management.

What is the BP?

The patient with resting or orthostatic hypotension should be managed as outlined in Chapter 18. Remember that a massive internal hemorrhage (such as a gastrointestinal [GI] bleed or a ruptured aortic aneurysm) can occasionally present with a syncopal attack.

Hypertension, if found in association with headache and neck stiffness, may indicate SAH. A brief loss of consciousness is common at the onset of an SAH and is often associated with dizziness, vertigo, or vomiting.

What is the temperature?

Patients with syncope are rarely febrile. If fever is present, it is usually due to a concomitant illness not related to the syncopal attack. However, especially if the syncopal attack was unwitnessed, be careful to exclude the possibility of a seizure secondary to meningitis, which may present as "fever + syncope."

Selective History and Chart Review

Has this ever happened before?

If it has, ask the patient if a diagnosis was made after the previous attack.

What does the patient or witnesses recall from the time immediately before the syncope?

- Syncope occurring while in the upright position after an emotional or a painful stimulus and preceded by nausea, diaphoresis, pallor, and a *gradual* loss of consciousness is typical of the common faint (vasodepressor syncope).
- Syncope occurring while changing from the supine or sitting *position* to the standing position suggests orthostatic hypotension.
- An *aura*, though rare, is helpful in pointing to a seizure as the cause of syncope in an unwitnessed attack.
- *Palpitations* preceding an attack may suggest a cardiac dysrhythmia as a cause of syncope.
- Syncope during or immediately after performance of *Valsalva's maneuver* such as a bout of *coughing, micturition, straining at stool, or sneezing* may occur because of transient reduction of venous return to the right atrium and neurally mediated reflex bradycardias.
- Syncope after *turning the head to one side* (especially if one is wearing a tight collar) or while *shaving* may represent carotid sinus syncope. This condition is seen most often in elderly men.
- Syncope occurring during *arm exercise* suggests subclavian steal syndrome.
- *Numbness and tingling* in the hands and feet are commonly experienced just before the presyncope or syncope due to hyperventilation or anxiety.

Is there any history of cardiac disease?

A patient with preexisting cardiac disease may have an increased risk of developing dysrhythmias.

Has the patient ever had a seizure?

An unwitnessed seizure may occur as a syncopal attack. Ask the patient if during the attack he bit his tongue or was incontinent of stool or urine. Either one is suggestive of seizure activity. *Hypoglycemia* should be suspected as a possible cause of seizure or syncope in the diabetic patient receiving oral hypoglycemic agents or insulin.

Has the patient ever had a stroke?

A patient with known cerebrovascular disease is a likely candidate for a brainstem TIA or stroke. However, because atherosclerosis is a diffuse process, the patient with a history of stroke may also have coronary atherosclerosis that may result in cardiac dysrhythmias.

What does the patient remember on waking from the syncopal attack?

Headache, drowsiness, and mental confusion are common sequelae of seizures but not of cardiac or orthostatic causes of syncope.

What are the medications?

Check the chart to see what medications the patient is being given.

Digoxin, beta blockers, and calcium channel blockers may result in bradycardias. Digoxin, if present in toxic amounts, may also precipitate ventricular tachycardia.

Quinidine, procainamide, disopyramide, sotalol, amiodarone, tricyclic antidepressants, phenothiazines, and some of the "nonsedating" antihistamines may prolong the QT interval, leading to ventricular tachycardia (torsades de pointes) (Fig. 26–1*A*) or the prolonged QT interval syndrome (see Fig. 26–1*B*).

Agents that reduce afterload and/or preload (angiotensin-converting enzyme [ACE] inhibitors, hydralazine, prazosin, nitroglycerin) may cause syncope, especially in the elderly or volume-depleted patient.

Phenothiazines, tricyclic antidepressants, alcohol, and cocaine lower the seizure threshold and may result in a seizure.

Oral hypoglycemic agents and insulin may cause hypoglycemic seizures or syncope. Many factors may contribute to erratic glucose levels in hospitalized diabetic patients, including coexisting illnesses, changing activity levels, poor appetite, and medication interactions.

Selective Physical Examination

Your physical examination is directed toward finding a cause for the syncope. However, a search for evidence of injuries sus-

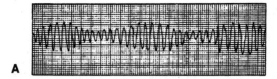

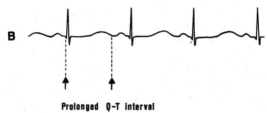

Prolonged Q-T interval
(usually ≈ 0.40 s)

Figure 26–1 □ *A*, Torsades de pointes. *B*, Prolonged QT interval.

tained if the patient fell during the syncopal attack is equally important at this time.

Vitals	Repeat now. At this time take the BP in both arms. A difference > 20 mm Hg may indicate subclavian steal syndrome.
HEENT	Fundoscopy—Look for subhyaloid hemorrhages (SAH). Blood diffuses between the retinal fiber layer and the internal limiting membrane, forming a pocket of blood with sharp borders and often a fluid level.
	Tongue or cheek laceration (seizure disorder)
	Neck stiffness (meningitis leading to a seizure, SAH)
	Supraclavicular or subclavicular bruit (subclavian steal syndrome)
Resp	Crackles, wheezes (aspiration during the syncopal episodes)
CVS	Pacemaker (pacemaker syncope)
	Flat JVP (volume depletion)
	Atrial fibrillation (vertebrobasilar embolism)
	Systolic murmur (aortic stenosis, pulmonic stenosis, hypertrophic obstructive cardiomyopathy)
GU	Urinary incontinence (seizure disorder)

Rectal	Fecal incontinence (seizure disorder)
MSS	Palpate bones for evidence of fracture that may have been sustained if patient fell.
Neuro	A complete neurologic examination must be done, looking for evidence of residual localizing signs that may indicate a TIA, completed stroke, SAH, a space-occupying intracranial lesion, or Todd's paralysis. Vertebrobasilar TIAs or strokes are frequently accompanied by other evidence of brainstem dysfunction (i.e., cranial nerve abnormalities) such as diplopia, nystagmus, facial paralysis, vertigo, dysphagia, dysarthria.

Management

An immediate cause for syncope frequently cannot be found. Because treatment of the various causes of syncope is so different, one must have *documented proof* of the cause of a syncopal episode before proceeding to definitive treatment. Investigations may take several days to complete. Your job, once you have assessed a patient with syncope, is to decide from the history, physical findings, and laboratory data what the most likely cause of syncope is and to arrange for further investigation, if necessary.

Cardiac Causes. If a cardiac cause of syncope is suspected, whether related to dysrhythmia, valvular, or pacemaker cause, the patient should be transferred to the CCU or to an intermediate care unit where continuous ECG monitoring is available. If there are no ECG monitored beds available and if there is no suspicion of ischemia-induced dysrhythmia, 24-hour Holter monitoring should be arranged for the patient first thing in the morning.

Always consider a silent myocardial infarction (MI) with subsequent transient AV block, ventricular tachycardia, or ventricular fibrillation as the cause for syncope of cardiac origin.

Treatment of specific dysrhythmia, if still present at the time you are assessing the patient, is discussed in Chapter 15.
1. Tachycardias
   a. Ventricular tachycardia (page 147)
   b. Supraventricular tachycardia (page 144)
2. Bradycardias
   a. Sinus bradycardia (page 154)
   b. AV blocks (page 154)
   c. SSS (page 154)

Pacemaker syncope will require cardiology consultation for reprogramming of the pacing rate, output, or mode or for an upgrade to AV sequential pacing.

If *aortic stenosis, pulmonic stenosis, or hypertrophic obstructive car-*

diomyopathy is thought to be responsible for exertional syncope, arrange for an echocardiogram in the morning to document the suspected cardiac lesion and ask for a cardiology consultation.

Neurologic Causes. Suspected *brainstem TIA or stroke* should be evaluated by a computed tomography (CT) scan of the head. Anticoagulation or platelet inhibitors should be started only after consultation with a neurologist.

If a *seizure* is suspected, you must first document the cause of the seizure, as outlined in Chapter 23, page 255.

If an *SAH* is suspected, arrange for an urgent noncontrast CT scan of the head, looking for evidence of aneurysm or blood in the subarachnoid space. A normal CT scan does not, however, exclude an SAH, and a lumbar puncture (LP) may be required to look for xanthochromic cerebrospinal fluid. If such a lesion is identified, a neurosurgeon should be consulted for further investigation and management.

Neurally Mediated (Reflex) Syncope. Most vasodepressor attacks can be managed without transfer to the ICU/CCU, as outlined in Chapter 18, page 177.

The definitive diagnosis of *carotid sinus syncope* requires potentially dangerous carotid sinus pressure, which must be done while the ECG is being monitored for cardiac dysrhythmia. Although the patient does not require ICU/CCU admission overnight, arrangements should be made in the morning to evaluate the cardiac rhythm during carotid sinus massage.

Orthostatic Hypotension. Syncope due to *volume depletion* can be managed with IV fluid replacement, as outlined in Chapter 18, page 180.

Drug-induced orthostatic hypotension and *autonomic failure* are complex treatment problems and, as long as the patient's volume status is normal, can be addressed in the morning through consultation with a neurologist or clinical pharmacologist.

Until the underlying problem responsible for orthostatic hypotension is corrected, instruct patients that if they must be out of bed during the night, they should (1) ask the RN for assistance and (2) move slowly from the supine to sitting position and then move slowly again from the sitting to standing position.

Miscellaneous. Syncope due to *hyperventilation* or *anxiety states* can be alleviated by instructing the patient to breathe into a paper bag when he or she begins to feel anxious or presyncopal. This step will correct hypocapnia and thereby prevent a syncopal attack.

■ REMEMBER

1. In the elderly patient, the main hazard of a syncopal attack

is not necessarily an underlying disease but rather a fracture or other injury sustained during a fall.

2. Except for the Stokes-Adams attack (third-degree AV block), true syncope rarely occurs when a patient is in the recumbent position.

27

TRANSFUSION REACTIONS

Blood transfusions are given around-the-clock in hospitals. Reactions to blood products may vary from severe to very mild. An organized approach will help you sort out both the nature of the reaction and what to do about it.

■ PHONE CALL
QUESTIONS

1. **What symptoms does the patient have?**
   Fever, chills, chest pain, back pain, diaphoresis, and shortness of breath (SOB) all can be manifestations of a transfusion reaction.
2. **What are the vital signs?**
3. **Which blood product is being transfused, and how long ago was it started?**
4. **What was the reason for admission?**

Orders

1. Stop the transfusion immediately if the patient has any of the following symptoms.
   a. Sudden onset of hypotension
   b. Chest or back pain, tachypnea
   c. Any symptom (even fever, chills, or urticaria) occurring within minutes of the start of the transfusion
   d. Fever in a patient who has never before received a blood transfusion or who has never been pregnant; this symptom may represent an acute hemolytic reaction

   An acute hemolytic transfusion reaction can appear with any of the aforementioned symptoms. Acute hemolytic reactions, although very rare, are associated with an extremely high mortality rate, which is proportionate to the volume of blood infused. In previously pregnant or transfused patients, fever may be a nonhemolytic febrile reaction.
2. If the blood transfusion has been stopped, keep the intravenous (IV) line open with normal saline (NS).

Inform RN

"Will arrive at bedside in . . . minutes."

Any suspected hemolytic or anaphylactic transfusion reaction requires you to see the patient immediately.

■ **ELEVATOR THOUGHTS**
(What causes transfusion reactions?)

1. Immune hemolysis. Mismatched red blood cells (RBCs) (ABO incompatibility) are errors in either identification of the patient or labeling of the blood. Mismatched RBCs result in an *acute hemolytic reaction*. They are exceedingly rare and usually occur in emergency situations (i.e., in the postanesthetic, operating, or emergency room) when the usual precautions in identification of the patient or labeling of the blood are breached. *Delayed hemolytic reactions* develop as a consequence of prior exposure to foreign red cell antigens (i.e., pregnancy or previous transfusion). Reexposure to these antigens results in an anamnestic rise in alloantibodies that were not detectable at the time of the original crossmatch. Hemolysis occurs 3 to 14 days after transfusion and may be accompanied by fever, jaundice, and increasing anemia.

2. Nonimmune hemolysis. Nonimmune hemolysis may occur if the blood has been overheated or has undergone trauma. Trauma to blood products occurs either by excessive hand squeezing or pumping of the infusion bag during the rapid administration of blood in an emergency or by being delivered through a needle that is too small.

3. Anaphylaxis (IgG response to IgA antibodies). Anaphylaxis may result from transmission of IgA antibodies from the donor's blood into a presensitized IgA-deficient patient.

   a. Congenital IgA deficiency is a common (1:1000), asymptomatic disorder. The first transfusion that an IgA-deficient patient receives will contain IgA antibodies, which are recognized by the patient's immune system as foreign antigens. Thus, the IgA-deficient patient becomes sensitized and develops anti-IgA antibodies, which may result in anaphylaxis or urticaria with subsequent transfusions.

   b. There are two known IgA *allotypes* (an allotype is simply a genetic variation in the structure of the immunoglobulin). Anaphylactic reactions are more common in patients who lack both allotypes of IgA, but they have been reported in patients who lack only one allotype. Individuals with IgA molecules of one allotype may develop antibodies against the other allotype, with subsequent transfusion reactions being exhibited as urticaria or, occasionally, anaphylaxis.

4. Urticaria. Transmission of the following antigens from the donor's blood can cause urticaria.

   a. Food allergens, e.g., shrimp (IgE response)

   b. Other plasma protein allergens

   c. IgA antibodies into an IgA-deficient patient (i.e., deficient

in one of the two allotypes); this is a very rare cause of urticaria
5. Fever
   a. Nonhemolytic febrile reaction. This is the most common cause of febrile transfusion reactions and does not require stopping the transfusion. It is usually seen in multiparous or multitransfused patients and is due to a white blood cell (WBC) antigen-antibody reaction.
   b. Early sign of acute hemolytic transfusion reaction—particularly in patients who have not had prior transfusions or pregnancies.
   c. Pulmonary leukoagglutinin reaction. The donor's blood (usually from a multiparous woman) contains antibodies to the patient's WBCs, resulting in the agglutinated WBCs lodging in the pulmonary capillaries, causing noncardiogenic pulmonary edema.
   d. Microbial contamination (very rare). Although many infectious agents can be transmitted via blood transfusions (causing, for example, non-A, non-B hepatitis, malaria, syphilis, cytomegalovirus [CMV], infectious mononucleosis, rubella, Rocky Mountain spotted fever), they do not result in reactions during infusion of the blood product.
   e. Blood banks in Canada screen for human immunodeficiency virus (HIV)-1, HIV-2, human T-cell lymphocytic virus type 1 (HTLV-1), hepatitis B virus (HBV), and hepatitis C virus (HCV) before blood is released for transfusion.
6. Pulmonary edema
   a. Congestive heart failure (CHF). Volume overload may be induced in the patient with a history of CHF because blood transfusions expand the intravascular volume.
   b. Pulmonary leukoagglutinin reaction (see previous section)

■ MAJOR THREAT TO LIFE

- Anaphylaxis
- Acute hemolytic reaction

Both of these reactions are very rare, but when they do occur, they can be fatal. *Anaphylaxis* may cause death either by severe laryngospasm or bronchospasm or by profound peripheral vasodilation and cardiovascular collapse. An *acute hemolytic reaction* is a medical emergency because of the possible development of renal failure, acute disseminated intravascular coagulation (DIC), or both.

■ BEDSIDE

Quick Look Test

Does the patient look well (comfortable), sick (uncomfortable or distressed), or critical (about to die)?
The patient with impending anaphylaxis may look sick (agitated, restless, or SOB). Patients with pulmonary edema secondary to a transfusion reaction may look critical, with severe SOB.

Airway and Vital Signs

What is the respiratory rate (RR)?
Tachypnea may be a manifestation of CHF or, particularly if associated with audible wheezing, may indicate impending anaphylaxis.

What is the blood pressure (BP)?
Hypotension is an ominous sign—ensure that the transfusion has been stopped. Hypotension is seen in acute hemolytic reactions and in anaphylactic reactions. However, if the transfusion is being given for volume depletion, such as in acute blood loss, hypotension may represent continued loss of intravascular volume from uncontrolled bleeding.

Tag and wristband check
Compare the identification tag on the blood with the patient's wrist band.

Selective Physical Examination

HEENT	Flushed face (hemolytic reaction or anaphylaxis)
	Facial or pharyngeal edema (anaphylaxis)
Resp	Wheezes (anaphylaxis)
Neuro	Decreased level of consciousness (anaphylaxis or hemolytic reaction)
Skin	Heat along the vein being used for the transfusion (hemolytic reaction)
	Oozing from IV sites may be the only sign of hemolysis in the unconscious or anesthetized patient. DIC is a late manifestation of an acute hemolytic transfusion reaction.
Urine	Check the urine color. Free Hb will turn urine red or brown and is indicative of a hemolytic reaction.

If there is evidence of anaphylaxis or hemolysis, *stop the transfusion* and immediately begin emergency treatment (see below).

Selective History

Ask about symptoms that the patient may have developed since the initial telephone call, as follows.

- Fever or chills (nonhemolytic febrile reaction)
- Headache, chest pain, back pain, or diaphoresis (hemolytic reaction)
- SOB (volume overload or pulmonary leukoagglutinin reaction). A leukoagglutinin reaction occurring in the elderly patient is often misdiagnosed as cardiogenic pulmonary edema.

Has the patient had previous transfusion reactions?

Chills and fever are most common in the patient who has received multiple transfusions or who has had several pregnancies.

Management

Anaphylaxis

1. Ensure that the transfusion has been stopped.
2. *Epinephrine* 3 to 5 ml (0.3 to 0.5 mg) of 1:10,000 solution IV by slow, direct injection; may repeat every 5 minutes as necessary. If epinephrine 1:10,000 solution is not immediately available, it can be made by adding 1 ml of a 1:1000 solution to 9 ml of NS.
3. *NS* 500 to 1000 ml IV to be given as fast as possible through a wide-open IV line
4. *Oxygen* by bag and mask if necessary
5. *Diphenhydramine* (Benadryl) 50 mg IV by slow, direct injection
6. *Hydrocortisone* (Solu-Cortef) 250 mg IV by slow, direct injection
7. Intubation if necessary

Acute Hemolytic Reaction

1. Ensure that the transfusion has been stopped.
2. Replace all IV tubing.
3. *NS* 500 ml IV to be given as fast as possible. Try to maintain the urine output over 100 ml/hr with IV fluids and diuretics.
4. *Furosemide* (Lasix) 40 mg IV by slow, direct injection at a rate not faster than 4 mg/min or *mannitol* 25 g IV over 5 minutes (to promote diuresis).
5. Draw 20 ml of the patient's blood and send for the following:
   a. Repeat crossmatch
   b. Coombs' test, free Hb
   c. Complete blood cell count (CBC), RBC morphology
   d. Platelets, prothrombin time (PT), activated partial thromboplastin time (aPTT), fibrin degradation products (FDP)

  e. Urea, creatinine levels

  f. Unclotted blood for a stat spin. Hemolysis is demonstrated when the plasma remains pink despite spinning for 5 minutes (i.e., hemoglobinemia).

6. Obtain a urine sample for free Hb. In addition, urine can be tested with dipsticks. If there is hemoglobinuria, the dipstick results will be positive for Hb and negative for RBCs.

7. Send the donor's blood back to the blood bank for the following:

  a. Repeat crossmatch

  b. Coombs' test

8. If oliguria develops despite adequate IV fluids and appropriate diuretics, *acute renal failure* should be suspected. (For management of acute renal failure, see Chapter 9, pages 76 to 77.)

Urticaria

1. Do not stop the transfusion. Hives alone are rarely serious, but "hives and hypotension" is an anaphylactic reaction until proved otherwise.

2. *Diphenhydramine* (Benadryl) 50 mg PO or IV

3. Before future transfusions, the patient should be premedicated with *diphenhydramine* 50 mg PO or IV (not IM). If this fails to prevent urticarial reactions, washed RBCs should be given.

Fever

1. Do not stop the transfusion unless a hemolytic reaction is suspected. Fever developing within minutes of the start of a blood transfusion is very likely to be a symptom of a hemolytic reaction.

2. Often no treatment is required. If the fever is high and the patient is distressed, however, an antipyretic drug, e.g., *acetaminophen* 650 mg PO, usually is effective.

3. If the patient has documented fever with two consecutive blood transfusions, premedication with an antipyretic before subsequent transfusions is indicated. If this step fails to prevent fever, washed RBCs can be given.

Pulmonary Edema

1. Stop the transfusion or slow the rate of transfusion, unless the patient urgently needs blood.

2. *Furosemide* (Lasix) 40 mg IV. If the patient is already receiving a diuretic or if there is renal insufficiency, a higher dose of furosemide may be required.

3. For the management of CHF refer to Chapter 24, page 273. Volume overload, with subsequent pulmonary edema, should be anticipated in a patient with a history of CHF. This problem may be prevented by administering a diuretic (e.g., *furosemide* 40 mg IV) during the transfusion.

LABORATORY-RELATED PROBLEMS: THE COMMON CALLS

28

ACID-BASE DISORDERS

Most cases of acidemia or alkalemia are first discovered by measurement of arterial pH.

ACIDEMIA (pH ≤ 7.35)

First decide whether the acidemia is a respiratory acidemia (i.e., due to hypoventilation) or a metabolic acidemia (i.e., due to acid gain or HCO_3 loss).

Respiratory Acidemia
- pH ≤ 7.35
- P_{CO_2} ↑
- HCO_3 normal or ↑

Metabolic Acidemia
- pH ≤ 7.35
- P_{CO_2} normal or ↓
- HCO_3 ↓

The normal response to respiratory acidemia is an increase in HCO_3. An immediate increase in HCO_3 occurs because the increase in P_{CO_2} results in the generation of HCO_3, according to the law of mass action.

$$CO_2 + H_2O \rightleftharpoons H + HCO_3$$

Later, renal tubular preservation of HCO_3 occurs to buffer the change in pH. The expected increase in HCO_3 in *acute respiratory acidemia* is 0.1 (ΔP_{CO_2}). The expected increase in HCO_3 in *chronic respiratory acidemia* is 0.4 (ΔP_{CO_2}). When the HCO_3 is less than expected, a mixed respiratory and metabolic acidemia should be suspected. An HCO_3 greater than expected suggests a combined respiratory acidemia and metabolic alkalemia.

The normal respiratory response to metabolic acidemia is hyperventilation, with a decrease in P_{CO_2}. The expected decrease in P_{CO_2} in uncomplicated metabolic acidemia is 1 to 1.5 (ΔHCO_3). When the P_{CO_2} is higher than this expected increase, a mixed metabolic and respiratory acidemia should be suspected. When the P_{CO_2} is lower than expected, a combined metabolic acidemia and respiratory alkalemia should be suspected.

315

Respiratory Acidemia

- pH $\leq$ 7.35
- P_{CO_2} ↑
- HCO_3 normal or ↑

Causes

1. Central nervous system (CNS) depression
   a. Drugs (e.g., morphine)
   b. Lesions of the respiratory center
2. Neuromuscular disorders
   a. Drugs (e.g., succinylcholine)
   b. Muscular disease
   c. Hypokalemia, hypophosphatemia
   d. Neuropathies
3. Respiratory disorders
   a. Acute airway obstruction
   b. Severe parenchymal lung disease
   c. Pleural effusion
   d. Pneumothorax
   e. Thoracic cage limitation

Manifestations

Respiratory acidemia occurs when there is a failure (either acute or chronic) in ventilation. The manifestations of respiratory acidemia are often overshadowed by those due to accompanying hypoxia. Symptoms and signs directly attributable to CO_2 retention are uncommon with P_{CO_2} < 70 mm Hg but include the following:

- Bradypnea
- Drowsiness
- Confusion
- Papilledema
- Asterixis

Management

Assess the Severity

Mild. pH 7.30–7.35. Patients with mild respiratory acidemia can be observed while reversible causes are searched for and corrected. Repeat arterial blood gases (ABGs) should be obtained depending on the patient's clinical condition and course. The exception here is the patient with an acute asthmatic attack, in whom even a normal and certainly an elevated P_{CO_2} is a warning sign of impending respiratory failure.

Moderate. pH 7.20–7.29. The patient with moderate respiratory acidemia is in the gray zone. Further decrease in pH puts the patient at risk for life-threatening ventricular dysrhythmias. If a readily reversible cause can be found, the patient can be carefully monitored while treatment measures are instituted. Such a patient should not be left alone until it is determined that he or she is improving. Sequential determinations of pH should be guided by the patient's clinical condition and course.

Severe. pH ≤ 7.19. This patient is at high risk for cessation of respiration, life-threatening ventricular dysrhythmias, or both. Call your resident for help now. This patient will most likely require transfer to the intensive care unit (ICU) for monitoring, intubation, and mechanical ventilation while reversible causes are searched for.

Metabolic Acidemia

- pH ≤ 7.35
- P_{CO_2} normal or ↓
- HCO_3 ↓

Causes

The metabolic acidemias are conveniently divided into *normal anion gap* and *high anion gap* varieties. The normal anion gap $(Na + K) - (Cl + HCO_3) = 10$ to 12 mmol/L. Most of the normal anion gap is accounted for by negatively charged plasma proteins. Remember that for every decline in serum albumin of 10 g/L, add 4 to the calculated anion gap. Failure to correct for hypoalbuminemia may lead to overlooking serious acidemias of the high anion gap type.

Normal Anion Gap Acidemia

1. Loss of HCO_3
   a. Diarrhea, ileus, fistula
   b. High-output ileostomy
   c. Renal tubular acidosis
   d. Carbonic anhydrase inhibitors
2. Addition of H^+
   a. NH_4Cl
   b. HCl

High Anion Gap Acidemia

1. Lactic acidemia
2. Ketoacidosis (type 1 diabetes, alcohol, starvation)
3. Renal failure

4. Drugs (aspirin, ethylene glycol, methyl alcohol, toluene, paraldehyde)
5. High-flux dialysis acetate buffer

The change in anion gap should equal the change in HCO_3. Any deviation from this reveals a mixed acid-base disorder. Always remember to *calculate the osmolar gap* (see Chapter 34, pages 366 to 367) in high anion gap acidemias to determine whether ingestions have contributed to the abnormalities.

Occasionally, the pH may be normal, but the presence of a wide anion gap may be a clue to underlying metabolic acidemia.

Manifestations

The signs and symptoms of metabolic acidemia are nonspecific and include the following:

- Hyperventilation (in an effort to blow off CO_2)
- Fatigue
- Confusion → stupor → coma
- Decreased cardiac contractility
- Peripheral vasodilation → hypotension

Management

Assess the Severity

Mild. pH 7.30–7.35

Moderate. pH 7.20–7.29

Severe. pH ≤ 7.19

For all causes of metabolic acidemia, management involves reversal of the underlying cause. In most cases of mild or moderate metabolic acidemia, the acid-base disorder can be treated effectively by reversing the underlying condition. However, in some conditions (e.g., chronic renal failure), the condition is not easily reversed. In this situation, mild or moderate metabolic acidemia does not require treatment. Severe metabolic acidemia from chronic renal failure can be treated with PO or IV $NaHCO_3$, being careful not to precipitate volume overload.

For other causes of metabolic acidemia, it is occasionally necessary to raise the blood pH by administering $NaHCO_3$, but this usually is reserved for severe metabolic acidemias only. Several important precautions should be considered.

1. The amount of $NaHCO_3$ given depends on the pH and how effective and rapid therapy for reversing the underlying cause is going to be. For instance, a metabolic acidemia with pH 6.9 is a medical emergency and may require an initial dose of 150 mmol of intravenous (IV) $NaHCO_3$ while other resuscitation measures are instituted. A metabolic acidemia

with pH 7.10 in a patient with diabetic ketoacidosis may require only 50 mmol of IV $NaHCO_3$ while insulin and fluids are administered. An estimate of the amount of bicarbonate required can be made by calculating the extracellular buffer deficit as follows:

$$\text{Buffer deficit} = (\text{normal serum HCO}_3 - \text{measured serum HCO}_3) (\text{body weight in kg}) (0.4)$$

where 0.4 is a correction factor representing the proportion of body weight composed of extracellular fluid (0.2) and for the buffering provided by intracellular components. The initial dose of HCO_3 should be approximately half of the calculated buffer deficit. Full correction should not be attempted within the first 24 hours because of the risk of delayed compensation and alkalemia with tetany, seizures, and ventricular dysrhythmias.

The HCO_3 should be diluted (50 to 150 mmol/L is achieved by adding one to three 50-mmol vials to 1 L of 5% dextrose in water [D5W]) and be given slowly because direct infusion of undiluted $NaHCO_3$ can result in fatal ventricular dysrhythmias.

2. In the presence of cardiac arrest, metabolic acidemia may be treated with HCO_3 but only after alveolar ventilation is ensured because there is a risk of further depression of respiration from a shift in intracellular pH in the respiratory control center in the CNS. When ventilation is ensured, an initial dose of 1 mmol/kg body weight of HCO_3 can be given by rapid IV injection with repeated doses of 0.5 mmol/kg body weight every 10 minutes during continued cardiac arrest.

Remember that IV $NaHCO_3$ is a significant sodium load and may put a patient in CHF. Do not substitute one problem for another!

ALKALEMIA (pH $\geq$ 7.45)

First decide whether the patient has a respiratory or a metabolic alkalemia.

Respiratory Alkalemia
- pH $\geq$ 7.45
- P_{CO_2} ↓
- HCO_3 ↓

Metabolic Alkalemia
- pH $\geq$ 7.45
- P_{CO_2} normal or ↑
- HCO_3 ↑

The normal response to respiratory alkalemia is a decrease in HCO_3. An immediate decrease in HCO_3 occurs because the decrease in PCO_2 results in a reduction of HCO_3 according to the law of mass action:

$$CO_2 + H_2O \rightleftharpoons H + HCO_3$$

Later, renal tubular loss of HCO_3 occurs to buffer the change in pH. The expected decrease in HCO_3 in acute respiratory alkalemia is 0.2 (ΔPCO_2). The expected decrease in HCO_3 in chronic respiratory alkalemia is 0.4 (ΔPCO_2). When the HCO_3 is greater than expected, a combined respiratory and metabolic alkalemia should be suspected. When the HCO_3 is less than expected, a combined respiratory alkalemia and metabolic acidemia should be suspected.

The normal response to metabolic alkalemia is hypoventilation with an increase in the PCO_2. The expected increase in uncomplicated metabolic alkalemia is 0.6 (ΔHCO_3). When the PCO_2 is greater than expected, a combined metabolic alkalemia and respiratory acidemia should be suspected. When the PCO_2 is less than expected, a combined metabolic and respiratory alkalemia should be suspected.

Respiratory Alkalemia

- pH ≥ 7.45
- PCO_2 ↓
- HCO_3 ↓

Causes

1. Physiologic conditions (pregnancy, high altitude)
2. CNS disorders (anxiety, pain, fever, tumor)
3. Drugs (aspirin, nicotine, progesterone)
4. Pulmonary disorders (CHF, pulmonary embolism, asthma, pneumonia)
5. Miscellaneous (hepatic failure, hyperthyroidism)

Manifestations

- Confusion
- Numbness, tingling, paresthesias (perioral, hands, feet)
- Lightheadedness
- Tetany in severe cases

Management

Assess the Severity

Mild. pH 7.45–7.55

Moderate. pH 7.56–7.69

Severe. pH $\geq$ 7.70

Mild respiratory alkalemia is commonly seen in physiologic conditions (pregnancy, high altitude) and in these cases requires no treatment. Any of the other causes listed may result in mild respiratory alkalemia, and many can be treated symptomatically (e.g., the febrile patient can be treated with antipyretics, the patient in pain can be treated with analgesics, and the anxious patient may be treated with reassurance or sedation). In addition to these measures, more pronounced degrees of respiratory alkalemia due to anxiety can be treated by rebreathing into a paper bag. The only effective treatment for the other causes listed is eliminating the underlying condition.

Metabolic Alkalemia

- pH $\geq$ 7.45
- P_{CO_2} normal or $\uparrow$
- HCO_3 $\uparrow$

Causes

1. With extracellular volume depletion and low (usually $<$ 10 mEq/L) urinary chloride
    a. Gastrointestinal (GI) losses
        (1) Vomiting
        (2) GI drainage (nasogastric [NG] suction)
        (3) Chloride-wasting diarrhea
        (4) Villous adenoma
    b. Renal losses
        (1) Diuretic therapy
        (2) Posthypercapnia
        (3) Nonreabsorbable anions
        (4) Penicillin, carbenicillin, ticarcillin
        (5) Bartter's syndrome
2. With extracellular volume expansion and presence (usually $>$ 20 mEq/L) of urinary chloride
    a. Mineralocorticoid excess
        (1) Endogenous
            (a) Hyperaldosteronism
            (b) Cushing's syndrome

      (2) Exogenous
        (a) Glucocorticoids
        (b) Mineralocorticoids
        (c) Carbenoxolone
        (d) Licorice excess
   b. Alkali ingestion
   c. Poststarvation feeding

Manifestations

There are no specific signs or symptoms of metabolic alkalemia. Severe alkalemia may result in

- Apathy
- Confusion/stupor

Management

Assess the Severity

Mild. pH 7.45–7.55

Moderate. pH 7.56–7.69

Severe. pH $\geq$ 7.70

Beyond correcting the underlying cause, mild or moderate metabolic alkalemia rarely requires specific treatment. *Metabolic alkalemia associated with extracellular fluid (ECF) volume depletion* usually responds to infusion of normal saline (NS), which will enhance renal HCO_3 excretion.

Note that associated electrolyte abnormalities (particularly hypokalemia) may be more threatening to the patient's well-being than the metabolic alkalemia. Attention to concomitant electrolyte disorders is very important.

In *diuretic-induced alkalemia*, administration of KCl may improve the alkalemia.

If the patient is *volume overloaded* and has a metabolic alkalemia, *acetazolamide* 250 to 500 mg PO or IV every 8 hours enhances the renal HCO_3 excretion and may be helpful.

In *Bartter's syndrome*, the alkalemia may respond to prostaglandin synthetase inhibitors, such as indomethacin.

It is very unusual to require acidifying agents, such as NH_4Cl or dilute HCl, even for severe metabolic alkalemia. Such agents should be given only under the direct guidance of your resident and the patient's attending physician.

29

ANEMIA

Serum hemoglobin (Hb) is one of the most common laboratory determinations made in hospitalized patients. Remember that Hb is a *concentration*, and its value can be modified by both a change in its *content* and a change in its *diluent* (plasma). For instance, a patient's Hb may be elevated (i.e., in the "normal" range) despite a sudden loss of intravascular volume, as is seen in an acute hemorrhage. Because of the possibility of transfusion-related illnesses, one must avoid the reflex administration of red blood cell (RBC) transfusions to correct a low Hb level. *Remember to treat the patient, not the laboratory value.*

Causes

1. Blood loss
   a. Acute
      (1) Gastrointestinal (GI) hemorrhage
      (2) Trauma
      (3) Concealed hemorrhage
         (a) Ruptured aortic aneurysm
         (b) Ruptured ectopic pregnancy
         (c) Retroperitoneal hematoma
         (d) Postsurgical bleeding
   b. Chronic
      (1) GI bleeding
      (2) Uterine bleeding
2. Inadequate production of RBCs
   a. Anemia of chronic disease (chronic inflammation, uremia, endocrine failure, liver disease)
   b. Iron deficiency
   c. Megaloblastic anemias (vitamin B_{12} and folate deficiency, drugs, inherited)
   d. Sideroblastic anemias (drugs, alcohol, malignancy, rheumatoid arthritis [RA], inherited)
   e. Acquired disorders of marrow stem cells (aplastic anemia, myelodysplastic syndromes, chemotherapy, drugs)
3. Hemolysis
   a. Extrinsic factors (immune hemolysis, splenomegaly, mechanical trauma, infections, microangiopathic hemolytic anemia)
   b. Membrane defects (e.g., hereditary spherocytosis, paroxysmal nocturnal hemoglobinuria)

c. Internal RBC defects (e.g., thalassemia, sickle cell disease)
d. Acute or delayed RBC transfusion reactions

Manifestations

The manifestations of anemia depend on underlying medical conditions, the severity of the anemia, and the rapidity with which it develops. The body's reaction to an acute reduction in RBC mass is usually manifested by (compensatory) alterations in the cardiovascular and respiratory systems.

Acute anemias due to hemorrhage will result in symptoms and signs of intravascular volume depletion, including the following:

- Pallor, diaphoresis, tachypnea
- Cold, clammy extremities
- Hypotension, tachycardia
- Shock

Anemias that develop slowly over weeks or months are not usually accompanied by signs of intravascular volume depletion. In these cases, symptoms and signs often are not so obvious and may vary depending on disease in other organ systems.

Common Symptoms

- Fatigue, lethargy
- Dyspnea
- Palpitations
- Worsening of symptoms in patients with angina pectoris or claudication, or presentation with a transient ischemic attack (TIA)
- GI disturbances (due to shunting of blood from the splanchnic bed)—anorexia, nausea, bowel irregularity
- Abnormal menstrual patterns

Signs

- Pallor
- Tachypnea
- Tachycardia, wide pulse pressure, hyperdynamic precordium
- Jaundice/splenomegaly (in hemolytic anemias)

Management

Assess the Severity. The severity of the situation should be determined according to the level of Hb, the patient's volume status, the rapidity with which the anemia developed, and the likelihood that the underlying process will continue unabated.

THE PATIENT WHO IS IN SHOCK OR WHO IS VOLUME DEPLETED. An

acute anemia due to blood loss (and, hence, intravascular volume depletion) will result in compensatory tachycardia and tachypnea. If full hemodynamic compensation is inadequate, hypotension or shock will result. Do not forget, in your assessment of the patient's volume status, to check for postural changes (see Chapter 3, page 10), which may be the earliest manifestation of an acute blood loss.

1. Notify your resident.
2. Ensure that at least one, and preferably two, large-bore (size 16 if possible) intravenous (IV) lines are in place.
3. If there is evidence of active bleeding, ensure that there is blood on hold. If not, order stat crossmatch for 2, 4, or 6 units of packed RBCs, depending on your estimate of blood loss.
4. **Replenish intravascular volume by giving IV fluids.** The best immediate choice is a crystalloid (normal saline [NS] or Ringer's lactate), which will at least temporarily stay in the intravascular space. Albumin or banked plasma can be given but is expensive, carries a risk of virus transmission, and is not always available. The assumption here, when the association of a new, severe anemia with intravascular volume depletion is seen, is that blood has been lost from the intravascular space—hence, blood is ideally what needs to be replaced. If there is no blood on hold for the patient, a stat crossmatch usually will take 50 minutes. If blood is on hold, it should be available at the bedside in 30 minutes. In an emergency, O-negative blood may be given, although this practice is usually reserved for the acute trauma victim. Transfusion-related infections can be minimized by transfusing only when necessary. *Rule-of-thumb*: Maintain the Hb level at 90 to 100 g/L.
5. **Order the appropriate IV rate**, which will depend on the patient's volume status. Shock will require IV fluid wide open through at least two large-bore IV sites. Elevating the IV bag, squeezing the IV bag, or using IV pressure cuffs may help speed the rate of delivery of the solution. *Mild or moderate volume depletion* can be treated with 500 to 1000 ml of NS given as rapidly as possible, with serial determinations of volume status and assessment of cardiac status. If blood is not at the bedside within 30 minutes, delegate someone to find out why there has been a delay.
   Note: Aggressive volume depletion in a patient with a history of CHF may result in pulmonary edema. Do not overshoot the mark!
6. **Determine the site of hemorrhage.**
   a. **Look for obvious signs of external bleeding**—bleeding from IV sites, skin lesions, hematemesis, menstrual bleeding.
   b. **Examine for signs of occult blood loss.**

    (1) Perform a rectal examination to look for melena.

    (2) Occult blood loss should be suspected if there is swelling at biopsy or surgical sites (e.g., flank swelling after renal biopsy, ascites after liver biopsy) or if there are flank or periumbilical ecchymoses (possible hemoperitoneum).

    (3) If the patient is a female in the childbearing years, a ruptured ectopic pregnancy must be considered. If indicated, a pelvic examination should be performed by an experienced physician.

    (4) If a ruptured thoracic or abdominal aortic aneurysm is likely, immediate surgical referral is necessary.

7. Review the chart for exacerbating factors that may contribute to ongoing hemorrhage, e.g., administration of **aspirin, heparin, warfarin, thrombolytic agents,** or **coagulopathies,** and for recent pertinent laboratory values (activated partial thromboplastin time [aPTT], prothrombin time [PT], and platelets).

8. Request **surgical consultation** when appropriate.

THE PATIENT WHO IS NORMOVOLEMIC. Patients can tolerate even severe (Hb < 70 g/L) anemia if the anemia develops slowly. Mild (Hb 100–120 g/L) chronic anemias in the context of normal intravascular volume often do not alter the vital signs. If the patient is normovolemic, transfusion therapy is seldom warranted on an urgent basis. If you have excluded the presence of active hemorrhage, the anemia must be due to (1) chronic blood loss, (2) inadequate production of RBCs, or (3) hemolysis.

1. An unexpected Hb of < 100 g/L merits a repeat measurement to exclude laboratory error while other assessment measures are taking place. Mild anemia (Hb 100 to 120 g/L) in an asymptomatic patient with normal vital signs usually can wait if other problems of higher priority exist. One must always keep in mind, however, that if active bleeding is responsible for the anemia, a stable patient may become unstable very quickly.

2. **What is the patient's usual Hb?** Look in the current or old chart to see if the anemia is a new finding. If the current Hb is more than 10 or 20 g/L lower than previous values, assume that the underlying cause of anemia has worsened or a second factor has developed (e.g., a patient with a chronic disease, such as systemic lupus erythematosus [SLE], may normally have an Hb of 90 g/L; a new value of 75 g/L may represent further marrow suppression, hemolysis, or new onset of bleeding).

3. If the patient is comfortable and has a normal cardiovascular examination and your examination reveals no suspicion of active bleeding, further investigation can take place in the morning. Several baseline studies are helpful in pointing you in the right direction to diagnose the cause of the anemia.

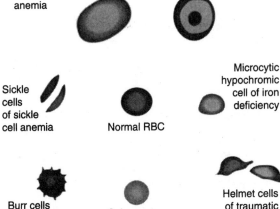

Oval macrocyte
of megaloblastic
anemia

Target cell of
liver disease

Sickle
cells
of sickle
cell anemia

Normal RBC

Microcytic
hypochromic
cell of iron
deficiency

Burr cells
of uremia

Spherocytes
seen in hemolysis

Helmet cells
of traumatic
hemolysis

Figure 29–1 □ Blood smear demonstrating examples of helpful diagnostic features associated with specific anemias.

a. **Measurement of RBC cell volume.** The mean corpuscular volume (MCV) is useful in classifying the anemias due to decreased RBC production (microcytic, normocytic, macrocytic).
b. **Examination of the blood smear** by an individual experienced in hematology often provides valuable clues helpful in diagnosing specific anemias (Fig. 29–1).
c. A **reticulocyte count** provides a measure of marrow erythropoiesis. An elevated reticulocyte count suggests hemolysis, recent hemorrhage, or a recently treated chronic anemia (e.g., recently treated vitamin B_{12} deficiency). An inappropriately low reticulocyte count suggests a failure to produce RBCs (e.g., untreated iron, vitamin B_{12}, or folate deficiency or anemia of chronic disease).

30

CALCIUM DISORDERS

HYPERCALCEMIA

Causes

1. Increased intake / absorption
   a. Vitamin D or A intoxication
   b. Excessive calcium supplementation
   c. Milk-alkali syndrome (excessive antacid ingestion)
   d. Sarcoidosis and other granulomatous disease
2. Increased production / mobilization from bone
   a. Primary hyperparathyroidism*
   b. Neoplasm.* There are four mechanisms for hypercalcemia of malignancy, as follows:
      (1) Bony metastasis (prostate, thyroid, kidney, breast, lung)
      (2) Parathyroid hormone (PTH)-like substance elaborated by tumor cells (lung, kidney, ovary, colon)
      (3) Prostaglandin E_2 increases bony resorption (multiple myeloma)
      (4) Osteoclast-activating factor (multiple myeloma, lymphoproliferative disorders)
   c. Severe secondary hyperparathyroidism associated with renal failure
   d. Paget's disease
   e. Immobilization
   f. Hyperthyroidism
   g. Adrenal insufficiency
   h. Acromegaly
   i. Sarcoidosis. In addition to sarcoidosis increasing absorption from the gastrointestinal (GI) tract, there is an increased conversion of 25(OH) vitamin D to the active form, $1,25(OH)_2$ vitamin D.
   j. Chronic lithium use
3. Decreased excretion
   a. Thiazide diuretics
   b. Familial hypocalciuric hypercalcemia

---

*Primary hyperparathyroidism and tumors account for 90% of cases of hypercalcemia.

Manifestations

The manifestations of hypercalcemia are numerous and nonspecific, e.g., "bones, stones, and groans."

HEENT	Corneal calcification (band keratopathy)
CVS	Short QT interval, prolonged PR interval (Fig. 30–1), dysrhythmias, digoxin sensitivity, hypertension
GI	Anorexia, nausea, vomiting, constipation, abdominal pain, pancreatitis ("groans")
GU	Polyuria, polydipsia, nephrolithiasis ("stones")
Neuro	Restlessness, delirium, dementia, psychosis, lethargy, coma
MSS	Muscle weakness, hyporeflexia, bone pain, fractures ("bones")
Misc	Hyperchlorhydric metabolic acidosis

Management

Assess the Severity. The severity of the situation should be determined according to the serum calcium concentration, the rate of progression, and the presence or absence of symptoms. It is important to recognize that most laboratories measure total serum calcium (ionized plus albumin bound), but the primary determinant of the physiologic effect is the ionized component.

If the patient is hypoalbuminemic, a correction factor can be used to estimate the total calcium concentration. For every 10 g/L of hypoalbuminemia, add 0.2 mmol/L to the serum calcium value—e.g., if the measured serum calcium value is 2.6 mmol/L (the upper limit of normal) but the serum albumin value is low at 30 g/L (with an anticipated normal concentration of 40 g/L),

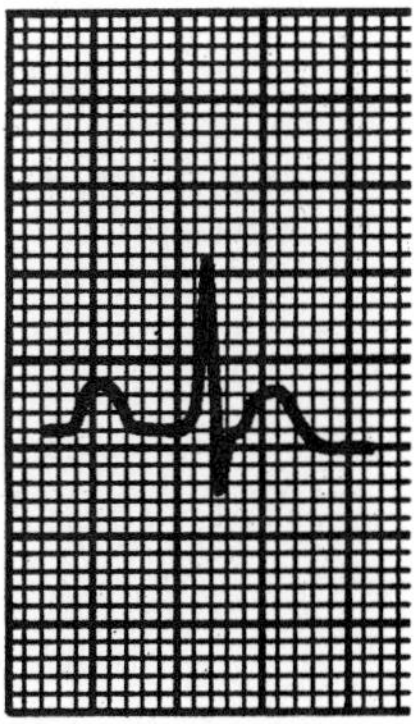

Figure 30–1 □ Hypercalcemia (short QT interval, prolonged PR interval).

the correct serum calcium value is 0.2 + 2.6 = 2.8 mmol/L (mild elevation).

How high is the serum calcium?
- Normal range = 2.2 to 2.6 mmol/L
- Mild elevation = 2.6 to 2.9 mmol/L
- Moderate elevation = 2.9 to 3.2 mmol/L
- Severe elevation > 3.2 mmol/L

Is there a progressive cause that is likely to result in further increases?

If the situation is progressive, the patient requires immediate treatment.

Is the patient symptomatic?

Any symptomatic patient requires immediate treatment.

Treatment

SEVERE HYPERCALCEMIA. Severe hypercalcemia (> 3.2 mmol/L) requires immediate treatment because of the danger of a fatal cardiac dysrhythmia.

1. *Correct volume depletion/expand extracellular volume.* Give normal saline (NS) 500 ml intravenous (IV) as fast as possible. Further NS boluses can be given dependent on the volume status. Titrate the NS IV maintenance rate to keep the patient slightly volume expanded. If the patient has a history of congestive heart failure (CHF), this volume expansion should be undertaken in the intensive care unit/cardiac care unit (ICU/CCU) because close monitoring of the volume status will be required. A reduction in the serum calcium level will be expected because of hemodilution and because an increased urinary sodium excretion is accompanied by an increased calcium excretion.

2. *Establish diuresis > 2500 ml/day.* If this cannot be achieved by volume expansion alone, *furosemide* (Lasix) 20 to 40 mg IV every 2 to 4 hours may be given. Care must be taken not to induce volume depletion with administration of furosemide. The patient may require 4 to 10 L of NS per day to maintain the volume expanded state. Furosemide inhibits the tubular reabsorption of calcium, thus increasing calcium excretion by the kidneys. Do not use thiazides to establish diuresis because they elevate the serum calcium level.

3. *Dialysis.* Occasionally, when the serum calcium level is extremely high, e.g., > 4.5 mmol/L, and a saline diuresis cannot be achieved, hemodialysis or peritoneal dialysis may be required.

4. *If hypercalcemia is secondary to neoplasm,* in addition to the administration of NS and furosemide (as previously discussed), one of the following medications may be of value.
   a. Corticosteroids. *Prednisone* 40 to 100 mg PO daily or *hy-*

drocortisone (Solu-Cortef) 200 to 500 mg IV daily in divided doses. Steroids antagonize the peripheral action of vitamin D (decreased absorption, decreased mobilization from bone, and decreased renal tubular reabsorption of calcium).

b. *Plicamycin* 25 μg/kg in 1 L of 5% dextrose in water (D5W) or NS IV over 4 to 6 hours. Plicamycin inhibits bone resorption. The onset of action is 48 hours.

c. Biphosphonates inhibit bone resorption and are effective agents in the control of cancer-associated hypercalcemia. *Disodium etidronate* may be given in a dose of 7.5 mg/kg IV daily for 3 days. Each daily dose should be diluted in 250 ml NS or D5W and given IV over a period of at least 2 hours. Alternatively, *pamidronate* 60 to 90 mg in 1 L NS or D5W may be given IV over 24 hours.

d. Indomethacin 50 mg PO every 8 hours. Indomethacin inhibits the synthesis of prostaglandin E_2, which is produced by some solid tumors, e.g., of the breast.

e. *Synthetic salmon calcitonin may* temporarily lower the serum calcium concentration but should not be initiated at night before first skin testing the patient for allergy (see package insert).

MODERATE HYPERCALCEMIA OR MILD SYMPTOMATIC HYPERCALCEMIA. Moderate hypercalcemia or mild symptomatic hypercalcemia (2.9 to 3.2 mmol/L or lesser elevations in the presence of symptoms) should be managed as follows.

1. *Correct volume depletion and expand extracellular fluid volume* with NS 500 ml IV given over 1 to 2 hours. Further NS can be given at a rate to keep the patient slightly volume expanded.

2. *Establish diuresis > 2500/day* if volume expansion alone is unsuccessful in lowering the serum calcium.

3. Oral phosphate 0.5 to 3 g/day depending on GI tolerance (flatulence, diarrhea) may be given for patients with a low or normal serum phosphate level.

MILD ASYMPTOMATIC HYPERCALCEMIA. Mild asymptomatic hypercalcemia (2.6 to 2.9 mmol/L) does not require immediate treatment. The appropriate investigations may be ordered in the morning.

HYPOCALCEMIA

Causes

1. Decreased intake/absorption
   a. Malabsorption

  b. Intestinal bypass surgery
  c. Short bowel syndrome
  d. Vitamin D deficiency
2. Decreased production/mobilization from bone
  a. Hypoparathyroidism (after subtotal thyroidectomy or para-thyroidectomy)
  b. Pseudohypoparathyroidism (PTH resistance)
  c. Vitamin D deficiency [decreased production of 25(OH) vitamin D or 1,25(OH)$_2$ vitamin D]
  d. Acute hyperphosphatemia (tumor lysis, acute renal failure, rhabdomyolysis)
  e. Acute pancreatitis
  f. Hypomagnesemia
  g. Alkalosis (hyperventilation, vomiting, fistulas)
  h. Neoplasm
     (1) Paradoxical hypocalcemia associated with osteoblastic metastasis (lung, breast, prostate)
     (2) Medullary carcinoma of the thyroid (calcitonin-producing tumor)
     (3) Rapid tumor lysis with phosphate release
3. Increased excretion
  a. Chronic renal failure
  b. Drugs (aminoglycosides, loop diuretics)

Manifestations

The earliest symptoms are paresthesias of the lips, fingers, and toes.

HEENT	Papilledema, diplopia
CVS	Prolonged QT interval without U waves (Fig. 30–2)
GI	Abdominal cramps

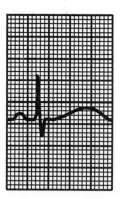

Figure 30–2 □ Hypocalcemia (long QT interval).

Neuro	Confusion, irritability, depression
	Hyperactive tendon reflexes
	Carpopedal spasm, laryngospasm (stridor), tetany
	Generalized tonic-clonic seizures
	Paresthesias of lips, fingers, toes
Special tests	
Chvostek's sign (Fig. 30–3)	Facial muscle spasm elicited by tapping the facial nerve immediately anterior to the ear lobe and below the zygomatic arch (this is a normal finding in 10% of the population)
Trousseau's sign (Fig. 30–4)	Carpal spasm elicited by occluding the arterial blood flow to the forearm for 3 to 5 minutes

Management

Assess the Severity. The severity of the situation should be determined according to the serum calcium and phosphate concentrations and the presence or absence of symptoms. If the serum albumin is not within the normal range, a correction factor can be used to estimate the total serum calcium (ionized plus albumin bound). See page 329 for a discussion of this correction factor.

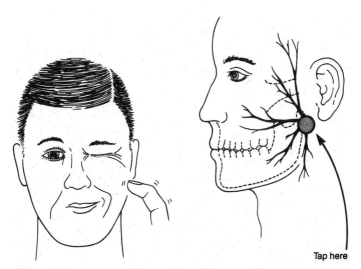

Figure 30–3 □ Chvostek's sign. Facial muscle spasm elicited by tapping the facial nerve immediately anterior to the earlobe and below the zygomatic arch.

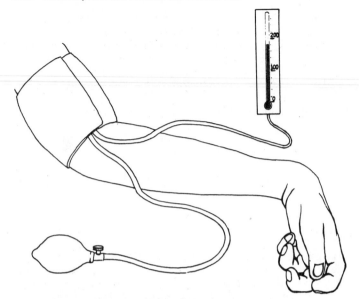

Figure 30–4 □ Trousseau's sign. Carpal spasm elicited by occluding the arterial blood flow to the forearm for 3 to 5 minutes.

How low is the serum calcium level?
- Normal range = 2.2 to 2.6 mmol/L
- Mild depletion = 1.9 to 2.2 mmol/L
- Moderate depletion = 1.5 to 1.9 mmol/L
- Severe depletion = < 1.5 mmol/L

What is the serum phosphate concentration?

If the serum phosphate concentration is markedly elevated (> 6 mmol/L) in severe hypocalcemia, correction of hyperphosphatemia must be carried out with IV glucose and insulin before calcium is given to avoid metastatic calcification.

Is the patient symptomatic?

Hypocalcemic patients who are asymptomatic do not require urgent correction with IV calcium.

Is the patient receiving digoxin?

Caution is required if the patient is receiving digoxin, since calcium potentiates the action of digoxin. Ideally, if IV calcium administration is required, the patient should have continuous electrocardiographic (ECG) monitoring.

Treatment

SEVERE, SYMPTOMATIC HYPOCALCEMIA. Severe, symptomatic hypocalcemia (< 1.5 mmol/L) requires immediate treatment because of the danger of respiratory failure from laryngospasm.

1. Provided the patient's PO_4 is normal or low, give 10 to 20 ml (93 mg elemental calcium/10 ml) of 10% solution of calcium gluconate IV in 100 ml D5W over 30 minutes. If the patient has evidence of tetany or laryngeal stridor, the same dose should be given over 2 minutes as a direct injection, i.e., calcium gluconate 10% solution 10 to 20 ml IV over 2 minutes. Oral calcium may be started immediately: 1 to 2 g of elemental calcium PO TID. If the corrected serum calcium value is < 1.9 mmol/L 6 hours after initiating this treatment, a calcium infusion is required. Add 10 ml (93 mg elemental calcium) of a 10% calcium gluconate solution to 500 ml D5W and infuse over 6 hours. If the serum calcium value is not within the normal range after 6 hours of this infusion, 5 ml (46.5 mg elemental calcium) of calcium gluconate can be added to the initial infusion dose every 6 hours until a satisfactory serum calcium level is achieved. The postparathyroidectomy patient may require 100 to 150 mg of elemental calcium per hour. Once a satisfactory response has been achieved with IV calcium gluconate, oral replacement may begin in doses of 0.5 to 2.0 g elemental calcium TID.

2. If the patient is hyperphosphatemic ($PO_4 > 6$ mmol/L), correction with glucose and insulin is required before administration of IV calcium. Consult the nephrology service immediately.

MILD AND MODERATE ASYMPTOMATIC HYPOCALCEMIA. Mild and moderate asymptomatic hypocalcemia does not require urgent IV calcium replacement. Oral calcium replacement with *elemental calcium* 1000 to 1500 mg/day may be started to achieve a corrected serum calcium level in the 2.2 to 2.6 mmol/L range. Long-term treatment with oral calcium or vitamin D depends on the etiology, which can be evaluated in the morning.

31

COAGULATION DISORDERS

You will be confronted on call by abnormal results of tests of hemostasis. These must always be interpreted in the clinical context in which the measurements were made. Bleeding is the most common clinical manifestation of a coagulation disorder, and the type of bleeding can alert you to the probable type of disorder present.

Patients with *vessel* or *platelet abnormalities* may have petechiae, purpura, or easy bruising. The bleeding characteristically occurs superficially (e.g., oozing from mucous membranes or intravenous [IV] sites). The bleeding of scurvy is seen only rarely in North America and is usually manifested by perifollicular hemorrhages, although gingival bleeding and intramuscular hematomas also may occur.

Bleeding due to *coagulation factor deficiencies* may occur spontaneously, in deeper organ sites (e.g., visceral hemorrhages and hemarthroses), and tends to be delayed and prolonged. Bleeding associated with *thrombolytic agents* is usually manifested by continuous oozing from IV sites.

Three tests are in common use to assess hemostasis—the prothrombin time (PT), the activated partial thromboplastin time (aPTT), and the platelet count. A fourth test, the bleeding time, is used infrequently because it rarely helps make a specific diagnosis, and it carries the risk of accidental exposure to hepatitis and human immunodeficiency syndrome (HIV). Laboratory features of the common coagulation disorders are listed in Table 31–1.

■ PROTHROMBIN TIME

The one-stage PT tests the *extrinsic coagulation system* (Fig. 31–1). It is affected by deficiencies in factors I, II, V, VII, and X. However, antagonists of the extrinsic system, including unfractionated heparin, activated antithrombin III, and fibrin degradation products, can prolong the PT.

Disorders Associated with Prothrombin Time Prolongation

- Coagulation factor abnormalities
- Oral anticoagulants
- Vitamin K deficiency

Table 31–1 □ LABORATORY FEATURES OF COMMON COAGULATION DISORDERS

Disorder	aPTT	PT	Platelets	Bleeding Time	Other
Vessel Abnormalities					
Vasculitis	Normal	Normal	Normal	Normal or ↑	C3 C4 C1Q binding
Increased vascular fragility	Normal	Normal	Normal	↑	
Hereditary connective tissue disorders	Normal	Normal	Normal	↑	
Paraproteinemias	Normal	Normal	Normal	↑	
Coagulation Factor Abnormalities					
Unfractionated heparin	↑	↑ or Normal	Normal or ↓	Normal or ↑	
Low-molecular-weight heparin	Normal	Normal	Normal	Normal or ↑	
Warfarin	Normal or ↑	↑	Normal	Normal	
Vitamin K deficiency	↑	↑	Normal	Normal	
DIC	↑	↑	↓	Normal or ↑*	↑ Fibrin degradation products; ↓ fibrinogen
Factor VIII deficiency	↑	Normal	Normal	Normal	↓ Factor VIII assay
Factor IX deficiency	↑	Normal	Normal	Normal	Normal factor IX assay
von Willebrand's disease	Normal or ↑	Normal	Normal	Normal or ↑	Normal or ↓ factor VIII assay; ↓ factor VIII antigen; ↓ Ristocetin cofactor
Liver disease	↑	↑	Normal or ↓	Normal or ↑	
Platelet Disorders					
Thrombocytopenia	Normal	Normal	↓	Normal or ↑*	
Impaired platelet function	Normal	Normal	Normal	↑	

*Depends on degree of thrombocytopenia.

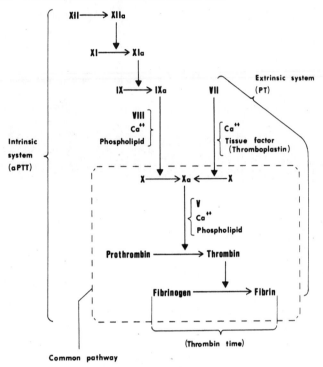

Figure 31–1 □ The coagulation cascade.

- Liver disease
- Disseminated intravascular coagulation (DIC)
- Unfractionated heparin (variable)

■ ACTIVATED PARTIAL THROMBOPLASTIN TIME

The aPTT is a test of the *intrinsic coagulation system* (see Fig. 31–1). It is most sensitive to deficiencies and abnormalities in the sequence of procoagulant activities that occur before factor X activation.

Disorders Associated with Activated Partial Thromboplastin Time Prolongation

- Circulating anticoagulant
- Unfractionated heparin

- Factor VIII, factor IX deficiency
- von Willebrand's disease (variable)
- DIC
- Vitamin K deficiency
- Oral anticoagulants (variable)

A frequent benign cause of prolongation of aPTT in hospital is the presence of an acquired anticoagulant, such as the lupus erythematosus anticoagulant. This situation can be differentiated from a factor deficiency by demonstrating failure to normalize the aPTT when a sample of the plasma of a patient with an acquired anticoagulant is mixed with normal plasma 50:50.

Note that low-molecular-weight heparin (LMWH) does not prolong the PT or aPTT. It exerts its anticoagulant effect by binding to antithrombin III, resulting in anti–factor Xa and IIa activity.

■ PLATELET COUNT

The platelet count is a reflection of production and destruction (sequestration) of platelets.

Disorders Associated with Low Platelets

Decreased Marrow Production
- Marrow replacement by tumor, granuloma (e.g., tuberculosis [TB], sarcoid), fibrous tissue
- Storage disease (e.g., Gaucher's disease)
- Marrow injury by drugs (e.g., sulfonamides, chloramphenicol)
- Defective maturation (e.g., vitamin B_{12} or folate deficiency)

Increased Peripheral Destruction

IMMUNE MEDIATED
- Drugs (e.g., quinine, quinidine, heparin)
- Connective tissue disorders (e.g., systemic lupus erythematosus [SLE])
- Lymphoproliferative disorders (e.g., chronic lymphocytic leukemia [CLL])
- HIV infection
- Idiopathic
- Posttransfusion purpura

NON–IMMUNE MEDIATED
- Consumption (e.g., DIC, thrombotic thrombocytopenic purpura [TTP], prosthetic valves)
- Dilutional (e.g., massive transfusion)

SEQUESTRATION
- For instance, any cause of splenomegaly

Factitious Thrombocytopenia

Some patients have platelets that are susceptible to clumping when exposed to disodium edetate (EDTA), a preservative used in the lavender-topped blood collection tubes. The platelet clumping will result in a falsely low platelet count when the blood specimen is read by an autoanalyzer. Factitious thrombocytopenia can be diagnosed by verifying platelet clumping by direct examination of the blood smear. An accurate platelet count in these patients can be obtained by recollecting a blood sample in a sodium citrate (blue top) tube.

■ VESSEL OR PLATELET FUNCTION ABNORMALITIES

If the patient has a normal PT, aPTT, and platelet count and is not receiving LMWH, bleeding can still occur. This may be a result of *vessel abnormalities* or *abnormal platelet function*.

Vessel Abnormalities (Vascular Factor)

Hereditary Disorders
- Hereditary hemorrhagic telangiectasia
- Ehlers-Danlos syndrome
- Marfan's syndrome
- Pseudoxanthoma elasticum
- Osteogenesis imperfecta

Acquired Disorders

VASCULITIS
- Schönlein-Henoch purpura
- SLE
- Polyarteritis nodosa
- Rheumatoid arthritis
- Cryoglobulinemia

INCREASED VASCULAR FRAGILITY
- Senile purpura
- Cushing's syndrome
- Scurvy

Impaired Platelet Function

Hereditary Disorders
- von Willebrand's disease

- Bernard-Soulier disease
- Glanzmann's thrombasthenia

Acquired Disorders
- Drugs (e.g., aspirin; nonsteroidal anti-inflammatory drugs [NSAIDs]; antibiotics, such as high-dose penicillin, cephalosporins, nitrofurantoin)
- Uremia
- Paraproteins (e.g., amyloidosis, multiple myeloma, Waldenström's macroglobulinemia)
- Myeloproliferative and lymphoproliferative disease (e.g., chronic granulocytic leukemia [CGL], essential thrombocytosis)
- Post–cardiopulmonary bypass

■ BLEEDING IN COAGULATION DISORDERS

Manifestations

Bleeding in the patient with a coagulation disorder is of concern for two reasons.
1. Progressive loss of intravascular volume, if uncorrected, may lead to hypovolemic shock, with inadequate perfusion of vital organs.
2. Hemorrhage into specific organ sites may produce local tissue or organ injury (e.g., intracerebral hemorrhage, epidural hemorrhage with spinal cord compression, hemarthrosis).

TTP characteristically occurs with a combination of hemolytic anemia, thrombocytopenia, fever, neurologic disorders, and renal dysfunction. The *hemolytic uremic syndrome* has a presentation similar to that of TTP but without the neurologic manifestations. These two syndromes can be distinguished from *DIC*, in which prolonged aPTT and PT, reduced fibrinogen level, and elevated fibrin degradation products are seen. DIC most often occurs in the context of infection (e.g., gram-negative sepsis), obstetric catastrophes, malignancy (e.g., prostatic cancer), and tissue damage/shock.

Management

1. **Vessel abnormalities**. Treatment of bleeding due to vessel abnormalities is usually treatment of the underlying disorder.
   a. Serious bleeding due to *hereditary disorders of connective tissue* and to hereditary hemorrhagic telangiectasia most often requires local mechanical or surgical measures at the site of hemorrhage to control blood loss. Bleeding in some patients with hereditary hemorrhagic telangiectasia may be controlled with aminocaproic acid.[1]

b. In the *vasculitides*, control of bleeding is best achieved by use of corticosteroids, other immunosuppressive agents, or a combination of both.

c. There is no good treatment for the increased vascular fragility that results in senile purpura. Purpura due to *Cushing's syndrome* is preventable with normalization of plasma cortisol levels. However, in the patient receiving therapeutic corticosteroids, the underlying indication for therapy often prevents significant reduction of steroid levels. Hemorrhages associated with *scurvy* will not recur after adequate dietary supplementation of ascorbic acid.

2. **Coagulation factor abnormalities**. Treatment of coagulation factor abnormalities is dependent on the specific factor deficiency or deficiencies.

a. *Specific factor deficiencies* should always be treated in consultation with a hematologist. Factor VIII deficiency (hemophilia A) can be treated with fresh frozen plasma or cryoprecipitate, but factor VIII concentrate is the treatment of choice. Nonblood products may also be of benefit, e.g., desmopressin acetate (DDAVP injection), aminocaproic acid. Factor IX deficiency (hemophilia B) may be treated with fresh frozen plasma or prothrombin complex concentrate, but factor IX concentrate is the treatment of choice.

b. *Liver disease*. Active bleeding in patients with liver disease and an elevated PT, aPTT, or INR should be managed with fresh frozen plasma. Because patients with liver disease frequently are also vitamin K deficient, it is worthwhile to also administer vitamin K 10 mg SC or IV daily for 3 days. IV vitamin K occasionally has caused anaphylactic reactions. Factor IX concentrates carry a risk of thrombosis and are contraindicated in liver disease.

c. *Vitamin K deficiency* may be treated in an identical manner to that subsequently outlined for correction of warfarin coagulopathy. Ideally, however, one should identify and treat the underlying cause of vitamin K deficiency.

d. The treatment of *DIC* is both complicated and controversial. All medical authorities agree, however, that definitive management involves treating the underlying cause. Additionally, a patient with DIC often requires coagulation factor and platelet support in the form of fresh frozen plasma, cryoprecipitate, and platelet transfusions. The role of heparin in the treatment of DIC is controversial and should not be instituted before hematologic consultation.

e. Bleeding due to *anticoagulant therapy* can be reversed slowly or rapidly depending on the clinical status of the patient and the site of bleeding.

(1) *Unfractionated heparin* has a half-life of only 1½ hours, and simply discontinuing a heparin infusion should

normalize the aPTT and correct the heparin-induced coagulopathy in minor episodes of bleeding. *LMWH,* however, has a longer half-life, and it may be necessary to reverse the heparin effect with protamine sulfate. This may also be necessary in serious bleeding in association with unfractionated heparin. The usual dose is *protamine sulfate* 1 mg/100 units (either fractionated or unfractionated) heparin (approximately) IV slowly. Dosage is determined by estimating the amount of circulating heparin—e.g., for a patient on a maintenance infusion of unfractionated heparin 1000 units/hr IV, the heparin infusion should be stopped and sufficient protamine should be given to neutralize approximately one half of the preceding hour's dose, i.e., a total protamine dose of 5 mg. No more than 50 mg per single dose in a 10-minute period should be given. Side effects of protamine include hypotension, bradycardia, flushing, and bleeding.

(2) Rapid reversal of *warfarin* effect, as may be required in life-threatening hemorrhages, can be achieved by administering *plasma* (e.g., 2 units at a time), with subsequent redetermination of PT. Although both fresh frozen plasma and banked plasma contain the vitamin K–dependent clotting factors, banked plasma is considerably less expensive and, hence, is preferred. Prothrombin complex concentrates, if available, may achieve a more rapid or complete reversal of warfarin effect than plasma alone. Severe bleeding (e.g., intracranial hemorrhage) requires urgent hematologic consultation. When prolonged reversal of anticoagulant effect is desired, *vitamin K* 10 mg PO, SC, or IV may be given daily for 3 days. Minor bleeding complications in patients on warfarin may require temporary discontinuation of this drug. IV vitamin K occasionally has caused anaphylactic reactions and, hence, should be given with caution.

f. *Bleeding due to thrombolytic agents.* Localized oozing at sites of invasive procedures often can be controlled by local pressure dressings or avoided in the first place by not doing invasive procedures. More serious hemorrhage requires discontinuation of the thrombolytic agent. Fibrinolytic agents that are not fibrin specific will cause systemic fibrinogenolysis, and therefore fresh frozen plasma may be required to replace fibrinogen. Cryoprecipitate may also be used to replace fibrinogen and factor VIII levels. *Aminocaproic acid,* which is an inhibitor of plasminogen activator, has also been used (20 to 30 g/day) but should not be initiated before hematologic consultation.

3. **Platelet abnormalities.** Treatment of bleeding in the thrombo-

cytopenic patient varies depending on the presence of either an abnormality in platelet production or an increase in platelet destruction.

a. *Decreased marrow production* of platelets is treated in the long term by identifying and, if possible, correcting the underlying cause (e.g., chemotherapy for tumor, removal of marrow toxins, vitamin B_{12} or folate supplementation when indicated). In the short term, however, a serious bleeding complication should be treated by platelet transfusion (e.g., 6–8 units at a time). One unit of platelets can be expected to increase the platelet count by 1000 in the patient with inadequate marrow production of platelets. Check the response to transfusion by ordering a 1-hour postplatelet transfusion count.

b. *Increased peripheral destruction* of platelets also is best managed by identifying and correcting the underlying problem. Often, this management involves the systemic use of corticosteroids or other immunosuppressive agents. The patient tends to have less serious bleeding manifestations than one with inadequate marrow production of platelets but may require platelet transfusion for life-threatening bleeding episodes. Significant bleeding in patients with *idiopathic thrombocytopenic purpura (ITP)* may respond to IV immune globulin followed by platelet transfusions.[2] There are exceptions to platelet transfusion therapy in thrombocytopenia in the patient with *TTP*. In this situation, platelet transfusions should be avoided because they actually may worsen the condition. The platelet abnormality in TTP is best treated with plasma infusion[3] or, preferably, plasma exchange.[4]

c. *Dilutional thrombocytopenia* due to massive red blood cell (RBC) transfusion and IV fluid therapy is treated with platelet transfusion as required. Dilutional thrombocytopenia can usually be prevented by remembering to transfuse 8 units of platelets for every 10 to 12 units of RBCs transfused. (Because massive transfusion may also result in consumption and dilution of coagulation factors in the recipient, plasma should also be administered if there is evidence of bleeding and a significantly elevated PT, aPTT, or INR.)

d. *von Willebrand's disease* may be treated with factor VIII concentrates or cryoprecipitate. Desmopressin acetate (DDAVP injection) is useful in type I von Willebrand's disease but may exacerbate thrombocytopenia in type II von Willebrand's disease.

e. Bleeding disorders resulting from *acquired platelet dysfunction* are best managed by identification and correction of the underlying problem. Temporary treatment of bleeding disorders due to these conditions may involve platelet transfusion or other more specialized measures (e.g., cryoprecipitate, desmopressin acetate [DDAVP injection], plasmapheresis, conjugated estrogens, or intensive dialysis in uremia).

References

1. Saba HI, Morelli GA, Logrono LA: Treatment of bleeding in hereditary hemorrhagic telangiectasia with aminocaproic acid. N Engl J Med 1994;330:1789–1790.
2. Baumann MA, Menitove JE, Aster RH, et al: Urgent treatment of idiopathic thrombocytopenic purpura with single-dose gammaglobulin infusion followed by platelet transfusion. Ann Intern Med 1986;104:808–809.
3. Byrnes JJ, Khurana M: Treatment of thrombotic thrombocytopenic purpura with plasma. N Engl J Med 1997;297:1386–1389.
4. Rock GA, Shumak KH, Buskard NA, et al: Comparison of plasma exchange with plasma infusion in the treatment of thrombotic thrombocytopenic purpura: Canadian Apheresis Study Group. N Engl J Med 1991;325:393–397.

GLUCOSE DISORDERS

HYPERGLYCEMIA

Causes

Patients with Documented Diabetes Mellitus
- Poorly controlled type 1 or type 2 diabetes mellitus
- Stress (surgery, infection, severe illness)
- Drugs (corticosteroids, thiazides, beta blockers, phenytoin, nicotinic acid, opiates)
- Total parenteral nutrition (TPN) administration
- Pancreatic injury (pancreatitis, trauma, surgical)

Patients Without Previously Documented Diabetes Mellitus
- New onset of diabetes mellitus
- Stress (surgery, infection, severe illness)
- Drugs (corticosteroids, thiazides, beta-blockers, phenytoin, nicotinic acid, opiates)
- TPN administration
- Pancreatic injury (pancreatitis, trauma, surgical)

Acute Manifestations

Mild Hyperglycemia (fasting blood glucose of 6.1 to 11.0 mmol/L)
- Polyuria, polydipsia, thirst

Moderate Hyperglycemia (fasting blood glucose of 11.1 to 22.5 mmol/L)
- Volume depletion (tachycardia, decreased jugular venous pressure [JVP], ± hypotension)
- Polyuria, polydipsia, thirst

Severe Hyperglycemia (fasting blood glucose > 22.5 mmol/L)

TYPE 1 DIABETES MELLITUS
- Musty odor on breath (ketone breath)
- Kussmaul's breathing (deep, pauseless respirations seen when pH is < 7.2)
- Volume depletion (tachycardia, decreased JVP, ± hypotension)
- Anorexia, nausea, vomiting, abdominal pain (may mimic a surgical abdomen)
- Ileus, gastric dilatation
- Hyporeflexia, hypotonia, delirium, coma

TYPE 2 DIABETES MELLITUS
- Polyuria, polydipsia
- Volume depletion
- Confusion, coma

Management

Many hyperglycemic patients will require SC or IV administration of insulin. Bovine, porcine, and human insulins are available, and each has different antigenicities. Bovine insulin is the most immunogenic, and human insulin is the least. Human insulin is derived from DNA recombinant techniques using either baker's yeast (Novolin ge insulins) or *Escherichia coli* bacteria (Humulin insulins). Human insulins are associated with fewer adverse reactions (e.g., insulin allergy, antibody-mediated insulin resistance, lipoatrophy) and should be considered especially when treatment is intermittent. If the patient is already receiving bovine or porcine insulin without complications, it is fine to make dosage adjustments with the same preparation the patient is receiving.

Assess the Severity. The severity of the situation should be determined according to the blood glucose level and the patient's symptoms (Table 32–1).

Treatment
MILD, ASYMPTOMATIC HYPERGLYCEMIA. Mild, asymptomatic hyperglycemia does not require urgent treatment. Order the following.
1. Fasting blood glucose in the morning: A fasting blood glucose of > 7.0 mmol/L on more than one occasion confirms the diagnosis of diabetes mellitus. Make sure the patient is not receiving glucose-containing IV solutions that will make these results invalid. In addition, the diagnosis of diabetes mellitus cannot be made in the setting of stress (e.g., infection, surgery, severe illness). Any one of the following criteria[1] is diagnostic for diabetes mellitus:
   a. Fasting blood sugar > 7.0 mmol/L $\times$ 2 (venous plasma)
   b. Random blood sugar > 11.1 mmol/L $\times$ 2 (venous plasma)

Table 32–1 □ **BLOOD GLUCOSE LEVELS**

	Fasting or AC Blood Glucose (mmol/L)	2-Hour PC Blood Glucose (mmol/L)
Normal range	3.5–6.0	< 11.0
Mild hyperglycemia	6.1–11.0	11.1–16.5
Moderate hyperglycemia	11.1–22.5	16.6–27.5
Severe hyperglycemia	> 22.5	> 27.5

    c. A glucose tolerance test (GTT) with a 2-hour PC blood sugar ≥ 11.1 mmol/L (venous plasma)

2. Chemstrip or Glucose meter readings before meals and at bedtime. If the readings are > 25 or < 2.8 mmol/L, a stat blood glucose sample should be drawn and a physician informed.

MODERATE HYPERGLYCEMIA. Moderate hyperglycemia may require an adjustment of the insulin being given. Examine the diabetic record for the past 3 days.

A sample adjustment in insulin dosage is given in Table 32–2. The Chemstrip or Glucose meter readings are in millimoles per liter, and the SC insulin dose given is indicated in parentheses (e.g., 20/10 indicates that 20 units of neutral protamine Hagedorn [NPH] and 10 units of regular insulin have been given).

You have been called at night because of a Chemstrip/Glucose meter reading of 25 mmol/L. Order the following:

1. Stat random blood glucose to confirm the Chemstrip or Glucose meter reading.

2. Regular insulin 5 to 10 units SC now. The main consideration now is not to devise a schedule that will achieve perfect blood glucose control for the rest of the patient's hospital stay. Short-term control of blood glucose levels has not been shown to decrease complications in the diabetic. When the blood glucose level is elevated at night, your aim is to prevent the development of ketoacidosis in the patient with type 1 diabetes mellitus or of the hyperosmolar state in the patient with type 2 diabetes mellitus without producing symptomatic hypoglycemia with your treatment.

3. Determining the reason for poor control of blood glucose AC breakfast may aid in an ongoing adjustment of the patient's insulin. This can be achieved by ordering an 0300 h Chemstrip or Glucose meter reading. Hypoglycemia documented at 0300 h would suggest that AC breakfast hyperglycemia is due to hyperglycemic rebound (the Somogyi effect), which is correctly managed by reducing the AC supper NPH insulin dose. Hyperglycemia documented at 0300 h would suggest that AC

Table 32–2 □ **SAMPLE INSULIN DOSAGE ADJUSTMENT**

	AC Breakfast (NPH/REG)	AC Lunch (NPH/REG)	AC Supper (NPH/REG)	QHS (NPH/REG)
August 1	16.7* (20/10)†	13.9 (0/0)	16.7 (10/10)	18.1 (0/0)
August 2	13.9 (20/10)	16.7 (0/4)	8.3 (10/10)	19.4 (0/0)
August 3	16.7 (20/10)	15.2 (0/0)	13.1 (10/10)	25.0 (0/0)

*Chemstrip or Glucose meter reading given in mmol/L.
†Indicates 20 units of NPH and 10 units of regular insulin.

breakfast hyperglycemia is due to inadequate insulin coverage overnight. This is correctly managed by increasing the AC supper NPH insulin dose.

SEVERE HYPERGLYCEMIA. Severe hyperglycemia requires urgent treatment.
1. **Diabetic ketoacidosis (DKA).** This complication may be seen in the patient with poorly controlled type 1 diabetes mellitus. It is due to an absolute insulin deficit, resulting in impaired resynthesis of long-chain fatty acids from acetate, with subsequent conversion to the acidic ketone bodies (ketosis).
    a. *Correct volume depletion.* Give 500 to 1000 ml NS IV over the first hour, with further IV rates guided by reassessment of volume status. Patients with DKA often have a 3- to 5-L volume deficit. It is therefore not unusual to require continued NS at rates of 500 ml/hr for an additional 2 to 8 hours to restore euvolemia. If the patient has a history of congestive heart failure (CHF), weight < 50 kg, or is ≥ 80 years of age, NS should be given cautiously to avoid iatrogenic CHF.
    b. *Begin an insulin infusion.* Give 5 to 10 units of IV regular insulin as a single dose by direct slow injection, followed by an infusion rate based on close monitoring of Chemstrip or Glucose meter readings. Start the insulin infusion at 0.1 U/kg/hr in NS. Regular insulin can bind to the plastic IV tubing. To ensure accurate insulin delivery, 30 to 50 ml of the infusion solution should be run through the IV tubing and discarded before connecting the IV tubing to the patient. Discontinue the standing order for SC insulin or oral hypoglycemics before beginning the insulin infusion.

    Monitor blood sugar hourly by Chemstrip or Glucose meter. When the blood sugar has fallen to 14 mmol/L, continue the insulin infusion but switch the delivery solution from NS to D5W. Continue the insulin infusion until the blood sugars remain stable at 8 to 10 mmol/L. As the blood sugar falls, the rate of insulin infusion should be slowed (e.g., 0.025 to 0.05 U/kg/hr). The rate of fall of blood sugar should be approximately 2.0 mmol/L/hr; more aggressive treatment of the hyperglycemia may result in severe hypokalemia and cerebral edema. When the sugars have stabilized at 8 to 10 mmol/L, restart SC insulin, remembering that the insulin infusion must be continued for 1 to 2 hours after the injection of SC insulin, or ketogenesis will be reactivated. Continue to monitor the bedside sugars every 4 hours, adding supplemental regular insulin to keep blood sugars between 8 and 10 mmol/L.
    c. *Monitor blood glucose, serum electrolytes, and arterial blood gases (ABGs).* Hyperglycemic patients can have metabolic

acidemia and hypokalemia. As NS and insulin are administered, the acidemia is corrected, and the potassium shifts
into the cells from the extracellular fluid. This can result
in worsening of the hypokalemia. Order baseline ABGs,
electrolytes, urea, creatinine, and glucose levels. Repeat the
ABGs and potassium level in 2 hours and thereafter as
required. When hypokalemia is first noted, add KCl to the
IV NS, provided the patient is passing urine and has normal
urea and creatinine levels. If the patient is in renal failure,
caution should be taken in adding any potassium to the IV,
to avoid iatrogenic hyperkalemia.

   d. *Search for the precipitating cause.* Common precipitating factors include the following.
   (1) Infection
   (2) Inadequate insulin dosage
   (3) Dietary indiscretion
   (4) Pancreatitis

2. **Hyperosmolar, hyperglycemic, nonketotic state.** This condition may be seen in a patient with poorly controlled type 2
diabetes mellitus. Typically, the patient is 50 to 70 years old.
Many have no prior histories of diabetes mellitus. The precipitating event is often stroke, infection, pancreatitis, or drugs.
The blood glucose level is often very high (e.g., > 55 mmol/
L), but significant ketosis is absent.

   a. *Correct volume depletion and water deficit.* The objective of
   fluid therapy in the nonketotic hyperosmolar state is to both
   correct the volume deficit and resolve the hyperosmolarity.
   These can be achieved by giving 500 to 1000 ml of NS IV
   over 1 to 2 hours, with further IV rates guided by reassess-
   ment of volume status. Once the volume deficit is corrected
   using NS, remaining water deficits, as indicated by persistent hypernatremia or hyperglycemia, are best corrected
   using hypotonic IV solutions, such as ½ NS.

   b. *Begin an insulin infusion.* See previous discussion of treatment of DKA. Rehydration alone often produces a substan-
   tial fall in blood glucose through renal excretion. As a result,
   patients with the hyperosmolar, hyperglycemic, nonketotic
   state generally require less insulin than the patient with
   type 1 diabetes and ketoacidosis.

   c. *Monitor blood glucose level and serum electrolytes.* Order baseline electrolytes, urea, creatinine, and glucose levels. Repeat
   the blood glucose level and the electrolytes determinations
   in 2 hours and thereafter as required.

   d. *Search for the precipitating cause.*
   (1) Infection
   (2) Inadequate fluid intake
   (3) Other acute illnesses (myocardial infarction [MI], stroke)

HYPOGLYCEMIA

Causes

Patients with Documented Diabetes Mellitus
- Excess insulin or oral hypoglycemic administration
- Decreased caloric intake
- Missed meals or missed snacks
- Increased exercise

Patients Without Documented Diabetes Mellitus
- Surreptitious intake of insulin or oral hypoglycemics
- Insulinoma
- Supervised 72-hour fasting for the investigation of hypoglycemia
- Drugs (ethanol, pentamidine, disopyramide, monoamine oxidase [MAO] inhibitors)
- Hepatic failure
- Adrenal insufficiency

Manifestations

Adrenergic Response (i.e., catecholamine release due to a rapid decrease in glucose level)
- Diaphoresis
- Palpitations
- Tremulousness
- Tachycardia
- Hunger
- Acral and perioral numbness
- Anxiety
- Combativeness
- Confusion
- Coma

CNS Response (slow response may develop over 1 to 3 hours)
- Headaches
- Diplopia
- Bizarre behavior
- Focal neurologic deficits
- Confusion
- Seizures
- Coma

The adrenergic response does not always precede the CNS response, and some patients may progress directly from confusion or inability to speak to seizures or coma.

Management

Assess the Severity. Any symptomatic patient with suspected hypoglycemia requires treatment. Symptoms may be precipitated by either a rapid fall in blood glucose level or an absolute low level of blood glucose.

1. *Draw 1 ml of blood* to be sent for blood glucose testing to confirm the diagnosis. If the cause of hypoglycemia is not clear, draw 10 ml, and ask the laboratory to save an aliquot for possible later insulin and C peptide measurement. Insulin produced endogenously includes the C peptide fragment, in contrast to commercial preparations of insulin. A high insulin level associated with a high C peptide fragment and hypoglycemia suggests endogenous production of excess insulin (e.g., insulinoma), whereas a high insulin level associated with a low C peptide level and hypoglycemia suggests surreptitious or therapeutic administration of exogenous insulin. **Do not wait for the blood glucose result to return from the lab before treating.**

2. In the cooperative awake patient, oral glucose in the form of sweetened fruit juice may be given. If the patient is unable to take oral fluids or is unconscious, *D50W* 50 ml IV should be given by direct, slow injection. If there is no IV access and the patient is unable to take oral fluids (e.g., unconscious), *glucagon* 1.0 mg SC or IM should be given. After glucagon administration, vomiting may develop, so the patient who is not fully conscious should be monitored carefully to prevent aspiration.

3. If ongoing hypoglycemia is anticipated or if the patient's symptoms were severe (e.g., seizure, coma), begin a maintenance IV of D5W or D10W at a rate of 100 ml/hr. Ask the RN to reassess the patient in 1 hour. In addition, remeasure the blood glucose level in 2 to 4 hours to ensure that hypoglycemic relapse has not occurred. Hypoglycemia due to oral hypoglycemics may require repeated doses of D50W because of the slow metabolism and excretion of these drugs.

Reference

1. Report of the Expert Committee on the Diagnosis and Classification of Diabetes Mellitus. Diabetes Care 1997;20:1183–1197.

33

POTASSIUM DISORDERS

HYPERKALEMIA

Causes

Excessive Intake
- K^+ supplements (oral [PO] or intravenous [IV])
- Salt substitutes
- High-dose IV therapy with K^+ salts of penicillin
- Blood transfusions

Decreased Excretion
- Renal failure (acute or chronic)
- Drugs
- K^+-sparing diuretics (spironolactone, triamterene, amiloride)
- Angiotensin-converting enzyme (ACE) inhibitors
- Nonsteroidal anti-inflammatory drugs (NSAIDs)
- Trimethoprim-sulfamethoxazole
- Pentamidine
- Cyclosporine
- Addison's disease, hypoaldosteronism
- Distal tubular dysfunction (i.e., type IV renal tubular acidosis [RTA])

Shift from Intracellular to Extracellular Fluid
- Acidemia (especially nonanion gap)
- Insulin deficiency
- Tissue destruction (hemolysis, crush injuries, rhabdomyolysis, extensive burns, tumor lysis)
- Drugs (succinylcholine, digoxin, arginine, beta blockers)
- Hyperkalemic periodic paralysis

Factitious
- Prolonged tourniquet placement for venipuncture
- Blood sample hemolysis
- Leukocytosis
- Thrombocytosis

Manifestations

Cardiac
- Fatal ventricular dysrhythmias
  The progressive electrocardiographic (ECG) changes seen in hyperkalemia are peaked T waves → depressed ST seg-

ments → decreased amplitude of R waves → prolonged PR interval → small or absent P waves → wide QRS complexes → biphasic sine wave pattern (Fig. 33–1). Dysrhythmias associated with hyperkalemia include bradycardias, complete heart block, ventricular fibrillation, and asystole.

Neuromuscular
- Weakness, often beginning in the lower extremities
- Paresthesias
- Depressed tendon reflexes

Management

ECG. Fatal ventricular dysrhythmias can occur at any time during treatment; hence, continuous ECG monitoring is required if the K^+ level is > 6.5 mmol/L.

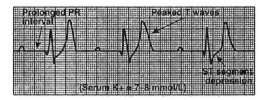

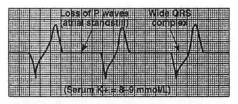

Figure 33–1 □ Progressive electrocardiographic manifestations of hyperkalemia.

Assess the Severity. The severity of the situation should be determined according to the serum K^+ concentration, the ECG findings, and whether the underlying cause is immediately remediable.

IF SEVERE
- Serum K^+ > 8.0 mmol/L
- ECG findings more advanced than peaked T waves alone
- Cause not immediately remediable

1. Notify your resident.
2. Place the patient on continuous ECG monitoring.
3. Correct contributing factors (acidemia, hypovolemia).
4. Give one or more of the following:
    a. *Calcium gluconate* 5 to 10 ml of a 10% solution given IV over 2 minutes. This will temporarily antagonize the cardiac and neuromuscular effects of hyperkalemia. The onset of calcium gluconate is immediate, and its effect lasts 1 hour. It will not, however, reduce the serum concentration of K^+. *Caution*: The administration of calcium to the patient on digoxin may precipitate ventricular dysrhythmias due to the combined effects of digoxin and calcium.
    b. *50% dextrose in water (D50W)* 50 ml IV followed by *regular insulin* 5 to 10 units IV will shift K^+ from the extracellular fluid (ECF) to the intracellular fluid (ICF). Its effect is immediate and lasts 1 to 2 hours. If the patient is already hyperglycemic, the D50W should be omitted. Serum glucose levels should be followed subsequently to determine whether additional doses of insulin are required and to ensure that hypoglycemia does not occur.
    c. *Sodium bicarbonate* 1 amp (44.6 mmol) IV will shift K^+ from the ECF to the ICF. Its effect is immediate and lasts 1 to 2 hours.
    d. Give a *glucose-insulin-HCO$_3$* cocktail: D10W 1000 ml with 3 ampules of $NaHCO_3$ and 20 units of regular insulin at 75 ml/hr until more definitive measures are taken.
    e. *Sodium polystyrene sulfonate* (Kayexalate) 15 to 30 g (4 to 8 teaspoonfuls) in 50 to 100 ml of 20% sorbitol PO every 3 to 4 hours or 50 g in 200 ml D20W PR by retention enema for 30 to 60 minutes every 4 hours. This is the only drug treatment that actually will remove K^+ from the total body pool. Watch carefully for evidence of volume overload because this resin works by exchanging Na for K^+.
    f. *β$_2$-adrenergic agonists* can temporarily reduce serum K^+ by stimulating cyclic AMP and shifting K^+ from the ECF to the ICF. *Salbutamol* 10 to 20 mg by nebulizer may be transiently effective in lowering serum K^+ in patients on hemodialysis.[1]
5. *Hemodialysis* should be considered on an urgent basis if the

aforementioned measures have failed or if the patient is in acute or chronic oliguric renal failure.
6. Monitor the serum K^+ concentration every 1 to 2 hours until it is < 6.5 mmol/L.

IF MODERATE
- Serum K^+ between 6.5 and 8.0 mmol/L
- ECG findings show peaked T waves only
- Cause is not progressive
1. Place the patient on continuous ECG monitoring.
2. Correct contributing factors (acidemia, hypovolemia).
3. Give one or more of the following in the dosages previously outlined.
   a. $NaHCO_3$
   b. Glucose and insulin
   c. Sodium polystyrene sulfonate
4. Monitor the serum K^+ concentration every 1 to 2 hours until it is < 6.5 mmol/L.

IF MILD
- Serum K^+ < 6.5 mmol/L
- ECG findings show peaked T waves only
- Cause is not progressive
   - Correct contributing factors (acidemia, hypovolemia).
   - Remeasure the serum K^+ concentration 4 to 6 hours later, depending on the cause.

HYPOKALEMIA

Causes

Renal Losses (urine K^+ > 20 mmol/day)
- Diuretics, osmotic diuresis
- Antibiotics (carbenicillin, ticarcillin, nafcillin, amphotericin, aminoglycosides)
- RTA (classic type I)
- Hyperaldosteronism
- Glucocorticoid excess
- Magnesium deficiency
- Chronic metabolic alkalosis
- Bartter's syndrome
- Fanconi's syndrome
- Ureterosigmoidostomy
- Vomiting, nasogastric (NG) suction. (Hydrogen ions are lost with vomiting and NG suction, inducing alkalosis that results in renal K^+ wasting.)

Extrarenal Losses (urine K$^+$ < 20 mmol/day)
- Diarrhea
- Intestinal fistula

Inadequate Intake
Over 1 to 2 weeks

Shift from Extracellular to Intracellular Space
- Acute alkalosis
- Drugs
- Insulin therapy
- Vitamin B$_{12}$ therapy
- Salbutamol
- Lithium
- Hypokalemic periodic paralysis
- Hypothermia

Manifestations

Cardiac
- Premature atrial contractions (PACs)
- Premature ventricular contractions (PVCs)
- Digoxin toxicity
- ECG changes (Fig. 33–2)
  - T wave flattening
  - U waves
  - ST segment depression

Neuromuscular
- Weakness
- Depressed deep tendon reflexes
- Paresthesias
- Ileus

Miscellaneous
- Nephrogenic diabetes insipidus
- Metabolic alkalosis
- Worsening of hepatic encephalopathy

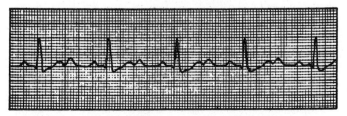

Figure 33–2 □ Electrocardiographic manifestations of hypokalemia.

Management

If possible, **correct the underlying cause**.

Assess the Severity. The severity of the situation should be determined according to the serum K^+ concentration, the ECG findings, and the clinical setting in which hypokalemia is occurring.

IF SEVERE. (Serum $K^+ < 3.0$ mmol/L with PVCs in the setting of myocardial ischemia or with digoxin toxicity)
1. Notify your resident.
2. Place the patient on continuous ECG monitoring.
3. IV replacement therapy may be required, i.e., 10 mmol KCl in 100 ml NS given IV over 1 hour. Repeat once or twice as necessary. KCl in small volumes should be given through central IV lines because these high concentrations of K^+ are sclerosing to peripheral veins. Further replacement can be achieved with maintenance therapy containing up to 40 to 60 mmol KCl/L of IV fluid at a maximum rate of 20 mmol/hr. K^+ can also be given by administration of the liquid salt by NG tube or by oral supplementation.
4. Recheck serum K^+ concentration after each 20 to 30 mmol IV KCl has been given.

IF MODERATE. (Serum $K^+ \leq 3.0$ mmol/L with PACs but no [or infrequent] PVCs and no digoxin toxicity)
1. Notify your resident.
2. Oral K^+ supplementation is usually adequate, e.g., Slow-K = 8 mmol KCl per tablet, Kay Ciel Elixir = 20 mmol/15 ml, and K-Lyte = 25 mmol/packet.
3. IV replacement therapy in this situation should be reserved for patients with marked hypokalemia or patients who are unable to take oral supplements (see previous recommendations).
4. Recheck serum K^+ concentration in the morning or sooner if clinically indicated.

IF MILD. (Serum K^+ between 3.1 and 3.5 mmol/L, no [or infrequent] PVCs, and patient asymptomatic)
1. Oral supplementation usually is adequate (see previous recommendations).
2. Recheck serum K^+ concentration in the morning or sooner if clinically indicated.

■ REMEMBER

1. Serious hyperkalemia has occurred as a result of K^+ supplementation. Hence, serum K^+ levels should be closely moni-

tored during treatment. Be particularly cautious in patients with renal impairment.

2. Hypokalemia and hypocalcemia may coexist. Correction of hypokalemia without accompanying correction of hypocalcemia may increase the risk of ventricular dysrhythmias.

3. Hypokalemia and hypomagnesemia may coexist. Correction of hypokalemia may be unsuccessful unless hypomagnesemia is corrected simultaneously.

Reference

1. Allon M, Dunlay R, Copkney C: Nebulized albuterol for acute hyperkalemia in patients on hemodialysis. Ann Intern Med 1989;110:426–429.

34

SODIUM DISORDERS

HYPERNATREMIA

Causes
1. Inadequate intake of water
   a. Coma
   b. Hypothalamic dysfunction
2. Excessive water losses
   a. Renal losses
      (1) Diabetes insipidus (nephrogenic or pituitary)
      (2) Osmotic diuresis (hyperglycemia, mannitol administration, urea)
   b. Extrarenal losses
      (1) Gastrointestinal (GI) losses (vomiting, nasogastric [NG] suction, diarrhea)
      (2) Insensible losses (burns, febrile illness, tachypnea)
3. Excessive sodium gain
   a. Iatrogenic (excessive sodium administration)
   b. Primary hyperaldosteronism

Manifestations

Hypernatremia most often results from extracellular fluid (ECF) volume depletion due to hypotonic fluid loss (e.g., vomiting, diarrhea, sweating, osmotic diuresis). Symptoms are dependent on the absolute increase in serum osmolality as well as the rate at which it develops. The manifestations of hypernatremia are due to acute brain cell shrinkage from an outward shift of intracellular water, which occurs as a result of increased ECF osmolality. They range from confusion and muscle irritability to seizures, respiratory paralysis, and death.

Management

1. **Assess the severity.** The severity of the situation should be determined according to the symptomatic state of the patient, the serum sodium concentration, the serum osmolality, and the ECF volume.
   a. Osmolality can be measured in the laboratory. However, sufficient information may be available to permit its calculation from knowledge of the major osmotically active substances in the ECF.

$$\text{Osmolality (mmol/kg)} = 2\,\text{Na (mmol/L)} + \text{urea (mmol/L)} + \text{glucose (mmol/L)}$$

The normal range is 281 to 297 mmol/kg.

  b. Most patients with hypernatremia have an accompanying extracellular volume deficit that can compromise perfusion of vital organs. Assess the volume status of the patient (see Chapter 3).

  c. Most patients with hypernatremia have relatively few symptoms and are not at immediate risk of dying!

2. If possible, **correct the cause**, which is usually evident from the history and physical findings.

3. **Correct volume and water deficits.** The choice of fluid is dependent on the severity of the extracellular volume deficit.

  a. In patients who are volume depleted, hypernatremia can be corrected by giving intravenous (IV) normal saline (NS) until the patient is hemodynamically stable and then changing to ½ NS or 5% dextrose in water (D5W) to correct the remaining water deficit.

  b. In patients who are not volume depleted, ½ NS or D5W can be used to correct the water deficit.

  An estimation of the volume of water required can be calculated, remembering that the deficit is in *total body water*, which is approximately 60% of body weight.

Water deficit =
$$\frac{[\text{serum Na (observed)} - \text{serum Na (normal)}] \times 0.6\ \text{weight (kg)}}{\text{Serum Na (normal)}}$$

EXAMPLE. A 65-year-old man is admitted to the hospital after being found in his apartment 2 days after falling and fracturing his hip. He is moderately volume depleted and has a serum sodium value of 156 mmol/L. His weight is 70 kg. To calculate the volume of water required to correct the serum sodium

Free water deficit =
$$\frac{[156\ \text{mmol/L} - 140\ \text{mmol/L}] \times 0.6\ (70\ \text{L})}{140\ \text{mmol/L}} = 4.8\ \text{L}$$

Remember to correct the osmolality abnormality at a rate similar to the rate at which it developed. Biological systems are more responsive to rates of change than to absolute amounts of change. It is safest to correct half the deficit and then reevaluate. More rapid corrections than 1 to 2 mmol/L in serum sodium can lead to brain swelling, resulting in the development of confusion, seizures, or coma.

  c. In the occasional patient with hypernatremia who is volume overloaded, the hypernatremia can be corrected by initiating a diuresis using *furosemide* (Lasix) 20 to 40 mg IV and repeating at intervals of 2 to 4 hours as necessary. Once the extracellular volume has returned to normal, if the serum sodium level is still elevated, diuresis should be continued, with urinary volume losses replaced with D5W until the serum Na repeat level is again in the normal range.

HYPONATREMIA

Causes

1. **Hyponatremia with decreased ECF volume**
   a. Renal loss of sodium
      (1) Diuretic excess
      (2) Na-losing nephropathies
      (3) Diuretic phase of acute tubular necrosis
      (4) Bartter's syndrome
      (5) Hypoaldosteronism
   b. Extrarenal losses of sodium
      (1) Vomiting, NG suction
      (2) Diarrhea
      (3) Sweating
      (4) Burns
      (5) Pancreatitis
2. **Hyponatremia with ECF volume excess and edema**
   a. Renal failure
   b. Nephrotic syndrome
   c. CHF
   d. Cirrhosis of the liver
3. **Hyponatremia with normal extracellular fluid volume**
   a. Syndrome of inappropriate antidiuretic hormone (SIADH)
      (1) Tumors
         (a) Small cell carcinoma of the lung
         (b) Pancreatic carcinoma
         (c) Duodenal adenocarcinoma
         (d) Lymphosarcoma
      (2) Central nervous system (CNS) disorders
         (a) Brain tumors
         (b) Brain trauma
         (c) Meningitis
         (d) Encephalitis
         (e) Subarachnoid hemorrhage
         (f) Guillain-Barré syndrome
      (3) Pulmonary disorders
         (a) Tuberculosis
         (b) Pneumonia

- (4) Drugs
  - (a) Hypoglycemic agents (chlorpropamide, tolbutamide)
  - (b) Neuroleptics (haloperidol, trifluoperazine, fluphenazine, and others)
  - (c) Antidepressants (amitriptyline, desipramine, tranylcypromine)
  - (d) Antineoplastic drugs (cyclophosphamide, vincristine)
  - (e) Narcotics
  - (f) Clofibrate
  - (g) Carbamazepine
  - (h) Nicotine
- (5) The postoperative state (particularly in premenopausal women)
- b. Primary polydipsia (water intoxication)
- c. Pseudohyponatremia
  - (1) Hyponatremia with normal serum osmolality
    - (a) Hyperlipidemia
    - (b) Hyperproteinemia
  - (2) Hyponatremia with increased serum osmolality
    - (a) Excess urea
    - (b) Hyperglycemia
    - (c) Mannitol
    - (d) Ethanol
    - (e) Methanol
    - (f) Ethylene glycol
    - (g) Isopropyl alcohol
- d. Endocrine disorders
  - (1) Hypothyroidism
  - (2) Addison's disease

Manifestations

Manifestations of hyponatremia depend on the absolute decrease in the serum osmolality, the rate of development of hyponatremia, and the volume status of the patient. When associated with a decreased serum osmolality, hyponatremia may cause the following.

- Confusion
- Lethargy
- Weakness
- Nausea and vomiting
- Seizures
- Coma

When hyponatremia develops gradually, a patient may tolerate a serum sodium concentration of less than 110 mmol/L with only moderate confusion or lethargy. However, a patient in whom the serum sodium concentration decreases rapidly from 140 to 115 mmol/L may experience a seizure.

Management

1. **Assess the severity.** The severity of the situation should be determined according to the symptomatic state of the patient, the serum sodium concentration, the serum osmolality, and the ECF.

   Remember that when attempting to correct disorders manifested by hyponatremia, brain cells try to maintain their volume in dilutional states by losing solutes (e.g., potassium). If the serum sodium level is corrected too rapidly (i.e., to levels greater than 120 to 125 mmol/L), the serum may become hypertonic relative to brain cells, resulting in an outward shift of water, with resultant CNS damage due to acute brain shrinkage.

2. If possible, **correct the cause** of the hyponatremia. Urinary electrolyte determination may be helpful in identifying the primary cause of hyponatremia when one or more possible etiologies exist. The renal response to salt and water loss differs depending on the cause of hyponatremia. When extrarenal losses of sodium and water occur through the skin (e.g., sweating, burns) or due to third-spacing (e.g., pancreatitis), the renal response is to conserve sodium (urine Na < 20 mmol/L) and to conserve water through secretion of antidiuretic hormone (ADH) (high urine osmolality). However, if volume loss is due to vomiting or NG suction, primarily HCl is lost from gastric secretions. The kidneys generate and excrete $NaHCO_3$ to maintain acid-base balance, resulting in a urine with a normal (> 20 mmol/L) Na but a low (< 20 mmol/L) Cl. If volume loss is due to diarrhea, primarily $NaHCO_3$ is lost in the stools. The kidneys generate and excrete NH_4Cl to maintain acid-base balance, resulting in a urine that is low in Na but not in Cl.

   Hyponatremia with ECF excess and edema may be accompanied by a low (< 20 mmol/L) urinary Na (e.g., nephrotic syndrome, CHF, cirrhosis of the liver) or a normal urinary Na (renal failure).

3. **Assess the volume status** of the patient (see Chapter 3).
   a. If the patient is volume depleted, correct the ECF volume using NS. Aim for a jugular venous pressure (JVP) of 2 to 3 cm H_2O above the sternal angle. In this case, the amount of sodium required to improve the serum sodium concentration can be calculated using the following formula.

$$\text{mmol Na} = [\text{serum Na (desired)} - \text{serum Na (observed)}] \times \text{TBW}$$

where

$$\text{TBW} = 0.6 \times \text{weight (in kg)}$$

Remember that biologic systems are more responsive to rates of change than to absolute amounts of change. Make corrections at a rate similar to the rate at which the abnormality developed. It is safest to correct half the deficit and reassess the situation.

EXAMPLE. For a 70-kg man in whom you want to raise the serum sodium level from 120 to 135 mmol/L, the amount of Na required

$$= (135 \text{ mmol/L} - 120 \text{ mmol/L}) (0.6 \times 70 \text{ L})$$
$$= (15 \text{ mmol/L}) (42 \text{ L})$$
$$= 630 \text{ mmol Na}$$

Because 1 L of NS contains 154 mmol of Na, you will require approximately 4 L of NS to raise the patient's serum level to 135 mmol/L.

b. If the patient has *extracellular volume excess and edema*, treat the volume excess and hyponatremia with water restriction and diuretics. Because most of these states are accompanied by secondary hyperaldosteronism, *spironolactone* is a reasonable choice of diuretic, as long as the patient is not hyperkalemic. Remember that the diuretic effect of spironolactone may be delayed for 3 to 4 days. The dose can range from 25 to 200 mg daily in adults and may be given once daily or in divided doses.

In this situation strict intake/output charts can be useful. To raise the serum sodium, the daily water intake should be less than the daily urine output.

c. If the patient has a normal ECF volume, SIADH, primary polydipsia, pseudohyponatremia, or endocrine disorders should be considered.

SIADH

The diagnosis of SIADH requires that stringent criteria be met.
1. Hyponatremia with serum hypo-osmolality
2. Urine that is less than maximally dilute when compared with serum osmolality (i.e., a simultaneous urine osmolality that is greater than the serum osmolality)
3. Inappropriately large amounts of urine Na ($U_{Na} > 20$ mmol/L)

4. Normal renal function
5. Normal thyroid function
6. Normal adrenal function
7. Patient not on diuretics

Management

SIADH should be treated by
1. Correcting the underlying cause or contributory factors (e.g., drugs), if present.
2. Water restriction, usually to less than insensible losses (e.g., 500 to 1000 ml/day).
3. In addition to the first two measures, patients with severe symptomatic hyponatremia (serum Na of <115 mmol/L) may benefit from furosemide-induced diuresis, with hourly replacement of urinary sodium and potassium losses using NS. Very rarely, 3% saline will be required.

   Too rapid correction of hyponatremia can result in central pontine myelinolysis and other undesirable side effects. Correct the serum sodium level slowly. Once the serum sodium level is greater than 120 to 125 mmol/L, many of the symptoms of hyponatremia will begin to lessen.
4. *Demeclocycline* 300 to 600 mg PO twice a day occasionally is useful in patients with chronic symptomatic SIADH in whom water restriction has been unsuccessful.

Primary Polydipsia

"Water intoxication" should be suspected in the patient with a psychiatric disorder, particularly when excessive drinking and polyuria interfere with sleep or are noticed by the ward staff. The hyponatremia is often exacerbated by effects of neuroleptic or antidepressant medication that the patient may be taking. Immediate treatment involves fluid restriction, but this is only temporarily effective if not coupled with psychiatric assessment. *Demeclocycline* 300 to 600 mg PO twice a day may reduce the severity of hyponatremic episodes in patients with this disorder.

Pseudohyponatremia

The diagnosis of pseudohyponatremia can be made by
1. Demonstrating a normal serum osmolality in the presence of hyperlipidemia or hyperproteinemia.
2. Demonstrating a significant (> 10 mmol/kg) osmolar gap, indicating the presence of additional osmotically active sol-

utes, which can falsely lower the serum sodium level. This can be done by first having the laboratory *measure* serum osmolality. You should then *calculate* serum osmolality using the following formula.

$$\text{Serum osmolality (mmol/kg)} = 2\,\text{Na (mmol/L)} \\ + \text{glucose (mmol/L)} + \text{urea (mmol/L)}$$

If the *measured* serum osmolality is more than 10 mmol/kg greater than the *calculated* serum osmolality, the hyponatremia is at least partially due to the presence of osmotically active solutes, such as excess lipids or plasma proteins.

Management

Treatment of pseudohyponatremia is restricted to correction of the underlying cause.

In cases of hyperglycemia, the true serum sodium concentration can be estimated by the following formula.

$$\frac{(\text{Observed glucose} - \text{normal glucose})(1.4)}{\text{Normal glucose}} + \text{serum Na (observed)}$$

The factor 1.4 is an arithmetic approximation to account for the shift of water that follows glucose into the extracellular compartment, thereby diluting sodium.

EXAMPLE. A 35-year-old woman in diabetic ketoacidosis is admitted with the following laboratory results.

- Glucose = 83 mmol/L
- Sodium = 127 mmol/L
- Urea = 25 mmol/L
- Creatinine = 274 mmol/L

The true serum Na, where normal glucose is taken as 5 mmol/L,

$$= \frac{(83\,\text{mmol/L} - 5\,\text{mmol/L})\,(1.4)}{5} + 127\,\text{mmol/L}$$

$$= 22\,\text{mmol/L} + 127\,\text{mmol/L}$$

$$= 149\,\text{mmol/L}$$

Endocrine Disorders

Hypothyroidism and *Addison's disease* can be diagnosed by their typical clinical features in association with confirmatory laboratory studies. Hyponatremia in either of these two conditions responds to treatment of the underlying endocrine disorder.

APPENDIX A

□ ☐ □

ADULT EMERGENCY CARDIAC
CARE ALGORITHMS*

THE ALGORITHM APPROACH TO
EMERGENCY CARDIAC CARE

These guidelines use algorithms as an educational tool. They are an illustrative method to summarize information. Providers of emergency care should view algorithms as a summary and a memory aid. They provide a way to treat a broad range of patients. Algorithms, by nature, oversimplify. The effective teacher and care provider will use them wisely, not blindly. Some patients may require care not specified in the algorithms. When clinically appropriate, flexibility is accepted and encouraged. Many interventions and actions are listed as "considerations" to help providers think. These lists should not be considered endorsements or requirements or "standard of care" in a legal sense. Algorithms do not replace clinical understanding. Although the algorithms provide a good "cookbook," the patient always requires a "thinking cook."

The following clinical recommendations apply to all treatment algorithms:

- First, treat the patient, not the monitor.
- Algorithms for cardiac arrest presume that the condition under discussion continually persists, that the patient remains in cardiac arrest, and that CPR is always performed.
- Apply different interventions whenever appropriate indications exist.
- The flow diagrams present mostly class I (acceptable, definitely effective) recommendations. The footnotes present class IIa (acceptable, probably effective), class IIb (acceptable, possibly effective), and class III (not indicated, may be harmful) recommendations.
- Adequate airway, ventilation, oxygenation, chest compressions, and defibrillation are more important than administration of medications and take precedence over initiating an intravenous line or injecting pharmacologic agents.
- Several medications (epinephrine, lidocaine, and atropine) can be administered via the endotracheal tube, but clinicians must use an endotracheal dose 2 to 2.5 times the intravenous dose.
- With a few exceptions, intravenous medications should always be administered rapidly, in bolus method.
- After each intravenous medication, give a 20- to 30-ml bolus of intravenous fluid and immediately elevate the extremity. This will enhance delivery of drugs to the central circulation, which may take 1 to 2 minutes.
- Last, treat the patient, not the monitor.

*Reproduced with permission from Journal of the American Medical Association: Guidelines for cardiopulmonary resuscitation and emergency cardiac care 1992, Vol. 268, CPR issue, pp 2199–2241, Copyrighted 1992, American Medical Association.

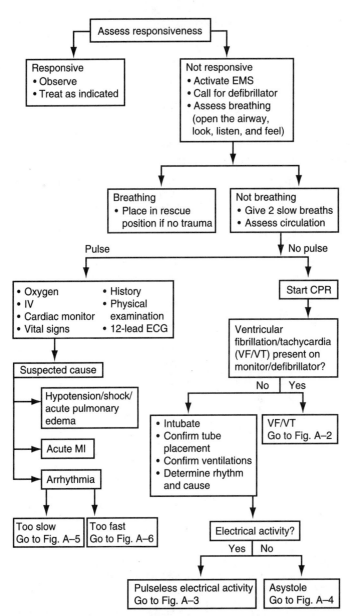

Figure A–1 □ Universal algorithm for adult emergency cardiac care (ECC). (Reproduced with permission from Journal of the American Medical Association: Guidelines for cardiopulmonary resuscitation and emergency cardiac care 1992, Vol. 268, CPR issue, pp 2199–2241, Copyrighted 1992, American Medical Association.)

Class I: definitely helpful
Class IIa: acceptable, probably helpful
Class IIb: acceptable, possibly helpful
Class III: not indicated, may be harmful

* Precordial thump is a class IIb action in witnessed arrest, no pulse, and no defibrillator immediately available.

† Hypothermic cardiac arrest is treated differently after this point. See section on hypothermia.

‡ The recommended dose of *epinephrine* is 1 mg IV push every 3–5 min. If this approach fails, several class IIb dosing regimens can be considered:
- Intermediate: *epinephrine* 2–5 mg IV push, every 3–5 min.
- Escalating: *epinephrine* 1 mg–3 mg–5 mg IV push (3 min apart)
- High: *epinephrine* 0.1 mg/kg IV push, every 3–5 min

§ *Sodium bicarbonate* (1 mEq/kg) is class I if patient has known preexisting hyperkalemia.

‖ Multiple sequenced shocks (200 J, 200–300 J, 360 J) are acceptable here (class I), especially when medications are delayed.

¶ • *Lidocaine* 1.5 mg/kg IV push. Repeat in 3–5 min to total loading dose of 3 mg/kg; then use.
- *Bretylium* 5 mg/kg IV push. Repeat in 5 min at 10 mg/kg.
- *Magnesium sulfate* 1–2 g IV in torsades de pointes or suspected hypomagnesemic state or severe refractory VF
- *Procainamide* 30 mg/min in refractory VF (maximum total 17 mg/kg)

• *Sodium bicarbonate* (1 mEq/kg IV):
Class IIa
- If known preexisting bicarbonate-responsive acidosis
- If overdose with tricyclic antidepressants
- To alkalinize the urine in drug overdoses
Class IIb
- If intubated and continued long arrest interval
- On return of spontaneous circulation after long arrest interval
Class III
- Hypoxic lactic acidosis

Figure A–2 □ Algorithm for ventricular fibrillation and pulseless ventricular tachycardia (VF/VT). (Reproduced with permission from Journal of the American Medical Association: Guidelines for cardiopulmonary resuscitation and emergency cardiac care 1992, Vol. 268, CPR issue, pp 2199–2241, Copyrighted 1992, American Medical Association.)

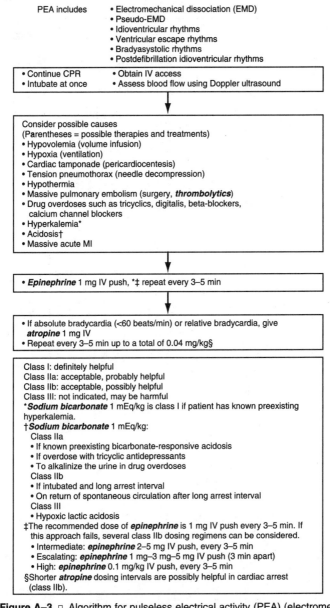

PEA includes
- Electromechanical dissociation (EMD)
- Pseudo-EMD
- Idioventricular rhythms
- Ventricular escape rhythms
- Bradyasystolic rhythms
- Postdefibrillation idioventricular rhythms

- Continue CPR
- Intubate at once
- Obtain IV access
- Assess blood flow using Doppler ultrasound

Consider possible causes
(Parentheses = possible therapies and treatments)
- Hypovolemia (volume infusion)
- Hypoxia (ventilation)
- Cardiac tamponade (pericardiocentesis)
- Tension pneumothorax (needle decompression)
- Hypothermia
- Massive pulmonary embolism (surgery, *thrombolytics*)
- Drug overdoses such as tricyclics, digitalis, beta-blockers,
  calcium channel blockers
- Hyperkalemia*
- Acidosis†
- Massive acute MI

- *Epinephrine* 1 mg IV push, *‡ repeat every 3–5 min

- If absolute bradycardia (<60 beats/min) or relative bradycardia, give
  atropine 1 mg IV
- Repeat every 3–5 min up to a total of 0.04 mg/kg§

Class I: definitely helpful
Class IIa: acceptable, probably helpful
Class IIb: acceptable, possibly helpful
Class III: not indicated, may be harmful
**Sodium bicarbonate* 1 mEq/kg is class I if patient has known preexisting
hyperkalemia.
†*Sodium bicarbonate* 1 mEq/kg:
  Class IIa
  - If known preexisting bicarbonate-responsive acidosis
  - If overdose with tricyclic antidepressants
  - To alkalinize the urine in drug overdoses
  Class IIb
  - If intubated and long arrest interval
  - On return of spontaneous circulation after long arrest interval
  Class III
  - Hypoxic lactic acidosis
‡The recommended dose of *epinephrine* is 1 mg IV push every 3–5 min. If
this approach fails, several class IIb dosing regimens can be considered.
  - Intermediate: *epinephrine* 2–5 mg IV push, every 3–5 min
  - Escalating: *epinephrine* 1 mg–3 mg–5 mg IV push (3 min apart)
  - High: *epinephrine* 0.1 mg/kg IV push, every 3–5 min
§Shorter *atropine* dosing intervals are possibly helpful in cardiac arrest
(class IIb).

Figure A–3 □ Algorithm for pulseless electrical activity (PEA) (electrome-chanical dissociation [EMD]). (Reproduced with permission from Journal of the American Medical Association: Guidelines for cardiopulmonary resuscitation and emergency cardiac care 1992, Vol. 268, CPR issue, pp 2199–2241, Copyrighted 1992, American Medical Association.)

Figure A–4 □ Asystole treatment algorithm. (Reproduced with permission from Journal of the American Medical Association: Guidelines for cardiopulmonary resuscitation and emergency cardiac care 1992, Vol. 268, CPR issue, pp 2199–2241, Copyrighted 1992, American Medical Association.)

Flowchart boxes:

- Continue CPR
- Intubate at once
- Obtain IV access
- Confirm asystole in more than one lead

↓

Consider possible causes
- Hypoxia
- Hyperkalemia
- Hypokalemia
- Preexisting acidosis
- Drug overdose
- Hypothermia

↓

Consider immediate transcutaneous pacing (TCP)*

↓

• *Epinephrine* 1 mg IV push, †‡ repeat every 3–5 min

↓

• *Atropine* 1 mg IV, repeat every 3–5 min up to a total of 0.04 mg/kg§‖

↓

Consider
• Termination of efforts¶

Class I: definitely helpful
Class IIa: acceptable, probably helpful
Class IIb: acceptable, possibly helpful
Class III: not indicated, may be harmful

* TCP is a class IIb intervention. Lack of success may be due to delays in pacing. To be effective TCP must be performed early, simultaneously with drugs. Evidence does not support routine use of TCP for asystole.

† The recommended dose of *epinephrine* is 1 mg IV push every 3–5 min. If this approach fails, several class IIb dosing regimens can be considered:
  • Intermediate: *epinephrine* 2–5 mg IV push, every 3–5 min
  • Escalating: *epinephrine* 1 mg–3 mg–5 mg IV push (3 min apart)
  • High: *epinephrine* 0.1 mg/kg IV push, every 3–5 min

‡ *Sodium bicarbonate* (1 mEq/kg) is class I if patient has known preexisting hyperkalemia.

§ Shorter *atropine* dosing intervals are class IIb in asystolic arrest.

‖ *Sodium bicarbonate* 1 mEq/kg:
Class IIa
  • If known preexisting bicarbonate-responsive acidosis
  • If overdose with tricyclic antidepressants
  • To alkalinize the urine in drug overdoses
Class IIb
  • If intubated and continued long arrest interval
  • On return of spontaneous circulation after long arrest interval
Class III
  • Hypoxic lactic acidosis

¶ If patient remains in asystole or other agonal rhythms after successful intubation and initial medications and no reversible causes are identified, consider termination of resuscitative efforts by a physician. Consider interval since arrest.

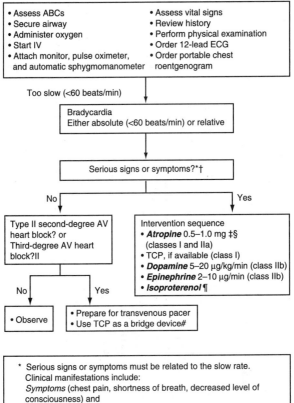

- Assess ABCs
- Secure airway
- Administer oxygen
- Start IV
- Attach monitor, pulse oximeter, and automatic sphygmomanometer

- Assess vital signs
- Review history
- Perform physical examination
- Order 12-lead ECG
- Order portable chest roentgenogram

Too slow (<60 beats/min)

Bradycardia
Either absolute (<60 beats/min) or relative

Serious signs or symptoms?*†

No ← | → Yes

Type II second-degree AV heart block? or
Third-degree AV heart block?II

Intervention sequence
- *Atropine* 0.5–1.0 mg ‡§ (classes I and IIa)
- TCP, if available (class I)
- *Dopamine* 5–20 µg/kg/min (class IIb)
- *Epinephrine* 2–10 µg/min (class IIb)
- *Isoproterenol* ¶

No | Yes

- Observe

- Prepare for transvenous pacer
- Use TCP as a bridge device#

* Serious signs or symptoms must be related to the slow rate. Clinical manifestations include:
 Symptoms (chest pain, shortness of breath, decreased level of consciousness) and
 Signs (low BP, shock, pulmonary congestion, CHF, acute MI).
† Do not delay TCP while awaiting IV access or for *atropine* to take effect if patient is symptomatic.
‡ Denervated transplanted hearts will not respond to *atropine*. Go at once to pacing, *catecholamine* infusion, or both.
§ *Atropine* should be given in repeat doses in 3–5 min up to total of 0.04 mg/kg. Consider shorter dosing intervals in severe clinical conditions. It has been suggested that atropine should be used with caution in AV block at the His-Purkinje level (type II AV block and new third-degree block with wide QRS complexes) (class IIb).
II Never treat third-degree heart block plus ventricular escape beats with *lidocaine*.
¶ *Isoproterenol* should be used, if at all, with extreme caution. At low doses, it is class IIb (possibly helpful); at higher doses, it is class III (harmful).
# Verify patient tolerance and mechanical capture. Use analgesia and sedation as needed.

Figure A–5 □ Bradycardia algorithm (with the patient not in cardiac arrest). (Reproduced by permission from Journal of the American Medical Association: Guidelines for cardiopulmonary resuscitation and emergency cardiac care 1992, Vol. 268, CPR issue, pp 2199–2241, Copyrighted 1992, American Medical Association.)

- Assess ABCs
- Secure airway
- Administer oxygen
- Start IV
- Attach monitor, pulse oximeter, and automatic sphygmomanometer
- Assess vital signs
- Review history
- Perform physical examination
- Order 12-lead ECG
- Order portable chest roentgenogram

Unstable, with serious signs or symptoms*

Yes

If ventricular rate >150 beats/min
- Prepare for immediate cardioversion (go to Fig. A–7)
- May give brief trial of medications based on arrhythmia
- Immediate cardioversion is seldom needed for heart rates <150 beats/min

No or borderline

Atrial fibrillation
Atrial flutter†

Consider use of
- *Diltiazem*
- *Beta-blockers*
- *Verapamil*
- *Digoxin*
- *Procainamide*
- *Anticoagulants*

Paroxysmal supraventricular tachycardia (PSVT)

Vagal maneuvers†

Adenosine
6 mg rapid IV push over 1–3 s

1–2 min

Wide-complex tachycardia of uncertain type

Lidocaine
1–1.5 mg/kg IV push

Lidocaine
0.5–0.75 mg/kg IV push, maximum total 3 mg/kg

Every 5–10 min

Ventricular tachycardia (VT)

Lidocaine
1–1.5 mg/kg IV push

Lidocaine
0.5–0.75 mg/kg IV push, maximum total 3 mg/kg

Every 5–10 min

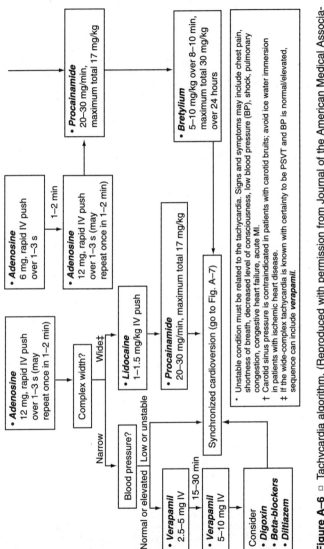

Figure A-6 □ Tachycardia algorithm. (Reproduced with permission from Journal of the American Medical Association: Guidelines for cardiopulmonary resuscitation and emergency cardiac care 1992, Vol. 268, CPR issue, pp 2199–2241, Copyrighted 1992, American Medical Association.)

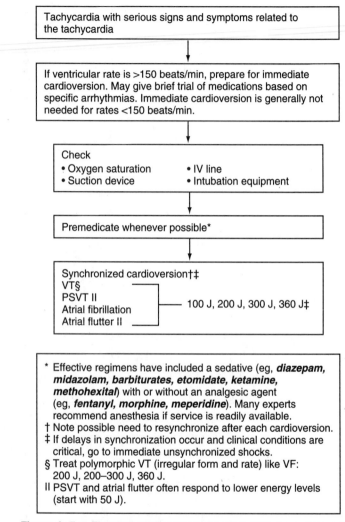

Tachycardia with serious signs and symptoms related to the tachycardia

↓

If ventricular rate is >150 beats/min, prepare for immediate cardioversion. May give brief trial of medications based on specific arrhythmias. Immediate cardioversion is generally not needed for rates <150 beats/min.

↓

Check
- Oxygen saturation
- Suction device
- IV line
- Intubation equipment

↓

Premedicate whenever possible*

↓

Synchronized cardioversion†‡
VT§
PSVT ‖
Atrial fibrillation
Atrial flutter ‖ —— 100 J, 200 J, 300 J, 360 J‡

---

* Effective regimens have included a sedative (eg, *diazepam, midazolam, barbiturates, etomidate, ketamine, methohexital*) with or without an analgesic agent (eg, *fentanyl, morphine, meperidine*). Many experts recommend anesthesia if service is readily available.
† Note possible need to resynchronize after each cardioversion.
‡ If delays in synchronization occur and clinical conditions are critical, go to immediate unsynchronized shocks.
§ Treat polymorphic VT (irregular form and rate) like VF: 200 J, 200–300 J, 360 J.
‖ PSVT and atrial flutter often respond to lower energy levels (start with 50 J).

Figure A–7 □ Electrical cardioversion algorithm (with the patient not in cardiac arrest). (Reproduced with permission from Journal of the American Medical Association: Guidelines for cardiopulmonary resuscitation and emergency cardiac care 1992, Vol. 268, CPR issue, pp 2199–2241, Copyrighted 1992, American Medical Association.)

APPENDIX B

ADVANCED CARDIAC LIFE SUPPORT DRUGS

Drug*	Indications/Precautions	Adult Dosage
ACE Inhibitors (Angiotensin-Converting Enzyme Inhibitors)	*Indications* • ACE inhibitors reduce mortality and improve LV dysfunction in post-AMI patients. They help prevent adverse LV remodeling, delay progression of heart failure, and decrease sudden death and recurrent MI.	*Approach* ACE inhibitor therapy should start with low-dose oral administration and increase steadily to achieve a full dose within 24 to 48 hours.
Enalapril maleate • 2.5-, 5-, 10-, and 20-mg tablets		*Enalapril maleate* • Start with a single dose of 2.5 mg PO. Titrate to 20 mg PO BID.
	Class I Recommendations • AMI associated with ST-segment elevation in two or more anterior precordial leads. • During AMI, development of LV ejection fraction <40%. • During AMI, development of clinical signs of heart failure due to systolic pump dysfunction.	
Captopril • 12.5-, 25-, 50-, and 100-mg tablets		*Captopril* • Start with a single dose of 6.25 mg PO. • Advance to 25 mg TID and then to 50 mg TID as tolerated.

Table continued on following page

Drug*	Indications/Precautions	Adult Dosage
Ramipril • 1.25-, 2.5-, 5-, and 10-mg capsules	**Precautions** • Contraindicated: — Pregnancy (may cause fetal injury or death). — Systolic BP <100 mm Hg. — History of bilateral stenosis of renal arteries. — Known allergy to ACE inhibitors. • Avoid hypotension, especially following initial dose and in relative volume depletion. • Generally not started in the ED but within the first 24 hours after thrombolytic therapy has been completed and blood pressure has stabilized.	**Ramipril** • Start with a single dose of 2.5 mg PO. Titrate to 5 mg PO BID as tolerated.
Adenosine • 3 mg/ml in 2-ml vial (total = 6 mg)	**Indications** • First drug for narrow-complex PSVT • May be used diagnostically (after lidocaine) in wide-complex tachycardias of uncertain type **Precautions** • Transient side effects include flushing, chest pain or tightness, brief periods of asystole or bradycardia, ventricular ectopy • Less effective in patients taking theophyllines; avoid in patients receiving dipyridamole	**IV Rapid Push** • Place patient in mild reverse Trendelenburg position before administration of drug • Initial bolus of 6 mg given *rapidly* over 1–3 s followed by normal saline bolus of 20 ml; then elevate the extremity • Repeat dose of 12 mg in 1–2 min if needed • A third dose of 12 mg may be given in 1–2 min if needed

Injection Technique

- Record rhythm strip during administration.
- Draw up adenosine dose and flush in two separate syringes.
- Attach both syringes to the IV injection port closest to patient.
- Clamp IV tubing above injection port.
- Push IV adenosine *as quickly as possible* (1 to 3 seconds).
- While maintaining pressure on adenosine plunger, push normal saline flush *as rapidly as possible* after adenosine.
- Unclamp IV tubing.

IV Loading Dose and Infusion

- 5 mg/kg given over 30–45 min
- Never exceed 500 mg loading dose
- Follow with infusion of 0.5–0.7 mg/kg/h

Table continued on following page

Aminophylline
- 25 mg/ml in 10-ml vial (total = 250 mg)
- 50 mg/ml in 10-ml vial (total = 500 mg)

Indications

- Third-line agent for acute pulmonary edema

Precautions

- May cause VT or other tachyarrhythmias
- Watch for toxicity in patients with congestive heart failure
- Avoid in patients with PSVT and acute ischemic heart disease
- Do not mix with other drugs

Drug*	Indications/Precautions	Adult Dosage
Amrinone • 5 mg/ml in 20-ml vial (total = 100 mg)	**Indications** • Severe congestive heart failure refractory to diuretics, vasodilators, and conventional inotropic agents **Precautions** • Do not mix with dextrose solutions or other drugs • May cause tachyarrhythmias, hypotension, or thrombocytopenia • Can increase myocardial ischemia	***IV Loading Dose and Infusion*** • 0.75 mg/kg, given over 10–15 min • Follow by infusion of 5–15 μg/kg/min titrated to clinical effect • Optimal use requires hemodynamic monitoring
Atropine sulfate • 0.1 mg/ml in 10-ml pre-loaded syringe (total = 1 mg) • Can be given via endotracheal tube	**Indications** • First drug for symptomatic bradycardia (class IIa) • Second drug (after epinephrine) for asystole or bradycardic pulseless electrical activity (class IIb) **Precautions** • Use with caution in the presence of myocardial ischemia and hypoxia • Increases myocardial oxygen demand • Avoid in hypothermia	***Asystole or Pulseless Electrical Activity*** • 1 mg IV push • Repeat every 3–5 min (if asystole persists) to maximum dose of 0.03–0.04 mg/kg ***Bradycardia*** • 0.5–1.0 mg IV every 3–5 min as needed; not to exceed total dose of 0.03–0.04 mg/kg • Use shorter dosing interval (3 min) and higher doses (0.04 mg/kg) in severe clinical conditions ***Endotracheal Administration*** • 2–3 mg diluted in 10 ml normal saline

- Seldom effective for infranodal (type II) AV block and new third-degree block with wide QRS complexes (class IIb) (In these patients may cause paradoxical slowing. Be prepared to pace or give catecholamines.)

Beta-Blockers

Metoprolol
- 1 mg/ml in 5-ml vial (total = 5 mg)

Atenolol
- 0.5 mg/ml in 10-ml ampule (total = 5 mg)

Propranolol
- 1 mg/ml in 1-ml ampule
- 4 mg/ml in 5-ml vial (total = 20 mg)

Esmolol
- 10 mg/ml in 10-ml ampule (total = 100 mg)

Indications

- To convert to normal sinus rhythm or to slow ventricular response (or both) in supraventricular tachyarrhythmias (PSVT, atrial fibrillation, or atrial flutter). Beta-blockers are second-line agents after adenosine, diltiazem, or digoxin
- To reduce myocardial ischemia and damage in AMI patients with elevated heart rates, blood pressure, or both
- For emergency antihypertensive therapy for hemorrhagic and acute ischemic stroke

Precautions

- Concurrent IV administration with IV calcium channel–blocking agents like verapamil or diltiazem can cause severe hypotension
- Avoid in bronchospastic diseases, cardiac failure, or severe abnormalities in cardiac conduction

Metoprolol
- 5 mg slow IV at 5-min intervals to a total of 15 mg

Atenolol
- 5 mg slow IV (over 5 min)
- Wait 10 min; then give second dose of 5 mg slow IV (over 5 min)
- In 10 min, if tolerated well, may start 50 mg PO, then give 50 mg PO twice a day

Propranolol
- 1–3 mg slow IV
- Do not exceed 1 mg/min
- Repeat after 2 min, if necessary

Esmolol
- 0.5 mg/kg over 1 min, followed by continuous infusion at 0.05 mg/kg/min
- Titrate to effect; esmolol has a short half-life (<10 min)

Table continued on following page

Drug*	Indications/Precautions	Adult Dosage
Labetalol • 5 mg/ml in 20-ml ampules	• Monitor cardiac and pulmonary status during administration • May cause myocardial depression	**Labetalol** • 10-mg labetalol IV-push over 1–2 min. May repeat or double labetalol every 10 min to a maximum dose of 150 mg, or give initial dose as a bolus, then start labetalol infusion 2–8 μg/min.
Bretylium • 50 mg/ml in 10-ml prefilled syringe (total = 500 mg) • 50 mg/ml in 10-ml vial (total = 500 mg)	*Indications* • Cardiac arrest from VF/VT after defibrillation shocks, epinephrine, lidocaine (class IIa) • Refractory/recurrent VT after full doses of lidocaine (class IIa) • Class IIa as first antiarrhythmic for hypothermic VF *Precautions* • Side effects include hypotension, nausea, and vomiting	*Cardiac Arrest* • 5 mg/kg IV bolus • May give 10 mg/kg in 5 min if needed • One 500-mg ampule IV bolus with a second dose of two 500-mg ampules in 5 min is acceptable *Stable VT* • 5–10 mg/kg IV over 8–10 min; wait 10–30 min before next dose • Maximum total dose, 30 mg/kg over 24 hours • Maintenance infusion: 1–2 mg/min

Calcium chloride
- 100 mg/ml in 10-ml vial (total = 1 g; a 10% solution)

Indications
- Known or suspected hyperkalemia (e.g., renal failure)
- Hypocalcemia (e.g., after multiple blood transfusions)
- As an antidote for toxic effects (hypotension and arrhythmias) from calcium channel blocker overdose
- Used prophylactically before IV calcium channel blockers to prevent hypotension

Precautions
- Do not use routinely in cardiac arrest
- Do not mix with sodium bicarbonate

IV Slow Push
- 8–16 mg/kg (usually 5 to 10 ml) IV for hyperkalemia and calcium channel blocker overdose
- 2–4 mg/kg (usually 2 ml) IV for prophylactic pretreatment before IV calcium channel blockers

Digibind (digoxin-specific antibody therapy)
- 40-mg vial (each vial binds about 0.6 mg digoxin.)

Indications
Digoxin toxicity with the following:
- Uncontrolled life-threatening arrhythmias
- Shock or congestive heart failure
- Hyperkalemia (potassium level is >5.0 mEq/L)
- Steady-state serum levels above 10–15 ng/ml

Precautions
- Serum digoxin levels rise after digibind therapy and should not be used to guide continuing therapy

Chronic Intoxication
- 3 to 5 vials may be effective

Acute Overdose
- IV dose varies according to amount of digoxin ingested
- Average dose is 10 vials (400 mg); may require up to 20 vials (800 mg)
- See package insert for details

Table continued on following page

Drug*	Indications/Precautions	Adult Dosage
Digoxin • 0.25 mg/ml or 0.1 mg/ml supplied in 1- or 2-ml ampule (total = 0.1–0.5 mg)	**Indications** • To slow ventricular response in atrial fibrillation or atrial flutter • Third-line choice for PSVT (after vagal maneuvers, adenosine, diltiazem, and verapamil) **Precautions** • Toxic effects are common and are frequently associated with serious arrhythmias • Avoid electrical cardioversion if patient is receiving digoxin unless condition is life threatening; use lower current settings (10–20 J)	**IV Infusion** • Loading doses of 10–15 μg/kg lean body weight provide therapeutic effect with minimum risk of toxic effects • Maintenance dose is affected by body size and renal function
Diltiazem • 5 mg/ml in 5- or 10-ml vial (total = 25 or 50 mg)	**Indications** • To control ventricular rate in atrial fibrillation and atrial flutter • Use after adenosine to treat refractory PSVT in patients with narrow QRS complex and adequate blood pressure • As an alternative, use verapamil **Precautions** • Do not use calcium channel blockers for wide-QRS tachycardias of uncertain origin	**Acute Rate Control** • 15–20 mg (0.25 mg/kg) IV over 2 min • May repeat in 15 min at 20–25 mg (0.35 mg/kg) over 2 min **Maintenance Infusion** • 5–15 mg/h, titrated to heart rate

Reproduced with permission. © 1997–99 *Handbook of Emergency Cardiovascular Care for Healthcare Providers*, 1997. Copyright American Heart Association.

- Avoid calcium channel blockers in patients with Wolff-Parkinson-White syndrome plus rapid atrial fibrillation or flutter, in patients with sick sinus syndrome, or in patients with AV block without a pacemaker
- Expect blood pressure drop resulting from peripheral vasodilation (greater drop with verapamil than with diltiazem)
- Avoid in patients receiving oral beta-blockers
- Concurrent IV administration with IV beta-blockers can cause severe hypotension

Dobutamine
- 12.5 mg/ml in 20-ml vial (total = 250 mg)

IV infusion
- Dilute 250 mg (20 ml) in 250 ml normal saline or 5% dextrose in water

Indications
- Consider pump problems (congestive heart failure, pulmonary congestion) with systolic blood pressure of 70–100 mm Hg and no signs of shock

Precautions
- Avoid when systolic blood pressure is <100 mm Hg and signs of shock are present
- May cause tachyarrhythmias, fluctuations in blood pressure, headache, and nausea

IV Infusion
- Usual infusion rate is 2–20 µg/kg per min
- Titrate so heart rate does not increase by >10% of baseline
- Hemodynamic monitoring is recommended for optimal use

Table continued on following page

Drug*	Indications/Precautions	Adult Dosage
Dopamine • 40 mg/ml in 5-ml ampule (total = 200 mg) • 160 mg/ml in 5-ml ampule (total = 800 mg) *IV infusion* • Mix 400–800 mg in 250 ml normal saline, lactated Ringer's solution, or 5% dextrose in water	*Indications* • Second drug for symptomatic bradycardia (after atropine) • Use for hypotension (systolic blood pressure ≤70–100 mm Hg) with signs and symptoms of shock *Precautions* • May use in patients with hypovolemia but only after volume replacement • Use with caution in cardiogenic shock with accompanying congestive heart failure • May cause tachyarrhythmias and excessive vasoconstriction • Taper slowly • Do not mix with sodium bicarbonate	*Continuous Infusions (Titrate to Patient Response)* *Low dose* • 1–5 µg/kg/min ("renal doses") *Moderate dose* • 5–10 µg/kg/min ("cardiac doses") *High dose* • 10–20 µg/kg/min ("vasopressor doses")
Epinephrine • 1.0 mg/10 ml in preloaded 10-ml syringe (total = 1 mg) • 1 mg/ml in glass 1-ml ampule (total = 1 mg) • 1 mg/ml in multidose 30-ml vial (total = 30 mg)	*Indications* • **Cardiac arrest:** VF, pulseless VT, asystole, pulseless electrical activity (class I) • **Symptomatic bradycardia:** after atropine and transcutaneous pacing (class IIb) • **Anaphylaxis, severe allergic reactions:** Combine with large fluid volumes, corticosteroids, and antihistamines	*Cardiac Arrest* • **First dose:** 1.0 mg IV push, may repeat every 3–5 min • **Alternative regimens for second dose (class IIb)** • *Intermediate:* 2–5 mg IV push, every 3–5 min • *Escalating:* 1 mg, 3 mg, 5 mg IV push, each dose 3 min apart • *High:* 0.1 mg/kg IV push, every 3–5 min

Reproduced with permission. © 1997–99 *Handbook of Emergency Cardiovascular Care for Healthcare Providers*, 1997. Copyright American Heart Association.

Endotracheal route

- 2.0–2.5 mg diluted in 10 ml normal saline

Profound Bradycardia

- 2–10 µg/min (Add 1 mg of 1:1000 to 500 ml normal saline; infuse at 1–5 ml/min)

First Dose

- 0.2 mg IV over 15 s

Second Dose

- 0.3 mg IV over 30 s. If no adequate response, give third dose

Third Dose

- 0.5 mg IV given over 30 s. If no adequate response, repeat once per min until adequate response or until total of 3 mg is given

IV Infusion

- 0.5–1.0 mg/kg given over 1–2 min
- If no response, double the dose to 2.0 mg/kg, slowly over 1–2 min

Table continued on following page

Precautions

- Raising blood pressure and increasing heart rate may cause myocardial ischemia, angina, and increased myocardial oxygen demand

Flumazenil
- 0.1 mg/ml in 5- and 10-ml vials (total = 0.5–1.0 mg)

Indications

- Reverse respiratory depression and sedative effects of benzodiazepines

Precautions

- Effects may not outlast effect of benzodiazepines
- Monitor for later respiratory depression
- Do not use in suspected tricyclic overdose
- Do not use in seizure-prone patients
- Do not use in unknown drug overdose

Furosemide
- 10 mg/ml in 2-, 4-, and 10-ml ampules or vials (total = 20 mg, 40 mg, and 100 mg)

Indications

- For adjunct therapy of acute pulmonary edema in patients with systolic blood pressure >90–100 mm Hg (without signs and symptoms of shock)
- Hypertensive emergencies
- Increased intracranial pressure

Drug*	Indications/Precautions	Adult Dosage
	Precautions	
	• Dehydration, hypovolemia, hypotension, hypokalemia, or other electrolyte imbalance may occur	
Glucagon	**Indications**	**IV Infusion**
• Powdered in 1- and 10-mg vials	• Adjuvant treatment of toxic effects of calcium channel blocker or beta-blocker	• 1–5 mg over 2–5 min
• Reconstitute with provided solution		
	Precautions	
	• Do not mix with saline	
	• May cause vomiting, hyperglycemia	
Heparin	**Indications**	**IV Infusion**
• 0.5- to 1.0-ml ampules, vials, and prefilled syringes	• Adjuvant therapy in acute MI	• Initial bolus 80 IU/kg
	• Benign heparin with alteplase	• Continue 18 IU/kg/h (round to the nearest 50 IU)
• 1-, 2-, 5-, and 30-ml multidose vials		• Adjust to maintain activated partial thromboplastin time (aPTT) 1.5–2.0 times the control values
• Concentrations range from 1000 to 40,000 IU/ml	**Precautions**	• Target range for aPTT after first 24 hours is 60–85 s (may vary with laboratory)
	• Same contraindications as for thrombolytic therapy, as follows:	• Check aPTT at 6, 12, 18, and 24 h
	• Active bleeding	• If aPTT is ≤60 s at 24 hours, repeat bolus with 20 IU/kg heparin; increase infusion by 3 IU/kg/h; recheck aPTT in 2 hours
	• Recent intracranial, intraspinal, or eye surgery	
	• Severe hypertension	
	• Bleeding disorders	
	• Gastrointestinal bleeding	

- Doses and laboratory targets appropriate when used in association with thrombolytic therapy
- Heparin reversal if necessary: Protamine 25 mg IV infusion over ≥10 min (Calculate dose as 1 mg protamine/100 IU of heparin remaining in the patient; heparin plasma half-life is 60 min)

Isoproterenol
- 1 mg/ml in 1-ml vial

IV infusion
- Mix 1 mg in 250 ml normal saline, lactated Ringer's solution, or 5% dextrose in water

IV Infusion
- Infuse at 2–10 µg/min
- Titrate to adequate heart rate
- In torsades de pointes titrate to increase heart rate until VT is suppressed

Indications
- Refractory torsades de pointes unresponsive to magnesium sulfate
- *Temporary* control of bradycardia in heart transplant patients
- Class IIb at low doses for symptomatic bradycardias

Precautions
- Do not use for treatment of cardiac arrest
- Increases myocardial oxygen requirements, which may increase myocardial ischemia. Do not give with epinephrine; can cause VF/VT

Lidocaine
- 20 mg/ml in preloaded 5-ml syringe (total = 100 mg)

Indications
- Cardiac arrest from VF/VT (class IIa)
- Stable VT, wide-complex tachycardias of uncertain type, wide-complex PSVT (class I)

Cardiac Arrest From VF/VT
- Initial dose: 1.0–1.5 mg/kg IV
- For refractory VF, may repeat 1.0–1.5 mg/kg IV in 3–5 min; maximum total dose of 3 mg/kg

Table continued on following page

Drug*	Indications/Precautions	Adult Dosage
• 10 mg/ml in 5-ml vial (total = 50 mg) • Can be given via endotracheal tube	**Precautions** • *Prophylactic* use in AMI patients is *not* recommended • Reduce maintenance dose (not loading dose) in the presence of impaired liver function or left ventricular dysfunction	• A single dose of 1.5 mg/kg IV in cardiac arrest is acceptable • Endotracheal administration: 2–4 mg/kg ***Perfusing Arrhythmia*** • For stable VT, wide-complex tachycardia of uncertain type, significant ectopy, use as follows: • 1.0–1.5 mg/kg IV push • Repeat 0.5–0.75 mg/kg every 5–10 min; maximum total dose, 3 mg/kg ***Maintenance Infusion*** • 2 to 4 mg/min (30 to 50 µg/kg per min)
Magnesium sulfate • 2- and 10-ml ampules of 50% MgSO₄ (total = 1 and 5 g) • 10 ml in preloaded syringe (total = 5 g/10 ml)	**Indications** • Cardiac arrest associated with torsades de pointes or suspected hypomagnesemic state • Refractory VF (after lidocaine and bretylium) • Torsades de pointes with a pulse • Life-threatening ventricular arrhythmias due to digitalis toxicity, tricyclic overdose • Consider prophylactic administration in hospitalized patients with AMI (class IIa)	***Cardiac Arrest*** • 1–2 g IV push (2–4 ml of a 50% solution) diluted in 10 ml of 5% dextrose in water ***Acute Myocardial Infarction*** • Loading dose of 1–2 g, mixed in 50–100 ml of 5% dextrose in water, over 5–60 min IV • Follow with 0.5–1.0 g/h IV for up to 24 hours

Mannitol
- 150-, 250-, and 1000-ml IV containers (strengths: 5%, 10%, 15%, 20%, and 25%)

Precautions
- Occasional fall in blood pressure with rapid administration
- Use caution if renal failure is present

Indications
- Increased intracranial pressure in management of neurologic emergencies

Precautions
- Monitor fluid status and osmolarity (not to exceed 310 mOsm/kg)
- Caution in renal failure, because fluid overload may result

Torsades de Pointes
- Loading dose of 1–2 g mixed in 50–100 mL of 5% dextrose in water, over 5–60 min IV
- Follow with 1 to 4 g/h IV (titrate dose to control the torsades)

IV Infusion
- Administer 0.5–1.0 g/kg over 5–10 min
- Additional doses of 0.25–2 g/kg can be given every 4–6 hours as needed
- Use in conjunction with mild hyperventilation

Morphine sulfate
- 2 to 10 mg/ml in 1-ml syringe

Indications
- Chest pain and anxiety associated with AMI or cardiac ischemia
- Acute cardiogenic pulmonary edema (if blood pressure is adequate)

IV Infusion
- 1–3 mg IV (over 1–5 min) every 5 to 30 min

Table continued on following page

Drug*	Indications/Precautions	Adult Dosage
	Precautions • Administer slowly and titrate to effect • May compromise respiration; therefore, use with caution in the compromised respiratory state of acute pulmonary edema • Causes hypotension in volume-depleted patients • Reverse, if needed, with naloxone (0.4–2.0 mg IV)	
Naloxone hydrochloride • 0.4- and 1-mg vials, ampules, and syringes	*Indications* • Respiratory and neurologic depression due to narcotic intoxication *Precautions* • May cause narcotic withdrawal • Effects may not outlast effect of narcotics • Monitor for later respiratory depression • Rare anaphylactic reactions have been reported	*IV Infusion* • 0.4–2.0 mg every 2 min • Use higher doses for complete narcotic reversal • Can administer up to 10 mg over short period (<30 min)
Nitroglycerin *Parenteral* • Ampules: 5 mg in 10 ml, 8 mg in 10 ml, 10 mg in 10 ml	*Indications* • Chest pain of suspected cardiac origin • Unstable angina • Complications of AMI, including congestive heart failure, and left ventricular failure • Hypertensive crisis or urgency with chest pain	*IV Infusion* • Infuse at 10–20 µg/min • Route of choice for emergencies • Use appropriate IV sets provided by pharmaceutical companies • Titrate to effect

- Vials: 25 mg in 5 ml, 50 mg in 10 ml, 100 mg in 10 ml
Sublingual tablets
- 0.3 and 0.4 mg
Aerosol spray
- 0.4 mg per dose

Sublingual Route
0.3–0.4 mg, repeat every 5 min

Aerosol Spray
Spray for 0.5–1.0 s at 5-min intervals

Precautions
- With evidence of AMI, limit systolic blood pressure drop to 10% if patient is normotensive, 30% drop if hypertensive, and avoid drop below 90 mm Hg
- Do not mix with other drugs
- Patient should sit or lie down when receiving this medication
- Do not shake aerosol spray because this affects metered dose

Norepinephrine
- 1 mg/ml in 4-ml ampule
- Mix 4 mg in 250 ml of 5% dextrose in water or 5% dextrose in normal saline
- Avoid dilution in normal saline alone

Indications
- For severe cardiogenic shock and hemodynamically significant hypotension (systolic blood pressure <70 mm Hg)
- This is an agent of last resort for management of ischemic heart disease and shock

IV Infusion (Only Route)
- 0.5–1.0 µg/min titrated to improve blood pressure up to 30 µg/min

Precautions
- Increases myocardial oxygen requirements because it raises blood pressure and heart rate
- May induce arrhythmias; use with caution in patients with acute ischemia; monitor cardiac output
- Extravasation causes tissue necrosis

Table continued on following page

Drug*	Indications/Precautions	Adult Dosage	
		Device	Flow Rate
Oxygen	**Indications**	Nasal prongs	1–6 L/min
• Delivered from portable tanks or installed, wall-mounted sources through delivery devices	• Any suspected cardiopulmonary emergency, especially (but *not* limited to) complaints of shortness of breath and suspected ischemic chest pain	Venturi mask	4–8 L/min
		Partial rebreather mask	6–10 L/min
		Bag-valve mask	15 L/min
			35–
			≈100
	• NOTE: Pulse oximetry provides a useful method to "dose" oxygen: aim to keep oxygen saturation level above 96%		
	Precautions		
	• Observe closely when using with pulmonary patients known to be dependent on hypoxic respiratory drive (very rare situation)		
	• Pulse oximetry is inaccurate in low cardiac output states or with vasoconstriction		
Procainamide	**Indications**	**Cardiac Arrest**	
• 100 mg/ml in 10-ml vial (total = 1 g)	• Recurrent VT not controlled by lidocaine	• 30 mg/min IV infusion (maximum total dose, 17 mg/kg)	
• 500 mg/ml in 2-ml vial (total = 1 g)	• Refractory PSVT	• In refractory VF/VT, 100 mg IV push doses given every 5 min are acceptable	
	• Refractory VF/pulseless VT	**Other Indications**	
	• Stable wide-complex tachycardia of unknown origin	• 20–30 mg/min IV until one of the following occurs:	
	• Atrial fibrillation with rapid rate in Wolff-Parkinson-White syndrome		

Precautions

- If cardiac or renal dysfunction is present, reduce maximum total dose to 12 mg/kg and maintenance infusion to 1–2 mg/min
- Proarrhythmic, especially in setting of AMI, hypokalemia, or hypomagnesemia

Indications

Specific indications for bicarbonate use are as follows:

- **Class I** if known preexisting hyperkalemia
- **Class IIa** if known preexisting bicarbonate-responsive acidosis (e.g., diabetic ketoacidosis); tricyclic antidepressant overdose; to alkalinize the urine in aspirin or other overdose
- **Class IIb** if prolonged resuscitation with effective ventilation; upon return of spontaneous circulation after long arrest interval
- **Class III** (not useful or effective) in hypoxic lactic acidosis or hypercarbic acidosis (e.g., cardiac arrest and CPR without intubation)

Sodium bicarbonate

- 50-ml preloaded syringe (8.4% sodium bicarbonate provides 50 mEq/50 ml)

- Arrhythmia suppression
- Hypotension
- QRS widens by >50%
- Total dose of 17 mg/kg is given

Maintenance Infusion

- 1–4 mg/min

IV Infusion

- 1 mEq/kg IV bolus
- Repeat half this dose every 10 min thereafter
- If rapidly available, use arterial blood gas analysis to guide bicarbonate therapy (calculated base deficits or bicarbonate concentration)

Blood Gas Interpretation Rules

- **Rule 1:** An acute change in $Paco_2$ of 1 mm Hg is associated with an increase or decrease in pH of 0.008 unit (relative to normal $Paco_2$ of 40 mm Hg and normal pH of 7.4)
- **Rule 2:** A pH change of 0.01 unit is the result of a base change of 0.67 mEq/L

Table continued on following page

Drug*	Indications/Precautions	Adult Dosage
	Precautions	• **Rule 3:** The total body bicarbonate deficit equals the base deficit (mEq/L) times the patient's weight (in kg) times 0.3 Complete buffer correction is seldom indicated; use one fourth to one half calculated dose
	• Adequate ventilation and CPR, not bicarbonate, are the major "buffer agents" in cardiac arrest	
	• Not recommended for routine use in cardiac arrest patients	
		IV Infusion
		• Begin at 0.10 μg/kg/min and titrate upward every 3–5 min to desired effect (up to 5.0 μg/kg/min)
Sodium nitroprusside	*Indications*	• Use with an infusion pump; use hemodynamic monitoring for optimal safety
• 10 mg/ml in 5-ml vial (total = 50 mg)	• Hypertensive crisis	• Action occurs within 1–2 min
• Mix 50 or 100 mg in 250 ml 5% dextrose in water only	• To reduce afterload in heart failure and acute pulmonary edema	• Cover drug reservoir and tubing with opaque material
	• To reduce afterload in acute mitral or aortic valve regurgitation	
	Precautions	
	• Light sensitive; therefore wrap drug reservoir in aluminum foil	
	• May cause hypotension, thiocyanate toxicity, and CO_2 retention	
	• Other side effects include headaches, nausea, vomiting, and abdominal cramps	

Thrombolytic Agents	Indications	
Alteplase, recombinant (Activase); tissue plasminogen activator (TPA) 50- and 100-mg vials reconstituted with sterile water to 1 mg/ml For all four agents, use two peripheral IV lines, *one line exclusively for thrombolytic administration.*	**For AMI in adults** • ST elevation (1 mm or more in at least two contiguous leads) or new or presumably new BBB; strongly suspicious for injury • In context of signs and symptoms of AMI • Time from onset of symptoms <12 hours **For acute ischemic stroke** (Alteplase is the only thrombolytic agent approved for acute ischemic stroke.) • Sudden onset of focal neurologic deficits or alterations in consciousness (e.g., language abnormality, motor arm, facial droop) • Absence of intracerebral or subarachnoid hemorrhage or mass effect on CT scan • Absence of variable or rapidly improving neurologic deficits • Alteplase can be started in <3 hours from symptom onset	**Alteplase, recombinant (TPA)** Recommended total dose is based on patient's weight. For AMI the total dose should not exceed 100 mg; for acute ischemic stroke the total dose should not exceed 90 mg. Note that there are two approved dose regimens for AMI patients, and a *different* regimen for acute ischemic stroke. **For AMI:** • Accelerated infusion (1.5 hours) — Give 15-mg IV bolus — Then 0.75 mg/kg over next 30 min (not to exceed 50 mg) — Then 0.50 mg/kg over next 60 min (not to exceed 35 mg) • 3-hour infusion — Give 60 mg in first hour (initial 6 to 10 mg is given as a bolus) — Then 20 mg/h for 2 additional hours *Table continued on following page*

Drug*	Indications/Precautions	Adult Dosage
	Precautions	**For acute ischemic stroke:**
	Specific exclusion criteria:	• Give 0.9 mg/kg (maximum 90 mg) infused over 60 min
	• Active internal bleeding (except menses) within 21 days	• Give 10% of the total dose as an initial IV bolus over 1 min
	• History of cerebrovascular, intracranial, or intraspinal event within 3 months (stroke, arteriovenous malformation, neoplasm, aneurysm, recent trauma, recent sugery)	• Give the remaining 90% over the next 60 min
	• Major surgery or serious trauma within 14 days	**Anistreplase (APSAC)**
	• Aortic dissection	• 30 IU IV over 2 to 5 min
	• Severe, uncontrolled hypertension	
	• Known bleeding disorders	
	• Prolonged CPR with evidence of thoracic trauma	**Reteplase, recombinant**
Anistreplase (Eminase) anisoylated plasminogen streptokinase activator complex (APSAC) Reconstitute 30 units in 50 ml sterile water or 5% dextrose in water	• Lumbar puncture within 7 days	• Give first 10-unit IV bolus over 2 min
	• Recent arterial puncture at noncompressible site	• 30 min later give second 10-unit IV bolus over 2 min (give NS flush before and after each bolus)
	• During the first 24 hours of thrombolytic therapy for ischemic stroke, do not administer aspirin or heparin	
Reteplase, recombinant (Retavase) 10-unit vials reconstituted with sterile water to 1 U/ml	*Adjuvant Therapy for AMI*	
	• 160–325 mg aspirin chewed as soon as possible	

Streptokinase (Streptase)
Reconstitute to 1 mg/ml

Verapamil
- 2.5 mg/ml in 2-, 4-, and 5-ml vials (total = 5, 10, and 12.5 mg)

- Begin heparin immediately and continue for 48 hours if alteplase or Retavase is used

Indications

- Drug of second choice (after adenosine) to terminate PSVT with narrow QRS complex and adequate blood pressure

Precautions

- Do not use calcium channel blockers for wide-QRS tachycardias of uncertain origin
- Avoid calcium channel blockers in patients with Wolff-Parkinson-White syndrome and atrial fibrillation; sick sinus syndrome; or second- or third-degree AV block without pacemaker
- Expect blood pressure drop caused by peripheral vasodilation; IV calcium can restore blood pressure, and some experts recommend prophylactic calcium administration before giving calcium channel blockers
- Concurrent IV administration with IV beta-blockers may produce severe hypotension
- Use with extreme caution for patients receiving oral beta-blockers

Streptokinase
- 1.5 million IU in a 1-hour infusion

IV Infusion

- 2.5–5.0 mg IV bolus over 1–2 min
- Second dose: 5–10 mg, if needed, in 15–30 min. Maximum dose: 30 mg
- Alternative: 5-mg bolus every 15 min to total dose of 30 mg
- Older patients: administer over 3 min

---

*Note: Most commonly available adult preparation.
Reproduced with permission. © 1997–99 *Handbook of Emergency Cardiovascular Care for Healthcare Providers*, 1997. Copyright American Heart Association.

APPENDIX C

BLOOD PRODUCTS

The maximum time over which blood products can be administered is 4 hours for 1 unit because of the danger of bacterial infection and red blood cell (RBC) hemolysis. For the same reasons, if the flow is interrupted for more than 30 minutes, the unit must be discarded.

PACKED RED BLOOD CELLS

- Volume: 300 ± 25 ml
- Maximum administration time: 4 hours
- Rate of infusion: dependent on patient's clinical condition
- Administration: standard blood set for each unit hung or Y-type set if blood is to be reconstituted
- Indications: active bleeding with loss of ≥15% of total blood volume; anemia that is adversely influencing another medical disorder (e.g., unstable angina); symptomatic chronic anemia unrelated to nutritional deficiency
- Outcome measurement: Hb level within 24 hours

DELEUKOCYTED RED BLOOD CELLS

- Volume: 300 ± 25 ml
- Maximum administration time: 4 hours
- Rate of infusion: dependent on the patient's clinical condition
- Administration: standard blood set for each unit hung plus a filter (filter not required if RBCs are washed)
- Indications: clinically significant transfusion reactions; to reduce sensitization to histocompatibility antigens

FROZEN RED BLOOD CELLS (DEGLYCEROLIZED)

- Volume: approximately 200 ml
- Maximum administration time: 4 hours
- Rate of infusion: dependent on the patient's clinical condition
- Administration: standard blood set for each unit hung
- Indications: storing of rare blood groups and autotransfusion
- *Note:* Use only in special situations

PLASMA

- Volume: approximately 200 ml
- Maximum administration time: 4 hours
- Rate of infusion: dependent on patient's clinical condition
- Administration: standard blood set
- Indications: plasma is indicated as a source of coagulation factors. *Frozen plasma* is frozen within 24 hours of collection and contains higher levels of labile coagulation factors (V and VIII). Nonlabile factors are well maintained in both frozen and *stored (banked) plasma*. Plasma may be used for
  - Significant hemorrhage due to a deficiency of coagulation factors
  - Immediate hemostasis in a patient on warfarin
  - A patient with severe liver disease or massive transfusion (whole blood volume replaced within 24 hours) with abnormal clotting tests and active bleeding
  - TTP
  - Prophylaxis before an invasive procedure associated with a significant bleeding risk
- Outcome measurement: PT, aPTT, or both within 4 hours of transfusion

PLATELETS

- Volume: approximately 50 ml
- Rate of infusion: as rapidly as is tolerated by the patient
- Administration: blood components recipient set
- Indications: the therapeutic aim of platelet transfusions is to improve hemostasis. Their use should be considered in the following situations.
  - Patients with platelet counts of less than 20 g/l on the basis of decreased platelet production
  - Patients with consumptive thrombocytopenia (e.g., immune thrombocytopenia, DIC only when there is significant bleeding
  - Patients with significant platelet dysfunction
- Outcome measurement: Platelet count 1 hour after transfusion
- *Note:* Platelet transfusion reactions are common. In patients with a history of reactions, the use of acetaminophen 650 mg PO and diphenhydramine (Benadryl) 50 mg IV may prevent reactions. Narcotics (morphine 5–10 mg IV) or steroids (hydrocortisone 100 mg IV) also may be helpful. If these measures fail, deleukocyted platelets are recommended.

  In patients who are unresponsive to random donor platelets (defined by less than a 5 g/l increment in platelets 1 hour after transfusion on two successive transfusions), platelets collected from a single donor by apheresis should be considered.

CRYOPRECIPITATE

- Volume: 5 to 10 ml
- Rate of infusion: as rapidly as possible
- Administration: blood component recipient set
- Indications: cryoprecipitate contains significant amounts of factor VIII (100 units/unit of cryoprecipitate), fibrinogen (250 mg/unit), and von Willebrand's factor. It is therefore useful in the treatment of mild hemophilia A and von Willebrand's disease and in the repletion of fibrinogen (e.g., DIC, dilutional coagulopathy). The dose is dependent on body mass, the indication for use, and the severity of the preexisting deficiency.
- Outcome measurement: factor VIII level and aPTT (hemophilia A); von Willebrand's factor antigen level, bleeding time, or both (von Willebrand's disease); fibrinogen level (DIC, dilutional coagulopathy)—within 4 hours of transfusion

FACTOR VIII CONCENTRATE

- Lyophilized, fractionated plasma product
- Specific activity and storage conditions stated on label
- Must be reconstituted before use
- Indications: moderate to severe factor VIII deficiency and low titer of factor VIII inhibitors
- *Note:* not for use in von Willebrand's disease. Consult with hematologist before administration.

FACTOR IX COMPLEX

- Lyophilized, fractionated plasma product
- Factor IX content and storage conditions stated on labels
- Must be reconstituted before use
- Indications: factor IX deficiency. Consult with hematologist before administration.

NORMAL SERUM ALBUMIN

- Concentrates of 25% in vials of 100 ml and 5% in vials of 250 and 500 ml
- Sodium content approximately 145 mmol/L
- Indications: hypoproteinemia with peripheral edema (give 25%); volume depletion where IV NS is contraindicated (give 5%); *not indicated* in the asymptomatic hypoproteinemic patient

BLOOD TUBES

Lavender Top (EDTA)
CBC and differential
Sickle cell
Reticulocyte count
Malaria stain
Direct Coombs' test
ACTH
G-6-PD

Red/Gray ("Tiger Top")
SMAC (glucose)*
C3, C4, cryoglobulins
Cardiac enzymes
Osmolality
Liver enzymes
Pregnancy test
Drug concentrations (alcohol, digoxin, gentamicin, and so on)
C peptide/insulin
Protein electrophoresis

Red Top
Crossmatch
RA latex
Haptoglobin
ANA
TCA concentrations

Green Top
Lactate*
Ammonia*

Blue Top (Citrate)
PT, aPTT
Fibrinogen
Circulating anticoagulants
Coagulation factor assays

Blue Top (for FDP only)
Fibrin degradation products

---

*These specimens must be delivered to the laboratory immediately or put on ice for transportation.

APPENDIX D

□☐□

READING ECGs

RATE

Multiply the number of QRS complexes in a 6-second period (30 large squares) by 10 = beats/min (Fig. D–1).
- Normal = 60–100 beats/min
- Tachycardia = >100 beats/min
- Bradycardia = <60 beats/min

RHYTHM

Is the rhythm regular?
Is there a P wave preceding every QRS complex? Is there a QRS complex following every P wave?
1. Yes = sinus rhythm.

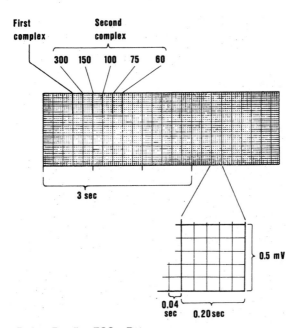

Figure D–1 □ Reading ECGs. Rate.

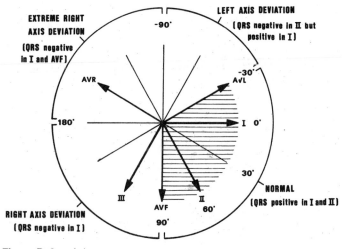

Figure D–2 □ Axis.

2. No P waves with irregular rhythm = atrial fibrillation.
3. No P waves with regular rhythm = junctional rhythm. Look for retrograde P waves in all leads.

AXIS

See Figure D–2.

P WAVE CONFIGURATION

Normal P wave. Look at all leads (Fig. D–3A).

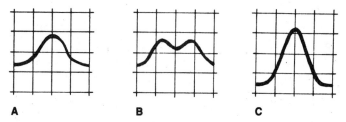

A   **B**   **C**

Figure D–3 □ Reading ECGs. P wave configuration in lead II. *A,* Normal P wave. *B,* Left atrial enlargement. *C,* Right atrial enlargement.

Left Atrial Enlargement (Fig. D–3*B*)

- Duration: 120 ms (three small squares in lead II); often notched indicates P mitrale.
- Amplitude: Negative terminal P wave in lead V_1 >1 mm in depth and >40 ms (one small square)

Right Atrial Enlargement (Fig. D–3C)

- Amplitude: 2.5 mm in leads II, III, or aVF (i.e., tall peaked P wave of P pulmonale); 1.5 mm in the initial positive deflection of the P wave in lead V_1 or V_2.

QRS CONFIGURATION
Left Ventricular Hypertrophy

1. Increased QRS voltage (S in lead V_1 or V_2 plus R in V5 >35 mm or R in aVL ≥11 mm)
2. ST-segment depression and negative T wave in left lateral leads are common.

Right Ventricular Hypertrophy

1. R > S in V_1
2. Right-axis deviation ($> +90$ degrees)
3. ST-segment depression and negative T wave in right precordial leads

CONDUCTION ABNORMALITIES
First-Degree Block

- PR interval ≥0.20 second (≥1 large square)

Second-Degree Block

- Occasional absence of QRS and T after a P wave of sinus origin
  1. Type I (Wenckebach's): progressive prolongation of the PR interval before the missed QRS complex (see Fig. 15–22)
  2. Type II: absence of progressive prolongation of the PR interval before the missed QRS complex (see Fig. 15–23)

Third-Degree Block

- Absence of any relationship between P waves of sinus origin and QRS complexes (see Fig. 15–24)

Left Anterior Hemiblock

- Left-axis deviation, Q in I and aVL; a small R in III, in the absence of left ventricular hypertrophy

Left Posterior Hemiblock

- Right-axis deviation, a small R in I, and a small Q in III, in the absence of right ventricular hypertrophy.

Complete Right Bundle Branch Block

See Figure D–4A.

Complete Left Bundle Branch Block

See Figure D–4B.

Ventricular Preexcitation

1. PR interval <0.11 second with widened QRS (>0.12 second) due to a delta wave indicates Wolff-Parkinson-White syndrome.
2. PR interval <0.11 second with a normal QRS complex indicates Lown-Ganong-Levine syndrome.

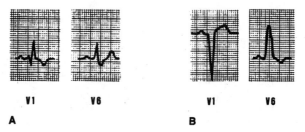

V1 **V6** **V1** **V6**

A **B**

Figure D–4 □ Reading ECGs. QRS configuration. *A*, Complete right bundle branch block. *B*, Complete left bundle branch block.

MYOCARDIAL INFARCTION PATTERNS

Type of Infarct	Patterns of Changes (Q Waves, ST Elevation or Depression, T Wave Inversion)*
Inferior	Q in II, III, aVF
Inferoposterior	Q in II, III, aVF, and V_6
	R > S and positive T in V_1
Anteroseptal	V_1 to V_4
Anterolateral to posterolateral	V_1 to V_5; Q in I, aVL, and V_6
Posterior	R > S in V_1, positive T, and Q in V_6

*A significant Q wave is >40 ms wide or more than one third of the QRS height. ST-segment or T wave changes in the absence of significant Q waves may represent a non–Q wave infarction.

APPENDIX E

MISCELLANEOUS

EMPIRIC AMINOGLYCOSIDE DOSING GUIDELINES FOR GENTAMICIN AND TOBRAMYCIN

- Loading dose: 2.0 to 2.5 mg/kg (IBW)
- Maintenance dose: 1.5 mg/kg (IBW) per dosing interval as suggested subsequently

Estimated Creatinine Clearance (CrCl)	Dosing Intervals
>1.25	q8h
0.8–1.25	q12h
0.7–0.8	q16h
0.6–0.7	q18h
0.4–0.6	q24h
0.3–0.4	q30h
0.25–0.3	q36h
0.2–0.25	q48h
<0.2	Once

CALCULATION OF CREATININE CLEARANCE

$$\text{CrCl (ml/s)} = \frac{(140 - \text{age in years}) \times 1.5}{\text{Serum creatinine } (\mu\text{mol/L})} \ (\times 0.85 \text{ in females})$$

CALCULATION OF THE ALVEOLAR-ARTERIAL OXYGEN GRADIENT [$P(A-a)O_2$]

The $P(A-a)O_2$ can be calculated easily from the ABG results. It is useful in confirming the presence of a shunt.

$$P(A-a)O_2 = P_{AO_2} - P_{aO_2}$$

- P_{AO_2} = the alveolar oxygen tension calculated as shown subsequently

- P_{aO_2} = the arterial oxygen tension measured by ABG determination

P_{AO_2} can be calculated by the following formula.

$$P_{AO_2} = (PB - PH_2O) (F_{IO_2}) P_{aCO_2}/R$$

- PB = barometric pressure (760 mm Hg at sea level)
- PH_2O = 47 mm Hg
- FIO_2 = the fraction of O_2 in inspired gas
- $PaCO_2$ = the arterial CO_2 tension measured by ABG determination
- R = the respiratory quotient (0.8)

Normal $P(A-a)O_2$ ranges from 12 mm Hg in the young adult to 20 mm Hg at age 70.

In pure ventilatory failure, the $P(A-a)O_2$ will remain 12 to 20 mm Hg. In oxygenation failure, it will increase.

INTERNATIONAL NORMALIZED RATIO (INR)

The INR has been developed to improve the consistency of oral anticoagulant therapy. It is calculated using the mean normal PT for a laboratory's system, not the PT of the "normal control material." The relation between PT and INR is

$$INR = (PT_{patient}/PT_{mean})^{ISI}$$

where $PT_{patient}$ is the patient's PT, PT_{mean} is the mean of the normal range for PT (measured by the laboratory), and ISI is the International Sensitivity Index, which is a measure of the responsiveness of the thromboplastin used to measure the PT to a reduction in vitamin K–dependent coagulation factors.

ANTIBIOTIC SUSCEPTIBILITY GUIDELINES (SENSITIVITIES MUST BE CHECKED)

Drug ++ Drug of Choice + Effective − Not Effective ± Depends on Sensitivities ? Clinical Efficacy Not Proved	Aerobe								Anaerobe	
	Pneumococci	Staphylococcus aureus (Penicillin Resistant)	Haemophilus influenzae	H. influenzae (Ampicillin Resistant)	Escherichia coli (Community Acquired)	Klebsiella	Pseudomonas	Coliforms	Above Diaphragm Excluding Bacillus fragilis	B. fragilis
Amikacin	−	?	−	−	+	+	+	++	−	−
Ampicillin/amoxicillin	+	−	++	−	++	−	−	±	+	−
Amoxicillin/clavulanate	+	+	++	+	++	+	−	±	+	+
Cefazolin	+	+	−	−	+	+	−	±	+	−
Cefotaxime	+	?	+	+	+	+	−	±	?	−
Cefoxitin	+	+	−	−	+	+	−	±	+	+

	1	2	3	4	5	6	7	8
Ceftazidime	?	+	+	+	+	+	+	−
Ceftriaxone	+	+	+	+	+	+	?	−
Cefixime	+	−	+	+	+	+	+	−
Cefuroxime	+	+	+	+	+	+	+	−
Chloramphenicol	+	+	+	+	+	−	−	+
Ciprofloxacin	−	+	+	+	+	+	+	−
Clindamycin	+	+ +/+	−	−	−	−	+	+
Cloxacillin	+	+/+	−	−	−	−	−	−
Cotrimoxazole	±	±	+	?	+	?	?	?
Erythromycin	+	+	?	+	+	+	+	−
Gentamicin	−	+	+	+	+	+	+	−
Imipenem	+	−	+	+	+	+	+	+
Metronidazole	+/+	−	−	−	−	−	+/+	+/+
Penicillin	+	−	−	+	+	+	+	+
Piperacillin	±	−	−	+	+	+	+	+
Tetracycline	+	+	+	+	+	+	+	+
Tobramycin	−	?	−	−	−	−	−	−
Vancomycin	+	+	−	−	−	−	−	−

Modified from *St. Paul's Formulary*, St. Paul's Hospital, Vancouver, British Columbia, Canada.

ANTIBIOTIC STANDARD DOSES FOR PATIENTS WITH NORMAL RENAL FUNCTION

Drug	Dosage Range (g/day) IV/IM*	Usual Dosage (g/dosing interval) IV/IM*	Special Comments Regarding Uses
Amikacin	15 mg/kg	7.5 mg/kg q12h	For infections due to gram-negative rods resistant to gentamicin and tobramycin
Amoxicillin	1–6	0.5–1.0 q8h	
Ampicillin	2–12	1 q6h	
Cefazolin	3–6	1 q8h	Useful first-generation cephalosporin for gram-positive aerobes
Cefotaxime	3–12	a. 1 q8h b. 2 q4h	a. For susceptible bacteria resistant to less expensive agents b. Meningitis due to gram-negative rods resistant to ampicillin
Cefoxitin	3–8	1 q6h	As a single agent in mixed infections including *Bacillus fragilis*
Ceftazidime	3–8	1 q8h	For *Pseudomonas aeruginosa* when aminoglycosides inappropriate
Ceftriaxone	1–4	1–2 q12–24h	a. For susceptible bacteria resistant to less expensive agents b. Meningitis due to gram-negative rods resistant to ampicillin
Cefuroxime	2.25–4.5	0.75 q8h	a. Mixed lung infections in penicillin-allergic patients b. *Haemophilus influenzae* resistant to ampicillin
Chloramphenicol	2–6	1 q6h	Rarely indicated (irreversible aplastic anemia 1/25,000)

Drug	Dose	Schedule	Comments
Clindamycin	0.6–2.4	a. 0.6 q8h b. 0.3 q6h	a. *B. fragilis* b. Other susceptible bacteria
Cloxacillin/methicillin	2–12	1 q6h	Effective for *Staphylococcus aureus* (penicillin sensitive), but penicillin is drug of choice
Cotrimoxazole†	—	—	
Erythromycin	1–4	0.5 q6h	IV drug of choice for *Legionella*
Gentamicin	3–5 mg/kg	1.5 mg/kg q8h	Initially for serious aerobic gram-negative rod infections
Imipenem	1–2	0.5 q6h	For susceptible bacteria resistant to less expensive agent
Metronidazole	1–2	0.5 q8h	Well absorbed orally
Penicillin	mu‡ 2–20	mu 1 q6h	Useful for *Clostridium difficile* pseudomembranous colitis
Piperacillin	a. 6–12 b. 8–18	a. 1.5 q4h b. 2.0 q4h	a. For susceptible bacteria resistant to less expensive agents b. With an aminoglycoside for leukopenic patients with *P. aeruginosa*
Tetracycline	1–2	0.5 q6h	
Tobramycin	3–5 mg/kg	1.5 mg/kg q8h	Better than gentamicin only for *P. aeruginosa*
Vancomycin	1–2	1 q12h	For cloxacillin-resistant staphylococci

*Unless otherwise specified.
†Trimethoprim and sulfamethoxazole.
‡Million units.
Courtesy of *St. Paul's Formulary*, St. Paul's Hospital, Vancouver, British Columbia, Canada.

ANTIBIOTIC DOSAGE ADJUSTMENTS RELATIVE TO RENAL FUNCTION

Drug	Creatinine Clearance		
	>0.8 ml/s >50 ml/min	0.8–0.4 ml/s 50–25 ml/min	<0.4 ml/s <25 ml/min
Parenteral Therapy			
Acyclovir	5–10 mg/kg q8h	5–10 mg/kg q12h	5–10 mg/kg q24h
Amikacin			
Ampicillin	1–2 g q6h	1–2 g q6–12h	1–2 g q12–16h
Cefazolin	1–2 g q8h	1–2 g q12h	1–2 g q12–24h
Cefotaxime	1–2 g q6–8h	1–2 g q6–8h	1–2 g q12h
Cefoxitin	1–2 g q6h	1–2 g q8–12h	1–2 g q12–24h
Ceftazidime	1–2 g q8h	1–2 g q12h	1–2 g q12–24h
Ceftriaxone	1–2 g q24h	1–2 g q24h	1–2 g q24h
Cefuroxime	750–1500 mg q8h	750–1500 mg q8–12h	750–1500 mg q12–24h
Clindamycin	600 mg q8h	NDN*	NDN
Cloxacillin	250–1000 mg q4–6h	NDN	NDN
Gentamicin			
Imipenem	500 mg q6–8h	500 mg q8h	500 mg q12h
Metronidazole	500 mg q8h	500 mg q8–12h	250–500 mg q12h
Piperacillin	2–4 g q4–6h	2–4 g q6–12h	2–4 g q12h
Oral Therapy			
Acyclovir	NDN	NDN	Increase to q12h
Amoxicillin	NDN	NDN	Increase to q12h
Ampicillin	NDN	NDN	Increase to q12h
Cephalexin	NDN	NDN	Increase to q12h
Cloxacillin	NDN	NDN	NDN
Clindamycin	NDN	NDN	NDN
Co-trimoxazole	NDN	NDN	Decrease by 50%
Doxycycline	NDN	NDN	Increase to q24h
Erythromycin	NDN	NDN	Decrease by 50%
Ketoconazole	NDN	NDN	NDN
Metronidazole	NDN	NDN	Increase to q12h
Nitrofurantoin	NDN	Avoid	Avoid
Norfloxacin	NDN	NDN	Increase to q24h
Tetracycline	NDN	Avoid	Avoid

NDN, no dosage adjustment needed.
Courtesy of St. Paul's Formulary, St. Paul's Hospital, Vancouver, British Columbia, Canada.

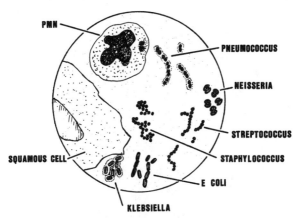

Figure E–1 □ Sputum Gram's stain. A useful sputum specimen for identification of the bacterial cause of pneumonia should have ≥25 PMNs and fewer than 10 squamous cells per low power field.

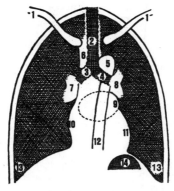

Figure E–2 □ Posteroanterior chest x-ray.

1. Clavicles
2. Trachea
3. Right mainstem bronchus
4. Left mainstem bronchus
5. Aortic knuckle
6. Superior vena cava
7. Right pulmonary artery
8. Left pulmonary artery
9. Left atrium
10. Right atrium
11. Left ventricle
12. Aortic stripe
13. Costophrenic angles
14. Gastric bubble

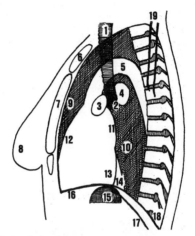

Figure E–3 □ Lateral chest x-ray.

1. Trachea
2. Left mainstem bronchus
3. Right pulmonary artery
4. Left pulmonary artery
5. Aortic arch
6. Manubrium
7. Sternum
8. Breast shadow
9. Retrosternal space
10. Retrocardiac space
11. Left atrium
12. Right ventricle
13. Left ventricle
14. Inferior vena cava
15. Gastric air bubble
16. Left hemidiaphragm
17. Right hemidiaphragm
18. Costophrenic angle
19. Scapular shadows

APPENDIX F

SI UNITS CONVERSION TABLE

SI units is the abbreviation for *le Système International d'Unites*. The SI is an outgrowth of the metric system and provides a uniform system of reporting laboratory data between nations. Most laboratory values in *On Call* are presented in SI units. Because some laboratories have not yet converted to this system of reporting, a conversion table for commonly measured laboratory parameters is provided.

Laboratory Test	Previous Reference Intervals	Previous Unit	Conversion Factor	SI Reference Intervals	SI Unit Symbol
Erythrocyte count					
Female	3.5–5.0	$10^6/mm^3$	1	3.5–5.0	$10^{12}/L$
Male	4.3–5.9	$10^6/mm^3$	1	4.3–5.9	$10^{12}/L$
Erythrocyte sedimentation rate (ESR)					
Female	0–30	mm/h	1	0–30	mm/h
Male	0–20	mm/h	1	0–20	mm/h
Hemoglobin					
Female	12.0–15.0	g/dl	10	120–150	g/L
Male	13.6–17.2	g/dl	10	136–172	g/L
Leukocyte count					
Number fraction (differential)		%	0.01	1	1
Platelet count	130–400	$10^3/mm^3$	1	130–400	$10^9/L$
Reticulocyte count	10,000–75,000	$/mm^3$	0.001	10–75	$10^9/L$
Number fraction	1–24	Number per 1000 RBCs	0.001	0.001–0.024	1
Albumin (serum)	0.1–2.4	%	0.001	0.001–0.024	1
Alkaline phosphatase	4.0–6.0	g/dl	10.0	40–60	g/L
Amylase (serum)	30–120	U/L	0.01667	0.5–2.0	μkat/L
Aspartate aminotransferase (AST)	0–130	U/L	0.01667	0–2.17	μkat/L
	0–35	U/L	0.01667	0–0.58	μkat/L

Bilirubin					
Total	0.1–1.0	mg/dl	17.10	2–18	μmol/L
Conjugated	0–0.2	mg/dl	17.10	0–4	μmol/L
Calcium (serum)					
Male	8.8–10.3	mg/dl	0.2495	2.20–2.58	mmol/L
Female (<50 years)	8.8–10.0	mg/dl	0.2495	2.20–2.50	mmol/L
Female (>50 years)	8.8–10.2	mg/dl	0.2495	2.20–2.56	mmol/L
Calcium ion (serum)	4.4–5.1	mEq/L	0.500	2.20–2.56	mmol/L
	2.00–2.30	mEq/L	0.500	1.00–1.15	mmol/L
CO_2 content (= $HCO_3 + CO_2$)	22–28	mEq/L	1.00	22–28	mmol/L
CO (proportion of Hb that is COHb)	<15	%	0.01	<0.15	1
Chloride (serum)	95–105	mEq/L	1.00	95–105	mmol/L
Cholesterol (plasma)					
<29 years	<200	mg/dl	0.02586	<5.20	mmol/L
30–39 years	<225	mg/dl	0.02586	<5.85	mmol/L
40–49 years	<245	mg/dl	0.02586	<6.35	mmol/L
>50 years	<265	mg/dl	0.02586	<6.85	mmol/L
Complement (serum)					
C3	70–160	mg/dl	0.01	0.7–1.6	g/L
C4	20–40	mg/dl	0.01	0.2–0.4	g/L
Creatine phosphokinase (CPK) (serum)	0–130	U/L	0.01667	0–2.16	μkat/L
MB fraction	>5 in MI	%	0.01	>0.05	1
Creatinine					
Serum	0.6–1.2	mg/dl	88.40	50–110	μmol/L
Urine	Variable	g/24 h	8.840	Variable	mmol/d

Table continued on following page

421

Laboratory Test	Previous Reference Intervals	Previous Unit	Conversion Factor	SI Reference Intervals	SI Unit Symbol
Creatinine clearance	75–125	ml/min	0.01667	1.24–2.08	ml/s
Digoxin (plasma)					
Therapeutic	0.5–2.2	ng/ml	1.281	0.6–2.8	nmol/L
	0.5–2.2	µg/L	1.281	0.6–2.8	nmol/L
Toxic	>2.5	ng/ml	1.281	>3.2	nmol/L
Electrophoresis, serum protein					
Albumin	60–65	%	0.01	0.60–0.65	1
Alpha-1 globulin	1.7–5.0	%	0.01	0.02–0.05	1
Alpha-2 globulin	6.7–12.5	%	0.01	0.07–0.13	1
Beta globulin	8.3–16.3	%	0.01	0.08–0.16	1
Gamma globulin	10.7–20.0	%	0.01	0.11–0.20	1
Albumin	3.6–5.2	g/dl	10.0	36–52	g/L
Alpha-1 globulin	0.1–0.4	g/dl	10.0	1–4	g/L
Alpha-2 globulin	0.4–1.0	g/dl	10.0	4–10	g/L
Beta gobulin	0.5–1.2	g/dl	10.0	5–12	g/L
Gamma globulin	0.6–1.6	g/dl	10.0	6–16	g/L
Ethanol (plasma)					
Legal limit [driving]	<80	mg/dl	0.2171	<17	mmol/L
Toxic	>100	mg/dl	0.2171	>22	mmol/L
Ferritin (serum)	18–300	ng/ml	1.00	18–300	µg/L
Fibrinogen (plasma)	200–400	mg/dl	0.01	2.0–4.0	g/L
Folate					
Serum	2–10	ng/ml	2.266	4–22	nmol/L
RBC	140–960	ng/ml	2.266	550–2200	nmol/L

Test	Reference range	Conversion factor	Units	SI range	SI units
Gases (arterial blood)					
Po₂	75–105	mm Hg (= Torr)	0.1333	10.0–14.0	kPa
Pco₂	33–44	mm Hg (= Torr)	0.1333	4.4–5.9	kPa
Gamma-glutamyltransferase (GGT) (serum)	0–30	U/L	0.01667	0–0.50	μkat/L
Glucose					
Serum (fasting)	70–110	mg/dl	0.05551	3.9–6.1	mmol/L
Spinal fluid	50–80	mg/dl	0.05551	2.8–4.4	mmol/L
Haptoglobin (serum)	50–220	mg/dl	0.01	0.50–2.20	g/L
Hemoglobin (blood)					
Male	14.0–18.0	g/dl	10.0	140–180	g/L
Female	11.5–15.5	g/dl	10.0	115–155	g/L
Iron (serum)					
Male	80–180	μg/dl	0.1791	14–32	μmol/L
Female	60–160	μg/dl	0.1791	11–29	μmol/L
Iron binding capacity (serum)	250–460	μg/dl	0.1791	45–82	μmol/L
Lactate dehydrogenase (LDH) (serum)	50–150	U/L	0.01667	0.82–2.66	μkat/L
LD1	15–40	%	0.01	0.15–0.40	1
LD2	20–45	%	0.01	0.20–0.45	1
LD3	15–30	%	0.01	0.15–0.30	1
LD4	5–20	%	0.01	0.05–0.20	1
LD5	5–20	%	0.01	0.05–0.20	1
LD1	10–60	U/L	0.01667	0.16–1.00	μkat/L
LD2	20–70	U/L	0.01667	0.32–1.16	μkat/L
LD3	10–45	U/L	0.01667	0.22–0.76	μkat/L
LD4	5–30	U/L	0.01667	0.08–0.50	μkat/L
LD5	5–30	U/L	0.01667	0.02–0.50	μkat/L
Lipase (serum)	0–160	U/L	0.01667	0–2.66	μkat/L

Table continued on following page

Laboratory Test	Previous Reference Intervals	Previous Unit	Conversion Factor	SI Reference Intervals	SI Unit Symbol
Lithium ion (serum) (therapeutic)	0.50–1.50	mEq/L	1.00	0.50–1.50	mmol/L
		µg/L	0.001441		mmol/L
		mg/dl	1.441		mmol/L
Magnesium (serum)	1.8–3.0	mg/dl	0.4114	0.80–1.20	mmol/L
	1.6–2.4	mEq/L	0.500	0.80–1.20	mmol/L
Osmolality					
Plasma	280–300	mOsm/kg	1.00	280–300	mmol/kg
Urine	50–1200	mOsm/kg	1.00	50–1200	mmol/kg
Phosphate (serum)	2.5–5.0	mg/dl	0.3229	0.80–1.60	mmol/L
Potassium ion					
Serum	3.5–5.0	mEq/L	1.00	3.5–5.0	mmol/L
Urine (diet dependent)	25–100	mEq/24 h	1.00	25–100	mmol/d
Protein, total					
Serum	6.0–8.0	g/dl	10.0	60–80	g/L
Urine	<150	mg/24 h	0.001	<0.15	g/day
Sodium ion					
Serum	135–147	mEq/L	1.00	135–147	mmol/L
Urine	Diet dependent	mEq/24 h	1.00	Diet dependent	mmol/day

	Reference range	Units	Factor	SI range	SI units
Theophylline (plasma)					
Therapeutic	10.0–20.0	mg/L	5.550	55–110	µmol/L
Thyroid tests (serum)					
TSH	2–11	µU/ml	1.00	2–11	mU/L
T$_4$	4.0–11.0	µg/dl	12.87	51–142	nmol/L
TBG	12.0–28.0	µg/dl	12.87	150–360	nmol/L
Free T$_4$	0.8–2.8	ng/dl	12.87	10–36	pmol/L
T$_3$	75–220	ng/dl	0.01536	1.2–3.4	nmol/L
T$_3$ uptake	25–35	%	0.01	0.25–0.35	1
Transferrin (serum)	170–370	mg/dl	0.01	1.70–3.70	g/L
Triglycerides (plasma)	<160	mg/dl	0.01129	<1.80	mmol/L
Urate (as uric acid)					
Serum	2.0–7.0	mg/dl	59.48	120–420	µmol/L
Urine	Diet dependent	g/24 h	5.948	Diet dependent	mmol/day
Urea (serum)	8–18	mg/dl	0.3570	3.0–6.5	mmol/L
Vitamin B$_{12}$	200–1000	pg/ml	0.7378	150–750	pmol/L
(plasma or serum)		ng/dl	7.378		pmol/L

THE ON CALL FORMULARY

The On Call Formulary is a quick reference for information on medications that are commonly encountered or prescribed by the student or resident on call.

Antibacterial susceptibility guidelines as well as doses for patients are presented in table format on pages 412–416. Drugs used in cardiopulmonary resuscitation are presented in table format on pages 377–399.

Doses listed are for adult patients with normal renal and hepatic function.

ACETAMINOPHEN (Tylenol, Paracetamol)   *Analgesic, antipyretic*

Indications:	Pain, fever.
Actions:	Raises the pain threshold; acts directly on the hypothalamic heat-regulating center.
Side effects:	Uncommon—rash, drug fever, mucosal ulcerations, leukopenia, and pancytopenia.
Comments:	Unlike aspirin, acetaminophen has no anti-inflammatory action, does not irritate the stomach, and does not affect the aggregation of platelets. It does, however, interact with oral anticoagulants.
Dose:	325–1000 mg PO q4–6h PRN, up to 4000 mg/24 h.

ACETYLSALICYLIC ACID (see Aspirin)

ACTIVASE r-tPA (see Alteplase)

ACYCLOVIR (Zovirax)   *Nucleoside analog*

Indications:	Herpes zoster.
Actions:	Inhibits viral replication and viral DNA synthesis. A nucleoside analog related to guanosine.
Side effects:	Nausea, vomiting, diarrhea, headache, rash, paresthesia.
Comments:	Drug of choice for herpes zoster.
Dose:	800 mg q4 h, 5 times a day.

ADALAT (see Nifedipine)

ADENOSINE (see Table page 378)

ALBUTEROL (see Salbutamol)

ALGINIC ACID COMPOUND (Gaviscon)

Indications:	Gastroesophageal reflux.
Actions:	Antacid demulcent.
Side effects:	Nausea, vomiting, eructation, flatulence.
Comments:	Contains significant amounts of sodium.
Dose:	10–20 ml of liquid or 2–4 tablets chewed 1–4 times daily after meals and QHS. May be followed by a drink of water.

ALLOPURINOL (Zyloprim)　　　　　　　　*Xanthine oxidase inhibitor*

Indications:	Gout, uric acid nephropathy, tumor lysis syndrome.
Actions:	Inhibits the formation of uric acid.
Side effects:	Rash, fever, gastrointestinal upset, hepatotoxicity.
Comments:	Reduce the dose in renal or hepatic insufficiency. Aminophylline, mercaptopurine, and azathioprine levels may be increased by allopurinol. Attacks of acute gout may occur shortly after starting allopurinol.
Dose:	100–300 mg PO QD after meals. Doses up to 800 mg/day (in divided doses) may be required in severe cases.

ALTEPLASE (Activase r-tPA, TPA,
Tissue Plasminogen Activator)　　　　　　　　*Thrombolytic agent*

Indications:	Acute MI, massive pulmonary embolism.
Actions:	Binds to fibrin and activates bound plasminogen to plasmin, initiating local fibrinolysis with little conversion of circulating plasminogen.
Side effects:	Intracranial, retroperitoneal, and internal bleeding.
Comments:	More expensive than streptokinase but may be more effective in young patients with a large MI (N Engl J Med 1993;329:673–682).
Dose:	For acute MI: 15 mg IV bolus, followed by 0.75 mg/kg (not to exceed 50 mg) over 30 min; then 0.5 mg/kg (not to exceed 35 mg) over the next 60 mins. For massive pulmonary embolism: 100 mg IV over 2 h.

ALUMINUM HYDROXIDE (Amphojel, Basaljel)　　　　　　　　*Antacid*

Indications:	Pain due to peptic ulcer disease, reflux esophagitis, prophylaxis for stress ulcers, reduction of urinary phosphate in patients with phosphate-containing renal calculi.
Actions:	Buffers gastric acidity, binds phosphate in the intestine.
Side effects:	Constipation, anorexia, nausea, hypophosphatemia, aluminum toxicity in patients in renal failure.
Comments:	May bind and reduce intestinal absorption of tetracycline, thyroxine, and other medications.
Dose:	30–60 ml PO q1–2h during the acute phase; 30–60 ml PO q1–4h PC and QHS for chronic therapy.

AMICAR (see Aminocaproic Acid)

AMINOCAPROIC ACID (Amicar)　　　　*Plasminogen activator inhibitor*

Indications:	Excessive bleeding due to fibrinolysis.
Actions:	Inhibits plasminogen activator, also has antiplasmin activity.
Side effects:	Increases the risk of DVT, pulmonary embolism, and cerebral vasospasm. Also, nausea, abdominal cramps, dizziness, rash, and headache.
Dose:	4–5 g IV over 1h, followed by a maintenance infusion of 1–1.25 g/h to achieve plasma levels of 0.130 mg/ml until bleeding has stopped.

AMINOPHYLLINE (Phyllocontin)   *Bronchodilator*

Indications:	Bronchospasm but no longer considered a first-line agent because in adults it may not improve the bronchodilation achieved with the safer aggressive use of inhaled bronchodilators.
Actions:	Phosphodiesterase inhibitor resulting in smooth muscle relaxation and bronchodilation. Also, stimulates the respiratory center.
Side effects:	Tachycardia, ventricular ectopy, nausea, vomiting, headaches, seizures, insomnia, and nightmares.
Comments:	Theophylline clearance is decreased by the addition of erythromycin, cimetidine, propranolol, allopurinol, and a number of other drugs.
Dose:	Aminophylline loading dose is 6 mg/kg IV followed by 0.6 mg/kg/h maintenance. Maintenance doses for patients in CHF, liver disease and the elderly should be reduced to 0.3 mg/kg/h while smokers require a larger dose of 0.9 mg/kg/h.

AMOXICILLIN (see Table page 414)

AMOXICILLIN/CLAVULANATE (see Table page 414)

Clavulanic acid binds to most bacterial beta-lactamases, thus protecting amoxicillin from enzymatic degradation and expanding the spectrum of activity to include beta-lactamase–producing bacteria.

AMOXIL (see Amoxicillin)

AMPHOJEL (see Aluminum Hydroxide)

AMPHOTERICIN B (Fungizone)   *Antifungal*

Indications:	Systemic fungal infections.
Actions:	A polyene antibiotic that disrupts fungal cell membranes.
Side effects:	Fever, chills, nausea, vomiting, diarrhea, hypotension, nephrotoxicity, hypokalemia, hypomagnesemia, thrombophlebitis.
Comments:	Premedication with antipyretics, antihistamines, antiemetics, and corticosteroids may reduce some of the side effects.
Dose:	Patients should receive a test dose of 1 mg in 100 ml D5W over 2 h. If the test dose is tolerated, a further dose of 10 mg can be given on the first day. The dose can then be increased by 5 mg every day until the desired dose of 0.5 mg/kg/day is reached. Infusion time should be 4–6 h.

AMPICILLIN (see Table page 414)

AMPICIN (see Ampicillin)

ANCEF (see Cefazolin)

ASPIRIN (Acetylsalicylic Acid)   *Analgesic, antipyretic, anti-inflammatory*

Indications: Pain due to inflammation, fever, antiplatelet agent in coronary syndromes.
Actions: Acts peripherally by interfering with the production of prostaglandins, thus reducing pain and inflammation and acts centrally to reduce pain perception and reduce temperature by increasing heat loss.
Side effects: Gastric erosion and bleeding, tinnitus, fever, thirst, diaphoresis. Severe allergic reactions can occur, including asthma.
Dose: 325–650 mg PO q4–6h for mild pain or fever; 650 mg PO QID for chest pain due to pericarditis; 80–325 mg/day for angina and antiplatelet effects; 2.6–5.2 g/day in divided doses for rheumatoid arthritis.

APRESOLINE (see Hydralazine)

ATENOLOL (Tenormin)   *Beta-1–selective blocker*

Indications: Angina pectoris, post-MI, treatment of SVTs, hypertension, thyrotoxicosis.
Actions: Beta-1–adrenergic blockade.
Side effects: Hypotension, bradycardia, CHF, nausea, fatigue, nightmares.
Comments: Should be chosen over a nonselective beta blocker when beta-2 blockade is undesirable (e.g., peripheral vascular disease).
Dose: 25–50 mg/day PO for most indications. 100 mg PO immediately and daily for hypertensive emergencies. 5 mg IV over 5 min for SVTs and, if tolerated, 5 mg 10 min later.

ATIVAN (see Lorazepam)

ATROPINE (see Table page 380)

AXID (see Nizatidine)

AZT (see Zidovudine)

BASALJEL (see Aluminum Hydroxide)

BECLOMETHASONE (Beclovent, Vanceril)   *Corticosteroid*

Indications: Bronchial asthma long-term treatment.
Actions: Topical anti-inflammatory
Side effects: Oral and pharyngeal candidiasis, laryngeal myopathy.
Comments: Has no role in the treatment of the acute asthma attack.
Dose: 2 inhalations BID to QID; may be more effective if inhaled 3–5 min after inhaled bronchodilator.

BECLOVENT (see Beclomethasone)

BENADRYL (see Diphenhydramine)

BISACODYL (Dulcolax) *Laxative*

Indications:	Constipation.
Actions:	Stimulates peristalsis.
Side effects:	Abdominal cramps, rectal bleeding.
Comments:	Onset PO in 6–10 h; onset PR 15–60 mins. Avoid in pregnancy, MI; may worsen orthostatic hypotension, weakness, and incoordination in the elderly.
Dose:	10–15 mg PO QHS PRN; 10 mg suppository PR PRN.

BISMUTH SUBSALICYLATE (Pepto-Bismol)

Indications:	Peptic ulcer disease, diarrhea.
Actions:	Acts locally at the ulcer site to promote healing of gastric and duodenal ulcers, has antibacterial activity, including against *Helicobacter pylori*. Neutralizes bacterial toxins and is useful in traveler's diarrhea.
Side effects:	Darkening of the tongue and stools, tinnitus.
Comments:	Avoid in patients with salicylate sensitivity. Used in combination with an antibiotic in the eradication of *H. pylori.*
Dose:	2 tablets or 30 ml PO QID (262 µg); for diarrhea 2 tabs q30min.

BRETYLIUM TOSYLATE (see Table page 382)

BREVIBLOC (see Esmolol)

BUMETANIDE (Bumex) *Loop diuretic*

Indications:	CHF.
Actions:	Inhibits the reabsorption of Na^+ and Cl^- in the ascending limb of the loop of Henle.
Side effects:	Electrolyte depletion, rash, hyperuricemia, reversible deafness.
Comments:	1 mg bumetanide = 40 mg furosemide. No advantage over furosemide, which is usually less expensive.
Dose:	0.5–1 mg PO or IV; if necessary, repeat dose every 20 min to a total dose of 3 mg.

BUMEX (see Bumetanide)

CALAN (see Verapamil)

CALCIUM GLUCONATE *Calcium supplement*

Indications:	Symptomatic hypocalcemia, hyperkalemia; adjunct in CPR protocol.
Actions:	Replacement; decreases cardiac automaticity, raises resting potential of cardiac cells.
Side effects:	Administration of Ca^{2+} to patients on digoxin may precipitate ventricular dysrhythmias due to the combined effects of digoxin and $Ca.^{2+}$
Comments:	500 mg of calcium gluconate = 2.3 mmol Ca^{2+} 10% solution contains 0.45 mmol Ca^{2+}/ml.
Dose:	1–15 g PO daily for control of hypocalcemia. 5–10 ml of a 10% solution for more rapid effects.

CANESTEN (see Clotrimazole)

CAPOTEN (see Captopril)

CAPTOPRIL (Capoten)   *Angiotensin-converting enzyme inhibitor*

Indications:	Hypertension, CHF.
Actions:	Inhibits the enzyme responsible for conversion of angiotensin I to angiotensin II.
Side effects:	Hypotension, dysgeusia, cough, rash, angioedema, neutropenia, proteinuria, renal insufficiency.
Comments:	May cause hyperkalemia if used in patients receiving potassium-sparing diuretics or potassium supplements.
Dose:	Begin with a test dose of 6.25 mg PO and monitor BP for 4 h. For hypertension: titrate up to 25–50 mg PO BID. For CHF: titrate to 25–50 mg PO TID.

CEFAZOLIN (Ancef, Kefzol) (see Table page 414)

CEFOTAXIME (Claforan) (see Table page 414)

CEFOXITIN (Mefoxin) (see Table page 414)

CEFTAZ (see Ceftazidime)

CEFTAZIDIME (Ceptaz, Fortaz) (see Table page 414)

CEFTIN (see Cefuroxime Axetil, Cefuroxime)

CEFTRIAXONE (Rocephin) (see Table page 414)

CEFUROXIME (Ceftin, Zinacef) (see Table page 414)

CEFUROXIME AXETIL (Ceftin) (see Table page 414)

Cefuroxime axetil is the ester form of cefuroxime; it is orally absorbed and then rapidly hydrolyzed to cefuroxime.

CEPTAZ (see Ceftazidime)

CHLORAL HYDRATE (Noctec and others)   *Hypnotic*

Indications:	Insomnia.
Actions:	Hypnotic.
Side effects:	Gastric irritation, rash.
Comments:	Do not use in patients with liver or kidney disease.
Dose:	0.5–1.0 g PO/PR.

CHLORAMPHENICOL (see Table page 414)

CHLORANASE (see Chlorpropamide)

CHLORDIAZEPOXIDE (Librium and others) *Benzodiazepine*

Indications:	Anxiety, alcohol withdrawal.
Actions:	Benzodiazepine sedative-antianxiety agent.
Side effects:	CNS depression.
Comments:	Unpredictable absorption after IM injection.
Dose:	5–25 mg PO TID for anxiety; 50–100 mg IV q2–6h PRN (maximum dose 500 mg for first 24 h) for alcohol withdrawal.

CHLORPROMAZINE (Largactil, Thorazine) *Antipsychotic phenothiazine*

Indications:	Agitation, nausea, vomiting, hiccoughs.
Actions:	Dopamine, histamine-1, muscarine, and alpha-1 adrenergic receptor antagonist.
Side effects:	CNS depression, hypotension, extrapyramidal effects, jaundice.
Comments:	In the acutely agitated patient, haloperidol may be a better choice because of its lesser effect on BP.
Dose:	30–75 mg for mild cases and 150 mg for severe cases daily PO; 25–50 mg IM repeated q6–8h; 10–25 mg PO/IM q6–8h for hiccoughs.

CHLORPROPAMIDE (Diabinese, Chloranase) *Oral hypoglycemic*

Indications:	Type 2 diabetes mellitus.
Actions:	Sulfonylurea, stimulates insulin secretion, increases the effect of insulin on the liver to increase gluconeogenesis and on muscle to increase glucose utilization.
Side effects:	Hypoglycemia, rash, blood dyscrasias, jaundice, hyponatremia, edema.
Comments:	Has a long duration of action (20–60 h) and is cleared largely by the kidneys. Hypoglycemic reactions may be prolonged in the elderly and in patients with renal impairment.
Dose:	100–500 mg/day PO in 1 or 2 doses.

CIMETIDINE (Tagamet) *Histamine-2 antagonist*

Indications:	Peptic ulcer disease, gastroesophageal reflux.
Actions:	Inhibits histamine induced secretion of gastric acid.
Side effects:	Gynecomastia, impotence, confusion, diarrhea, leukopenia, thrombocytopenia, increase in serum creatinine.
Comments:	Reduces microsomal enzyme metabolism of drugs including oral anticoagulants, phenytoin, and theophylline.
Dose:	300 mg PO/IV q6–8h. 800 mg QHS PO is effective in peptic ulcer disease and 400 mg PO BID in reflux.

CISAPRIDE (Propulsid) *GI prokinetic agent*

Indications:	Gastroesophageal reflux.
Actions:	Enhances the release of acetylcholine at the myenteric plexus, thus increasing esophageal peristalsis and low-

ering esophageal tone, as well as increasing gastric and duodenal contractility.

Side effects:	Diarrhea, abdominal discomfort, QT interval prolongation, torsade de pointes.
Comments:	Expensive; preferred over metaclopropamide because of fewer central nervous system effects.
Dose:	5–10 mg 3–4 times per day 15 min PC and QHS with a beverage.

CLAFORAN (see Cefotaxime)

CLAVULIN (see Amoxicillin/Clavulanate)

CLINDAMYCIN (see Table page 415)

CLOTRIMAZOLE (Canesten and others)   *Antifungal*

Indications:	Esophageal, vaginal, and intertrigonal candidiasis.
Actions:	Damages fungal cell membranes.
Side effects:	Local irritation, although generally well tolerated.
Dose:	10 mg troche PO QID for esophageal candidiasis; 100 mg intravaginally QHS ×7 nights for vaginal candidiasis; 1% cream or solution BID for intertrigonal candidiasis.

CLOXACILLIN (see Table page 415)

CODEINE   *Narcotic analgesic*

Indications:	Pain, cough, diarrhea.
Actions:	Narcotic analgesic, depresses the medullary cough center; decreases propulsive contractions of the small bowel.
Side effects:	Dysphoria, agitation, pruritus, constipation, lightheadedness, sedation.
Comments:	Useful in mild to moderate pain.
Dose:	30–60 mg PO/SC/IM q4–6h for analgesia; 8–20 mg Q4H for diarrhea and cough.

COLACE (see Docusate)

CORGARD (see Nadolol)

CO-TRIMOXAZOLE (see Trimethoprim/Sulfamethoxazole)

COUMADIN (see Warfarin)

DDAVP INJECTION (see Desmopressin)

ddC (Dideoxycytidine, Hivid)   *Nucleoside analog*

Indications:	Advanced HIV disease.
Actions:	Inhibition of reverse transcriptase, thus inhibiting retrovirus replication. Cytidine analog.
Side effects:	Mucosal ulcers and rash, peripheral neuropathy.
Comments:	Used in combination therapy with AZT.
Dose:	0.01 mg/kg PO q8h.

ddl (Dideoxyinosine, Didanosine, Videx)   *Nucleoside analog*

Indications:	Advanced HIV disease.
Actions:	Inhibition of reverse transcriptase thus inhibition of retrovirus replication. Purine analog.
Side effects:	Headache, insomnia, increase in uric acid, pancreatitis, increase in triglycerides, peripheral neuropathy.
Dose:	167–325 mg PO BID.

DEMEROL (see Meperidine)

DESMOPRESSIN (DDAVP Injection)

Indications:	To maintain hemostasis in patients with hemophilia A and factor VIII levels greater than 5% or with mild to moderate von Willebrand's disease (Type I).
Actions:	A synthetic analog of antidiuretic hormone with identical actions on water reabsorption in the renal tubule. Has additional action to release factor VIII complex and plasminogen activator from endothelial cell storage sites. This action peaks in 1 h and lasts 8–12 h. It may also have a direct effect on the vessel wall, decreasing bleeding at an injury site.
Side effects:	Facial flushing, tachycardia, mild hypotension. Water retention. Headache, nausea, abdominal pain. Allergic reactions.
Comments:	Should not be used in hemophilia B because it has no effect on factor IX. Should not be used in severe type I Von Willebrand's disease or type IIB because severe disease is least likely to respond and severe thrombocytopenia may develop.
Dose:	10.0 μg/m^2 (maximum dose 20 μg) by slow IV infusion.

DIABINESE (see Chlorpropamide)

DIAZEPAM (Valium)   *Benzodiazepine*

Indications:	Anxiety, seizure disorders, alcohol withdrawal.
Actions:	Benzodiazepine sedative–antianxiety agent.
Side effects:	Sedation, hypotension, respiratory depression, paradoxical agitation.
Comments:	IM administration is not recommended because of unpredictable absorption. Patients have a wide variability in tolerance to the benzodiazepines: always start with a conservative dose in patients who have not previously received them.
Dose:	For anxiety: 2–10 mg PO BID to QID. For status epilepticus: 2 mg/min IV until the seizures stop or to a total dose of 20 mg. For acute alcohol withdrawal or delirium tremens: 5–10 mg IV at a rate of 2–5 mg/min q30–60 min until the patient is sedated; then follow with a maintenance dose of 10–20 mg PO QID.

DIFLUCAN (see Fluconazole)

DIGOXIN (Lanoxin)   *Digitalis glycoside*

Indications:	Supraventricular tachycardia, CHF.
Actions:	Slows AV conduction; increases the force of cardiac contraction; Na^+,K^+-ATPase inhibitor.
Side effects:	Dysrhythmias, nausea, vomiting, neuropsychiatric disturbances.
Comments:	80% renally excreted: dose must be reduced in patients with renal impairment and the elderly. Avoid hypokalemia, which can predispose to digitalis-induced arrhythmias.
Dose:	IV: 0.125–0.5 mg q6h to a total of 1 mg; then 0.125–0.25 mg/day. PO: 0.125–0.5 mg q6h to a total of 1.5 mg; then 0.125–0.25 mg/day. Higher doses may be required to control SVTs.

DILANTIN (see Phenytoin)

DILTIAZEM (see Table page 384)

DIMENHYDRINATE (Dramamine, Gravol)   *Antihistamine*

Indications:	Nausea, vomiting, labyrinthine and vestibular disturbances.
Actions:	Antihistamine and anticholinergic.
Side effects:	Drowsiness, dizziness, dry mouth, urinary retention.
Comments:	Anticholinergic effect is additive to that of other drugs such as the tricyclic antidepressants.
Dose:	50 mg PO or 25 mg IM/IV q4–6h PRN.

DIPHENHYDRAMINE (Benadryl)   *Antihistamine*

Indications:	Allergic reactions.
Actions:	Antihistamine and anticholinergic.
Side effects:	Drowsiness, dizziness, dry mouth, urinary retention.
Comments:	Anticholinergic effect is additive to that of others.
Dose:	25–50 mg PO/IM/IV q6–8h PRN.

DIPHENOXYLATE HYDROCHLORIDE/ATROPINE
SULFATE (Lomotil)   *Antidiarrheal*

Indications:	Diarrhea.
Actions:	Synthetic narcotic with little or no CNS actions combined with an anticholinergic. Reduces peristalsis.
Side effects:	Nausea, cramps, sedation, dry mouth, toxic megacolon.
Comments:	Onset of action in 2–4 h.
Dose:	5 mg/0.05 mg PO TID or QID.

DOCUSATE (Colace, Dioctyl Sodium Sulfosuccinate)   *Laxative*

Indications:	Prevention of constipation.
Actions:	Stool softener: lowers surface tension.
Side effects:	Nausea, bitter taste.
Dose:	100 mg PO QD to TID.

DOPAMINE HYDROCHLORIDE (see Table page 386)

DRAMAMINE (see Dimenhydrinate)

DULCOLAX (see Bisacodyl)

EDECRIN (see Ethacrynic Acid)

ENALAPRIL (Vasotec)   *Angiotensin-Converting Enzyme Inhibitor*

Indications:	Hypertension, CHF.
Actions:	Inhibits the enzyme responsible for conversion of angiotensin I to angiotensin II.
Side effects:	Hypotension, headache, nausea, diarrhea.
Comments:	May cause hyperkalemia if used in patients receiving potassium-sparing diuretics or potassium supplements.
Dose:	Begin with a test dose of 2.5 mg PO and monitor BP for 4 h. For hypertension: titrate up to 2.5–40 mg/day PO. For CHF: titrate to 10–25 mg PO BID.

EPINEPHRINE (see Table page 386)

ERYTHROMYCIN (see Table page 415)

ESIDRIX (see Hydrochlorothiazide)

ESMOLOL (Brevibloc)   *Nonselective beta blocker*

Indications:	Any situation in which a short-duration beta blockade is desired (e.g., aortic dissection).
Actions:	Nonselective beta blockade.
Side effects:	Exacerbation of CHF.
Comments:	Not compatible with normal saline, administer in D/W or dextrose in Ringer's.
Dose:	500 μg/kg over 1–4 min; then 50–300 μg/kg/min by maintenance infusion.

ETHACRYNIC ACID (Edecrin)   *Loop diuretic*

Indications:	CHF.
Actions:	Inhibition of the reabsorption of Na^+ and Cl^- in the ascending limb of the loop of Henle.
Side effects:	Electrolyte depletion; hyperuricemia, hyperglycemia anorexia, nausea, vomiting, diarrhea, sensorineural hearing loss.
Comments:	Associated with more side effects than other loop diuretics.
Dose:	50 mg IV 1 or 2 doses.

FAMOTIDINE (Pepcid)   *Histamine-2 antagonist*

Indications:	Peptic ulcer disease; gastroesophageal reflux.
Actions:	Inhibits histamine-induced secretion of gastric acid.
Side effects:	Headache, dizziness, constipation, diarrhea.
Comments:	Generally well tolerated. Does not have the same effects

as cimetidine on microsomal enzymes or androgen blocking.

Dose: 40 mg PO QHS or 20 mg IV BID for acute conditions. 20 mg PO QHS for maintenance.

FERROUS SULFATE   *Iron supplement*

Indications: Iron deficiency.
Actions: Replaces iron stores.
Side effects: Constipation, nausea, diarrhea, abdominal cramps.
Comments: Stools may turn black but do not have the typical tarry appearance of melena.
Dose: 325 mg/day PO to TID.

FLUCONAZOLE (Diflucan)   *Antifungal*

Indications: Oropharyngeal, esophageal, and systemic candidiasis; cryptococcal meningitis.
Actions: Inhibition of cell membranes of yeasts and fungi.
Side effects: Nausea, vomiting, headache, rash, abdominal pain, diarrhea, hepatic necrosis.
Comments: Many drug interactions due to microsomal enzyme inhibition: sulfonylureas, phenytoin, warfarin, cyclophosphamide.
Dose: 200 mg PO followed by 100 mg/day PO. For systemic candidiasis and cryptococcal meningitis: 200–400 mg QD. Reduce doses in patients with renal impairment.

FLUMAZENIL   *Benzodiazepine antagonist*

Indications: Reversal of benzodiazepine sedation.
Side effects: Seizures, nausea, dizziness, agitation, pain at injection site.
Comments: Onset of reversal within minutes. Contraindicated in patients with cyclic antidepressant overdose (risk of precipitating seizures).
Dose: 0.2 mg IV over 15 secs. Wait 1 min. If ineffective, this may be followed with additional doses of 0.2 mg IV every 60 secs to a maximum dose of 1 mg. If patient becomes resedated, this regimen may be repeated again in 20 mins. No more than 3 mg total dose should be given in 1 h.

FORTAZ (see Ceftazidime)

FUNGIZONE (see Amphotericin B)

FUROSEMIDE (Lasix)   *Loop diuretic*

Indications: CHF, edema, hyperkalemia, hypercalcemia.
Actions: Inhibition of the reabsorption of Na^+ and Cl^- in the ascending limb of the loop of Henle.
Side effects: Electrolyte depletion; hyperuricemia, hyperglycemia, reversible deafness.
Comments: Loop diuretics are well absorbed orally with a prompt onset of action.

Dose: For acute pulmonary edema: 40 mg PO or IV repeated in 60 to 90 min if required. Higher doses may be required in patients with life-threatening pulmonary edema or renal impairment.

GAVISCON (see Alginic Acid Compound)

GELUSIL (Aluminum Hydroxide/Magnesium Hydroxide)   *Antacid*

Indications: Pain due to peptic ulcer disease; reflux esophagitis; prophylaxis of stress ulcers.
Actions: Buffers gastric acidity.
Side effects: Diarrhea, hypermagnesemia in renal failure.
Comments: Aluminum salts cause constipation and magnesium salts diarrhea. The mixture attempts to balance these effects. May bind and reduce absorption of tetracycline, thyroxine, and other medications.
Dose: 30–60 ml PO q1–2h during the acute phase; 30–60 ml PO q1–4h PC and QHS for chronic therapy.

GENTAMICIN (see Table page 415)

GRAVOL (see Dimenhydrinate)

HALDOL (see Haloperidol)

HALOPERIDOL (Haldol)   *Antipsychotic*

Indications: Psychotic disorders; acute agitation.
Actions: Antipsychotic neuroleptic butyrophenone.
Side effects: Extrapyramidal reactions, postural hypotension, sedation, galactorrhea, jaundice, blurred vision, bronchospasm, neuroleptic malignant syndrome.
Comments: Extrapyramidal effects are more pronounced, but hypotension is less frequent than with phenothiazines.
Dose: 0.5–2 mg PO TID; 2–5 mg IM up to q1h for control of acute psychotic crises.

HEPARIN (Low Molecular Weight)   *Anticoagulant*

Indications: Prophylaxis and treatment of DVT.
Actions: Enhances the activity of antithrombin III. The heparin–antithrombin III complexes inactivate several coagulation enzymes, particularly thrombin and factor Xa.
Side effects: Hemorrhage, thrombocytopenia (although less than standard heparin).
Comments: Compared with standard heparin has less plasma protein binding, is almost completely excreted by the renal route, and has a longer half-life. The dose is more predictable, and the kinetics are not dose dependent.
Dose: Commercial preparations differ in the ratio of IIa and Xa inhibitory activity, and dose recommendations vary. Check the manufacturer's information. The drug is administered SC, QD or BID depending on the preparation. Note that the dose for *treatment* of arterial and venous

thrombosis is considerably higher than the dose used for *prophylaxis* of DVT.

HEPARIN (Unfractionated)   *Anticoagulant*

Indications:	Prophylaxis and treatment of DVT, pulmonary embolism, embolic CVA; adjunct in treatment of unstable angina, thrombolytic therapy.
Actions:	Enhances the activity of antithrombin III. The heparin–antithrombin III complexes inactivate several coagulation enzymes, particularly thrombin and factor Xa.
Side effects:	Hemorrhage, thrombocytopenia.
Comments:	Monitor aPTT closely when using IV.
Dose:	For treatment of DVT or pulmonary embolism: 5000–10,000 units IV bolus followed by 1000–2000 units/h maintenance, according to desired aPTT.

HYDRALAZINE (Apresoline)   *Arteriolar vasodilator*

Indications:	Hypertension.
Actions:	Arteriolar vasodilator.
Side effects:	Tachycardia, SLE reaction at higher doses (>200 mg/day).
Comments:	Very limited effect on veins, so little postural hypotension.
Dose:	10–25 mg PO q6h.

HYDROCHLOROTHIAZIDE (HydroDIURIL, Esidrix)   *Thiazide diuretic*

Indications:	Hypertension, CHF, edema.
Actions:	Blocks Na^+ and Cl^- reabsorption in the cortical diluting segment of the loop of Henle.
Side effects:	Electrolyte depletion, hyperuricemia, hyperglycemia, hypercalcemia, pancreatitis, jaundice.
Comments:	Despite the long list of side effects, thiazides are generally well tolerated when used in appropriate doses.
Dose:	12.5–50 mg/day PO.

HYDROCORTISONE   *Corticosteroid*

Indications:	Severe bronchospasm, anaphylaxis, hypercalcemia.
Actions:	Anti-inflammatory effects result in an improvement in air flow after several hours.
Side effects:	Na^+ retention, hyperglycemia, potassium loss.
Comments:	Side effects are few during short-term use.
Dose:	250 mg IV followed by 100 mg IV q6h.

HYDRODIURIL (see Hydrochlorothiazide)

IBUPROFEN (Motrin and others)   *NSAID*

Indications:	Inflammation due to arthritis, soft tissue injuries; analgesia.
Actions:	Proprionic acid derivative. Interferes with the production of prostaglandins.
Side effects:	Nausea, diarrhea. May compromise renal function in pa-

tients with renal impairment. Contraindicated in the syndrome of ASA sensitivity, nasal polyps, and bronchospasm.

Comments: Available as an analgesic in many countries without prescription.

Dose: For analgesia: 200 mg PO TID to QID. For anti-inflammatory effects: 200–400 mg TID to QID.

IMIPENEM (see Table page 415)

IMIPENEM/CILASTATIN (Primaxim) (see Table page 415)

Cilastatin prevents the metabolism of imipenem by dehydropeptidase in the proximal renal tubular cells and therefore decreases the rate of loss of imipenem.

IMITREX (see Sumatriptan Succinate)

IMODIUM (see Loperamide)

INDERAL (see Propranolol)

INDOCIN (see Indomethacin)

INDOMETHACIN (Indocin)   *NSAID*

Indications: Inflammation due to arthritis, soft tissue injury, pericarditis.

Actions: Indole acetic acid derivative. Interferes with the production of prostaglandins.

Side effects: Headaches, dizziness, and lightheadedness, epigastric pain. May compromise renal function in patients with renal impairment.

Comments: Contraindicated in the syndrome of ASA sensitivity, nasal polyps, and bronchospasm. May increase the risk of GI bleeding if used in patients receiving oral anticoagulants.

Dose: 25–50 mg PO TID.

INSULIN   *Hypoglycemic*

Indications: Diabetes mellitus.

Actions: Enhances hepatic glycogen storage, enhances the entry of glucose into cells, inhibits the breakdown of protein and fat. Enhances the entry of K^+ into cells.

Side effects: Hypoglycemia, local skin reactions, lipohypertrophy.

Comments: Less immunogenicity with human insulin than with insulin from natural sources.

Dose: Extremely variable.

Insulin	Example	Onset	Peak	Duration
Regular	Humulin-R	15–60 min	2–4 h	5–7 h
NPH	Humulin-N	1.5–4 h	6–16 h	12–28 h
Lente	Humulin-L	1–4 h	6–16 h	14–28 h

ISOPROTERENOL (see Table page 389)

ISOPTIN (see Verapamil)

ISORDIL (see Isosorbide Dinitrate)

ISOSORBIDE DINITRATE (Isordil, Sorbitrate)   *Vasodilator*

Indications:	Angina pectoris, CHF.
Actions:	Venous, coronary, and arteriolar vasodilator.
Side effects:	Headache, hypotension, flushing.
Comments:	Nitrate tolerance may develop with prolonged continuous administration.
Dose:	5–30 mg PO QID.

ITRACONAZOLE (Sporanox)   *Antifungal*

Indications:	Oral and esophageal candidiasis, aspergillosis, and a variety of other fungal infections.
Actions:	Inhibits the synthesis of ergosterol, thus interfering with the synthesis of fungal and yeast cell membranes.
Side effects:	Nausea, pruritus, rash, headache.
Comments:	More expensive than ketoconazole.
Dose:	100–200 mg QD with food.

KAYEXALATE (see Sodium Polystyrene Sulfonate)

KEFZOL (see Cefazolin)

KETOCONAZOLE (Nizoral)   *Antifungal*

Indications:	Esophageal candidiasis, pulmonary histoplasmosis.
Actions:	Inhibition of yeast and fungal cell membranes.
Side effects:	Nausea, anorexia, vomiting, rash, pruritus. Inhibits microsomal enzymes: gynecomastia, impotence; interacts with warfarin and cyclophosphamide.
Comments:	Absorption is impaired in patients receiving drugs reducing gastric acidity.
Dose:	200–400 mg/day PO.

LABETALOL (Trandate)   *Alpha-1 and beta blocker*

Indications:	Hypertensive emergencies.
Actions:	Alpha-1–blocking action is predominant in acute use but is accompanied by nonspecific beta blockade.
Side effects:	Postural hypotension, bronchospasm, jaundice, bradycardia, negative inotropic effect.
Comments:	Effect is largely due to alpha-1 adrenergic–blocking activity. Contraindications are the same as for those of "pure" beta blockers.
Dose:	20 mg IV q10–15 min in incremental doses (e.g., 20, 20, 40, 40 mg). Alternatively, an infusion beginning at 2 mg/min and titrating to BP response may be given with a maximum daily dose of 2400 mg.

LANOXIN (see Digoxin)

LARGACTIL (see Chlorpromazine)

LASIX (see Furosemide)

LEVODOPA-CARBIDOPA (Sinemet)   *Dopamine agonist*

Indications:	Parkinson's disease.
Actions:	Levodopa is converted to dopamine in the basal ganglia. Carbidopa inhibits the peripheral destruction of levodopa.
Side effects:	Anorexia, nausea, vomiting, abdominal pain, dysrhythmias, behavioral changes, orthostatic hypotension, involuntary movements.
Comments:	Side effects are common.
Dose:	Begin with 1 tablet 100 mg/10 mg PO BID increasing the dose until desired response is obtained, with a maximum dose of 8 tablets (800 mg/80 mg) per day.

LIBRIUM (see Chlordiazepoxide)

LIDOCAINE (Xylocaine)   *Class IB antiarrhythmic*

Indications:	Prophylaxis and treatment of ventricular tachycardia.
Actions:	Lengthens the effective refractory period in ventricular conducting system. Decreases ventricular automaticity.
Side effects:	Nausea, vomiting, hypotension, confusion, seizures, perioral paresthesias.
Comments:	Lower maintenance doses are required in the elderly and in patients with CHF, liver disease, and hypotension.
Dose:	1 mg/kg IV loading dose in 2–3 min. A further dose of 50 mg may be given at 5–10-min intervals to a total dose of 300 mg, followed by a maintenance dose of 1–4 mg/min IV. For prophylaxis: a loading dose of 200 mg given as 50 mg q 5 min followed by a maintenance infusion of 3 mg/min IV.

LOMOTIL (see Diphenoxylate Hydrochloride/Atropine Sulfate)

LOPERAMIDE (Imodium)   *Antidiarrheal*

Indications:	Diarrhea.
Actions:	Interacts directly with the nerve endings and ganglia in the intestinal wall, decreasing muscle action and peristalsis.
Side effects:	Constipation, drowsiness.
Comments:	No more effective in short-term treatment than codeine.
Dose:	4 mg, then 2 mg after each loose stool to a total of 16 mg/day.

LORAZEPAM (Ativan)   *Benzodiazepine*

Indications:	Insomnia, anxiety.
Actions:	Benzodiazepine sedative-hypnotic.
Side effects:	Sedation, respiratory depression.
Comments:	Peak effect in 1–6 h.
Dose:	0.5–1.0 mg PO QHS for hypnosis. 1.0 mg PO TID for anxiety.

LOSEC (see Omeprazole)

LOW-MOLECULAR-WEIGHT HEPARIN (see Heparin,
Low Molecular Weight)

MAALOX (Aluminum Hydroxide/Magnesium Hydroxide)   *Antacid*

Indications:	Pain due to peptic ulcer disease, reflux esophagitis, prophylaxis of stress ulcer.
Actions:	Buffers gastric acidity.
Side effects:	Diarrhea, hypermagnesemia in renal failure.
Comments:	Aluminum salts cause constipation and magnesium salts diarrhea. The mixture attempts to balance these effects. May bind and reduce absorption of tetracycline, thyroxine, and other medications.
Dose:	30–60 ml PO q1–2h during the acute phase; 30–60 ml PO q1–3h PC and QHS for chronic therapy.

MAGNESIUM SULFATE (see Table page 390)

MANNITOL   *Osmotic diuretic*

Indications:	Cerebral edema, hemolytic transfusion reactions.
Actions:	Osmotic diuretic.
Side effects:	Volume overload, hyperosmolality, hyponatremia.
Comments:	Contraindicated in renal failure.
Dose:	25 g IV over 15–30 min q2–3h PRN.

MEDROL (see Methylprednisolone)

MEPERIDINE (Demerol, Pethidine)   *Narcotic analgesic*

Indications:	Moderate to severe pain.
Actions:	Narcotic analgesic.
Side effects:	Respiratory depression, hypotension, nausea, vomiting constipation, agitation, rash.
Comments:	100 mg meperidine SC/IV = 10 mg morphine SC/IV; antidote is naloxone.
Dose:	50–100 mg SC/IM q4h.

METHYLPREDNISOLONE (Medrol)   *Glucocorticoid*

Indications:	Treatment of acute asthma when the patient is unable to take or absorb oral corticosteroids.
Actions:	Anti-inflammatory effects result in an improvement in air flow after several hours.

Side effects: Na$^+$ retention, hyperglycemia, potassium loss.
Comments: Side effects are few during short-term use. More expensive than hydrocortisone and much more expensive than oral prednisolone, which is efficiently absorbed.
Dose: 100–200 mg IV.

METOLAZONE (Zaroxolyn)   *Thiazide diuretic*

Indications: Hypertension, CHF, edema, some forms of renal failure.
Actions: Blocks Na$^+$ and Cl$^-$ reabsorption in the proximal and distal convoluted tubule.
Side effects: Electrolyte depletion, hyperuricemia, hyperglycemia, hypomagnesemia.
Comments: Only difference from hydrochlorothiazide is the longer duration of effect. When given in combination with furosemide, metolazone should be administered 30 min before the furosemide for maximum diuretic effect.
Dose: 2.5–10 mg/day PO.

METRONIDAZOLE (see Table page 415)

MIDAZOLAM (Versed)   *Benzodiazepine*

Indications: Premedication before surgery or diagnostic procedure.
Action: Benzodiazepine sedative/hypnotic.
Side effects: Sedation, paradoxical agitation, respiratory depression.
Comments: Should be used only in the presence of individuals equipped to provide resuscitation. Benzodiazepine effects can be reversed with the antagonist flumazenil.
Dose: 0.20–0.35 mg/kg PRN IV in 20–30 sec as an induction dose in the unpremedicated healthy adult. Smaller doses in the elderly, debilitated, and premedicated patient.
                   Always inject IV slowly to avoid respiratory depression and hypotension.

MORPHINE SULFATE   *Narcotic analgesic*

Indications: Moderate to severe pain. Pulmonary edema.
Actions: Narcotic analgesic. Splanchnic venodilation.
Side effects: Respiratory depression, hypotension, nausea, vomiting.
Comments: 10 mg morphine IM/SC = 100 mg meperidine IM/SC.
Dose: For pulmonary edema or chest pain due to coronary ischemia: 2–4 mg IV q5–10min to a maximum dose of 10–12 mg. For pain: 2–15 mg IV/IM/SC q4h PRN.

MOTRIN (see Ibuprofen)

MYCOSTATIN (see Nystatin)

MYLANTA (Aluminum Hydroxide/Magnesium Hydroxide)   *Antacid*

Indications: Pain due to peptic ulcer disease, reflux esophagitis, prophylaxis of stress ulcer.
Actions: Buffers gastric acidity.
Side effects: Diarrhea, hypermagnesemia in renal failure.
Comments: Aluminum salts cause constipation and magnesium salts

diarrhea. The mixture attempts to balance these effects. May bind and reduce absorption of tetracycline, thyroxine, and other medications.

Dose: 30–60 ml PO q1–2h during the acute phase; 30–60 ml PO q1–3h PC and QHS for chronic therapy.

NADOLOL (Corgard) *Nonselective beta blocker*

Indications: Angina pectoris; post-MI treatment of SVTs, hypertension; thyrotoxicosis.
Actions: Nonspecific beta adrenergic blockade.
Side effects: Hypotension, bradycardia, bronchospasm, CHF, nausea, vomiting, fatigue; may mask symptoms of hypoglycemia.
Comments: Less lipid soluble than propranolol and less likely to cause insomnia.
Dose: 10–40 mg/day PO. Begin with a low dose and adjust to desired effect.

NALOXONE HYDROCHLORIDE (Narcan) *Narcotic antagonist*

Indications: Narcotic antagonism.
Actions: Competitive antagonist of narcotics.
Side effects: Nausea, vomiting, may precipitate withdrawal in narcotic addicts.
Comments: Effect is shorter than many narcotics.
Dose: 0.2–2.0 mg IV/IM/SC q5min to a maximum dose of 10 mg.

NAPROXEN (Naprosyn) *NSAID*

Indications: Inflammation due to arthritis, soft tissue injury, pericarditis.
Actions: Proprionic acid derivative. Interferes with the production of prostaglandins.
Side effects: Headaches, dizziness, and lightheadedness, epigastric pain. May compromise renal function in patients with renal impairment.
Comments: Should be used with caution in anticoagulated patients; contraindicated in the syndrome of ASA sensitivity, nasal polyps, and bronchospasm.
Dose: 250–500 mg PO BID.

NARCAN (see Naloxone)

NIFEDIPINE (Adalat, Procardia) *Calcium channel blocker*

Indications: Angina pectoris, coronary spasm, hypertension.
Actions: Calcium channel blocker, arterial vasodilator.
Side effects: Hypotension, flushing, dizziness, headaches, peripheral edema.
Comments: The edema is due to vasodilation and does not respond to diuretics. Nifedipine has a greater effect than verapamil and diltiazem on peripheral vasculature.
Dose: The long-acting preparation is preferable, e.g., nifedipine PA (or CC, CR, LA) 30–90 mg/day PO.

NITROGLYCERIN

Vasodilator

Indications:	Angina pectoris, CHF.	
Actions:	Venous, coronary, and arteriolar vasodilator.	
Side effects:	Headache, hypotension, flushing.	
Comments:	Nitrate tolerance may develop with prolonged continuous administration.	
Dose:	Sublingual:	0.15–0.6 mg.
	Lingual aerosol:	One or two doses sprayed on or under the tongue q3–5 min to a maximum of 3 times/15 min.
	Transdermal patch:	0.2 mg/h increasing to 0.8 mg/h. Patch should be left on 10–12 h, then off for 12–14 h to avoid tolerance.
	Transdermal ointment:	0.5–4 inches q4–8h. Rotate sites. Leave off for at least 6 h/day to avoid tolerance.
	Oral sustained release:	2–9 mg BID to TID.

NIZATIDINE (Axid)

Histamine-2 antagonist

Indications:	Peptic ulcer disease; gastroesophageal reflux.
Actions:	Inhibits histamine-induced secretion of gastric acid.
Side effects:	Sweating, urticaria, somnolence, elevation of hepatic enzymes.
Comments:	Does not have the same effects as cimetidine on microsomal enzymes and androgen receptors. Expensive.
Dose:	150 mg BID for reflux and 300 mg QD for peptic ulcer. Maintenance dose 150 mg QHS.

NIZORIL (see Ketoconazole)

NOCTEC (see Chloral Hydrate)

NOREPINEPHRINE (see Table page 393)

NYSTATIN (Mycostatin)

Antifungal

Indications:	Oral and esophageal candidiasis.
Actions:	Disruption of fungal cell membranes.
Side effects:	Nausea, vomiting.
Comments:	Not absorbed orally.
Dose:	400,000–600,000 units PO (swish and swallow) QID.

OCTREOTIDE ACETATE (Sandostatin)

Somatostatin analog

Indications:	Mainly used in the carcinoid syndrome and in tumors secreting vasoactive intestinal peptide. Used in bleeding esophageal varices.
Actions:	Suppresses the secretion of serotonin, pancreatic peptides, gastrin, vasoactive intestinal peptide, insulin, glu-

cagon, secretin, and motilin. Reduces collateral splanchnic blood flow.

Side effects: Abdominal pain, transient hypoglycemia and hyperglycemia. May decrease GFR and increase intestinal transit time.

Comments: Expensive

Dose: 25 μg/hr IV for 5 days.

OMEPRAZOLE (Losec, Prilosec)   *Na^+,K^+-ATPase inhibitor*

Indications: Peptic ulcer, gastroesophageal reflux.

Actions: Inhibition of gastric proton pump, thus inhibiting basal and stimulated gastric acid secretion.

Side effects: Abdominal pain, nausea, headache.

Comments: Expensive.

Dose: 20–40 mg QD.

OXAZEPAM (Serax)   *Benzodiazepine*

Indications: Insomnia, anxiety.

Actions: Benzodiazepine sedative/hypnotic.

Side effects: Sedation, respiratory depression, confusion.

Comments: Peak effect in 1–4 h, and relatively short duration.

Dose: 10–30 mg PO QHS PRN for sleep, 30–100 mg/day in divided doses for anxiety.

PARACETAMOL (see Acetaminophen)

PENBRITIN (see Ampicillin)

PENICILLIN (see Table page 415)

PENTACARINAT (see Pentamidine Isethionate)

PENTAMIDINE ISETHIONATE (Pentacarinat)   *Anti-PCP agent*

Indications: *Pneumocystis carinii* pneumonia (PCP).

Action: Unknown.

Side effects: Hypotension, renal failure, cardiac arrhythmia, hypoglycemia, pancreatitis.

Comments: Reduce dose in renal impaired patients.

Dose: 4 mg/kg in 50–250 ml D5W IV given over 2 h QD.

PEPTO-BISMOL (see Bismuth Subsalicylate)

PHENAZOPYRIDINE (Pyridium)   *Urinary analgesic*

Indications: Urethritis, cystitis.

Actions: Analgesic effect on inflamed urinary tract mucosa.

Side effects: Orange discoloration of urine. Nausea.

Comments: Has no antibacterial effect.

Dose: 200 mg PO TID after meals.

PHENYTOIN (Dilantin)   *Anticonvulsant, antiepileptic*

Indications:	Seizure disorders.
Actions:	Anticonvulsant. Reduces Na^+ transport across cerebral cell membranes.
Side effects:	Hypotension, cardiac dysrhythmias, ataxia, nystagmus, dysarthria, hepatotoxicity, gingival hypertrophy, hirsutism, megaloblastic anemia, lymphadenopathy, fever, rash.
Comments:	At therapeutic doses, the drug is metabolized in the liver at 0 order (a fixed absolute amount per unit time). Relatively small changes in dose can cause major changes in serum concentrations over the long term.
Dose:	For status epilepticus: 18 mg/kg loading dose IV in NS at a rate of ≤25–50 mg/min. For epilepsy: 300 mg/day.

PHYTONADIONE (Vitamin K₁)   *Vitamin K*

Indications:	Vitamin K deficiency, reversal of warfarin effect.
Actions:	Essential for hepatic synthesis of factors II, VII, IX, and X.
Side effects:	Hematoma formation with SC/IM administration.
Comment:	Avoid IV administration because of hypotension and anaphylaxis. Serious hemorrhage due to excessive warfarin is better treated with fresh frozen plasma.
Dose:	2.5–10 mg PO/SC/IM.

PIPERACILLIN (see Table page 415)

PITRESSIN (see Vasopressin)

POTASSIUM   *Potassium supplements*

Indications:	Hypokalemia.
Actions:	Potassium supplement.
Side effects:	Nausea, vomiting, diarrhea, abdominal discomfort, hyperkalemia.
Comments:	Danger of hyperkalemia in patients with renal impairment and those on angiotensin-converting enzyme inhibitors.

Dose:	Micro-K-Extencaps:	8 mmol K^+
	Micro-K-10 Extencaps:	10 mmol K^+
	Slow-K:	8 mmol K^+
	Kay Ciel Elixir:	20 mmol/15 ml
	Prevention:	24–40 mmol/day.
	Treatment:	60–120 mmol/day or more.

PREPULSID (see Cisapride)

PRESSYN (see Vasopressin)

PRIMAXIN (see Imipenem/cilastatin)

PROCAINAMIDE (Pronestyl, Procan)   *Class Ia antiarrhythmic*

Indications:	Atrial and ventricular tachydysrhythmias.
Actions:	Reduces the maximum rate of depolarization in atrial

and ventricular conducting tissue. Class Ia antiarrhythmic.

Side effects:	Hypotension, anorexia, nausea, vomiting, heart block, proarrhythmia, rash, fever, SLE-like syndrome, arthralgias.
Comments:	Similar to quinidine except that it does not have an atropinic effect. Cross-allergy to procaine.
Dose:	1 g load PO followed by 250–500 mg PO q3h; delayed release preparations may be given q6h. For life-threatening tachydysrhythmias, give 100 mg IV over 2 min repeatedly until the arrhythmia has abated or until a total dose of 1 g has been given. If successful, follow with a maintenance dose of 2–4 mg/min IV.

PROCAN (see Procainamide)

PROCARDIA (see Nifedipine)

PROMETHAZINE (Phenergan)   *Antihistamine*

Indications:	Sedation, nausea, vomiting.
Actions:	Antihistamine and anticholinergic.
Side effects:	Drowsiness, dizziness, constipation, dry mouth, urinary retention.
Comments:	Anticholinergic effects are additive with those of other drugs such as the tricyclic antidepressants.
Dose:	25–50 mg PO/PR/IM q4–6h PRN or 12.5–25 mg IV q4–6h PRN.

PROPRANOLOL (Inderal)   *Nonspecific beta blocker*

Indications:	Angina pectoris; post-MI treatment of SVTs, hypertension; thyrotoxicosis.
Actions:	Nonspecific beta adrenergic blockade.
Side effects:	Hypotension, bradycardia, bronchospasm, CHF, nausea, vomiting, fatigue, insomnia, nightmares; may mask symptoms of hypoglycemia.
Comments:	Abrupt withdrawal may precipitate angina in patients with coronary heart disease.
Dose:	10–80 mg PO BID to QID. Begin with a low dose and adjust to desired effect. In aortic dissection: 0.5 mg IV followed by 1 mg IV q5min to a total dose of 0.15 mg/kg in 4 h.

PROPULSID (see Cisapride)

PROTAMINE SULFATE   *Heparin antagonist*

Indications:	Reversal of heparin anticoagulation.
Actions:	Binds to and inactivates heparin.
Side effects:	Hypotension, bradycardia, flushing.
Comments:	Overdosage may paradoxically result in worsening hemorrhage because protamine possesses anticoagulant activity.
Dose:	1 mg/100 units of heparin, IV slowly, based on an estima-

tion of the circulating heparin. Do not give more than 50 mg in a 10-min period.

PROVENTIL (see Salbutamol)

PYRIDIUM (see Phenazopyridine)

QUININE SULFATE   *Antimalarial*

Indications:	Nocturnal leg cramps.
Actions:	Unknown.
Side effects:	Nausea, visual disturbances, hemolytic anemia, thrombocytopenia.
Comments:	Side effects are unusual at this dose, which is 1/10th that used in malaria.
Dose:	200–300 mg PO QHS PRN.

RANITIDINE (Zantac)   *Histamine-2 antagonist*

Indications:	Peptic ulcer disease; gastroesophageal reflux.
Actions:	Inhibits histamine-induced secretion of gastric acid.
Side effects:	Jaundice, gynecomastia, headache, confusion, leukopenia.
Comments:	Generally well tolerated. Does not have the same effect as cimetidine on microsomal enzymes or androgen blocking.
Dose:	50 mg IV q8h or 150 mg PO BID or 300 mg PO QD. Maintenance therapy 150 mg QD QHS.

ROCEPHIN (see Ceftriaxone)

SALBUTAMOL (Ventolin, Albuterol, Proventil)   *Beta-2 agonist*

Indications:	Bronchospasm.
Actions:	Beta-2–adrenergic agonist.
Side effects:	Headache, dizziness, nausea, tremor, palpitations.
Comments:	Larger doses cause tachycardia.
Dose:	2.5–5 mg in 3 ml NS by nebulizer q4h PRN. In severe bronchospasm may be required q 3–5 min initially.

SANDOSTATIN (see Octreotide)

SERAX (see Oxazepam)

SINEMET (see Levodopa-Carbidopa)

SODIUM BICARBONATE (see Table page 395)

SODIUM POLYSTYRENE SULFONATE
(Kayexalate)   *Cation exchange resin*

Indications:	Hyperkalemia.
Actions:	Nonabsorbable cation exchange resin.
Side effects:	Nausea, vomiting, gastric irritation, sodium retention.
Comments:	20 mmol of Na^+ is exchanged for 20 mmol of K^+ for each 15 g PO. Mg^{2+} and Ca^{2+} may also be exchanged.

Dose:	15–30 g in 50–100 ml of 20% sorbitol PO q3–4h or 50 g in 200 ml of 20% sorbitol or D20W PR by retention enema for 30–60 min q6h PRN.

SORBITRATE (see Isosorbide Dinitrate)

SPIRONOLACTONE (Aldactone)   *Diuretic-aldosterone antagonist*

Indications:	Ascites, edema, hypertension, hyperaldosteronism.
Actions:	Aldosterone antagonist.
Side effects:	Hyponatremia, gynecomastia, confusion, headache, hyperkalemia.
Comments:	Most effective in states of hyperaldosteronism, but equipotent to thiazides in hypertension.
Dose:	50–100 mg PO QD. Higher doses are required in states of hyperaldosteronism.

SPORANOX (see Itraconazole)

STREPTASE (see Streptokinase)

STREPTOKINASE (Streptase)   *Thrombolytic agent*

Indications:	Acute MI, massive pulmonary embolism.
Actions:	Binds to fibrin and activates bound plasminogen to plasmin initiating local fibrinolysis with little conversion of circulating plasminogen.
Side effects:	Intracranial, retroperitoneal, and internal bleeding.
Comments:	Should not be used in patients with streptococcal infections or patients who have received streptokinase in the preceding 12 months because these patients are likely to have streptokinase antibodies and be resistant.
Dose:	For acute MI: 1.5 million IU given IV over 60 min. For massive pulmonary embolism: 250,000 IU in 45 ml of diluent IV over 30 min, followed by 100,000 IU/h for 24 h.

SUMATRIPTAN SUCCINATE (Imitrex)   *5-Hydroxytryptamine antagonist*

Indications:	Intermittent treatment of migraine.
Actions:	Selective 5-hydroxytryptamine–like receptor agonist. Causes vasoconstriction particularly of the dilated carotid arterial circulation in migraine.
Side effects:	Can cause coronary artery spasm, contraindicated in coronary artery disease, concomitant use of ergot alkaloids, uncontrolled hypertension, use of MAOI's, SSRI's, lithium, and hemiplegic migraine. Flushing, dizziness, feelings of heat, pressure, malaise, fatigue, drowsiness, nausea, vomiting.
Comments:	SC injection accompanied by local pain. Peak effects after SC dose in 15 min, after PO dose in 0.5–5 h.
Dose:	100 mg PO. Do not repeat if first dose has not had an effect. If successful, recrudescences can be treated with further doses not to exceed 300 mg PO in 24 h. 6 mg SC.

SUPRAX (see Cefixime)

TENORMIN (see Atenolol)

TETRACYCLINE (see Table page 415)

THEOPHYLLINE (see Aminophylline)

THIAMINE (Vitamin B₁)   *Vitamin B₁*

Indications:	Thiamine deficiency, prophylaxis of Wernicke's encephalopathy.
Action:	Vitamin B_1 replacement.
Side effects:	IV administration may result in hypotension or, rarely, anaphylactic shock. Well absorbed orally.
Comments:	Consider the oral route even in "emergencies."
Dose:	100 mg/day PO/IM/IV for 3 days. If given IV, give slowly over 5 min.

THORAZINE (see Chlorpromazine)

TOBRAMYCIN (see Table page 415)

TPA (see Alteplase)

TRANDATE (see Labetalol)

TRIAZOLAM (Halcion)   *Benzodiazepine*

Indications:	Insomnia.
Actions:	Benzodiazepine hypnotic.
Side effects:	Sedation, respiratory depression, confusion.
Comments:	Possible link to suicidal ideation. May be a greater risk of anterograde amnesia than with other benzodiazepines.
Dose:	0.125–0.25 mg PO QHS PRN.

TRIMETHOPRIM-SULFAMETHOXASOLE (Cotrimazole)
(see Table page 415)

TYLENOL (see Acetaminophen)

VALIUM (see Diazepam)

VANERIL (see Beclomethasone)

VANCOMYCIN (see Table page 415)

VASOPRESSIN (Pitressin, Pressyn)   *Antidiuretic agent*

Indications:	Principal use is to replace endogenous antidiuretic hormone in deficiency states. Used in bleeding esophageal varices.
Actions:	Increase water reabsorption by the renal tubules. Causes contraction of smooth muscle of the GI tract and all parts

of the vascular bed with a lesser effect on large veins. Reduces portal pressure.

Side effects:	Water intoxication. Nausea, cramps, myocardial ischemia.
Comments:	Care must be taken to control water balance.
Dose:	100 units in 250 ml of D5W at the rate of 0.4 unit/min (60 ml/h).

VASOTEC (see Enalapril)

VENTOLIN (see Salbutamol)

VERAPAMIL (Isoptin, Calan)   *Calcium channel blocker*

Indications:	Angina pectoris; treatment or SVTs; hypertension, left ventricular diastolic dysfunction.
Actions:	Calcium channel blocker, depresses AV conduction.
Side effects:	CHF, bradycardias, hypotension, headaches, dizziness, constipation.
Comments:	Calcium gluconate 1–2 g IV may reverse the negative inotropic and hypotensive effects but not the AV block.
Dose:	80–120 mg PO TID; IV administration should take place only in monitored patients. 2.5–5 mg IV may be given for rate control to "break" an SVT. This dose may be repeated in 5–10 min.

VERSED (see Midazolam)

VITAMIN B (see Thiamine)

VITAMIN K (see Phytonadione)

WARFARIN (Coumadin)   *Oral anticoagulant*

Indications:	Prophylaxis and treatment of DVT, pulmonary embolism, and embolic CVA.
Actions:	Inhibits vitamin K–dependent clotting factors.
Side effects:	Hemorrhage, nausea, vomiting, skin necrosis, fever, rash.
Comments:	Individualize dosage to maintain PT in the desired range. Many drugs interact to increase or decrease the effect of warfarin: always look up new medications before starting them in patients on warfarin to see whether they interact. Fresh frozen plasma is the treatment of choice to rapidly reverse the effect of warfarin. An alternative is vitamin K.
Dose:	Give 10 mg daily for 2 days; then an estimated maintenance dose of 5–7.5 mg/day modified according to PT or INR.

XYLOCAINE (see Lidocaine)

ZANTAC (see Ranitidine)

ZAROXOLYN (see Metolazone)

ZIDOVUDINE (AZT, Azidothymidine, Retrovir)   *Nucleoside analog*

Indications:	Advanced HIV disease.
Actions:	Inhibition of reverse transcriptase, thus inhibiting virus replication. Thymidine analog.
Side effects:	Headache, anorexia, nausea, vomiting, myalgias, anemia, leukopenia.
Comments:	Mild anemia (macrocytic and megaloblastic) is common but readily reversible on stopping the drug.
Dose:	100 mg q4h or 200 mg q8h.

ZINACEF (see Cefuroxime)

ZOVIRAX (see Acyclovir)

ZYLOPRIM (see Allopurinol)

INDEX

Note: Page numbers in *italics* refer to illustrations; page numbers followed by t refer to tables.

455